YOGA
A Gem for Women

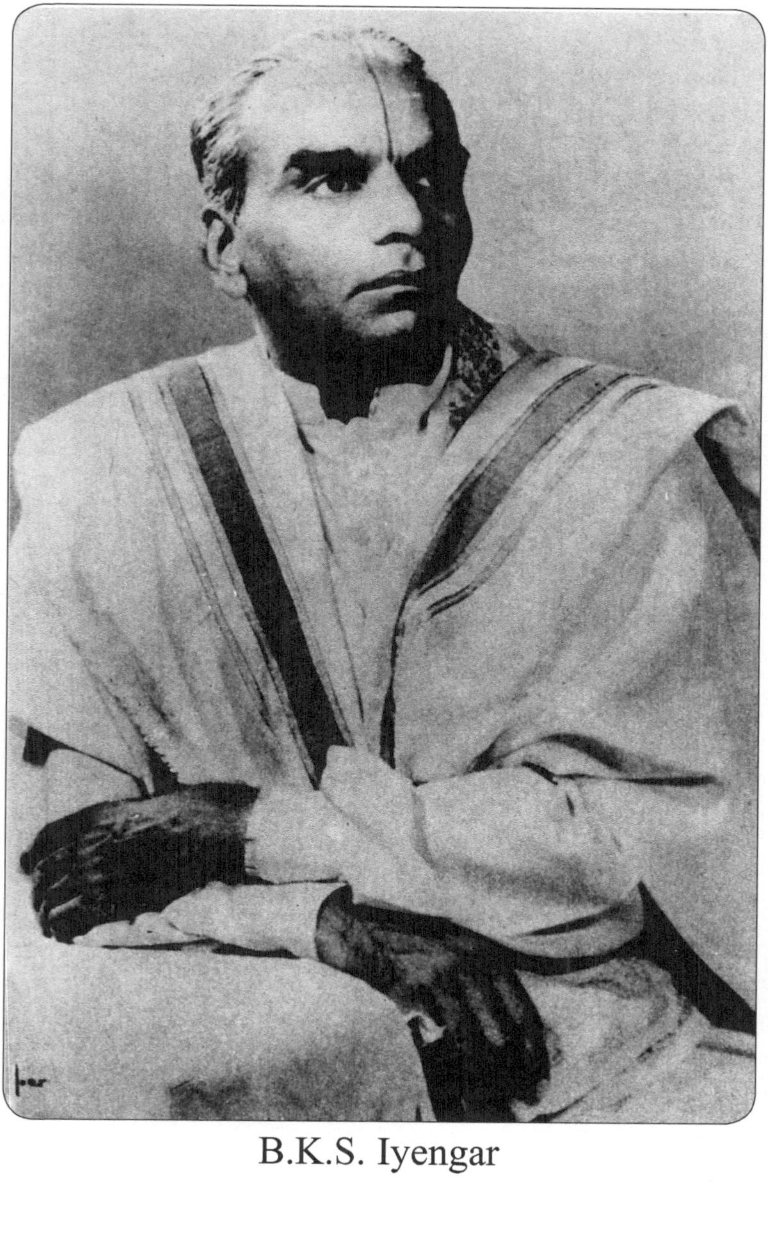

B.K.S. Iyengar

YOGA
A Gem for Women

Geeta S. Iyengar

ALLIED PUBLISHERS PVT. LTD.

New Delhi • Mumbai • Kolkata • Chennai • Bangalore • Hyderabad

ALLIED PUBLISHERS PRIVATE LIMITED

D-5, Sector-2, **Noida**–201 301
Ph. Nos.: 0120-4320295/2542557/4352866
E-mail: delhi.books@alliedpublishers.com

17 Chittaranjan Avenue, **Kolkata**–700072
Ph.: 033-22129618 • E-mail: cal.books@alliedpublishers.com

15 J.N. Heredia Marg, Ballard Estate, **Mumbai**–400001
Ph.: 022-42126969 • E-mail: mumbai.books@alliedpublishers.com

No. 25/10, Commander-in-Chief Road, Ethiraj Lane (Next to Post Office)
Egmore, **Chennai**–600008
Ph.: 044-28223938 • E-mail: chennai.books@alliedpublishers.com

P.B. No. 9932, No. 15, 3rd Floor (Next to Vijaya Bank), 5th Cross, Gandhinagar,
Karnataka, **Bangalore**–560009,
Ph.: 080-41530285 / 22386239
E-mail: bngl.journals@alliedpublishers.com / apsabng@airtelmail.in

Sri Jayalakshmi Nilayam, No. 3-4-510, 3rd Floor (Above More Super Market)
Barkatpura, **Hyderabad**–500027
Ph.: 040-27551811, 040-27551812 • E-mail: hyd.books@alliedpublishers.com

Website: www.alliedpublishers.com

First Published, 1983
Second Edition, 1997
Twelfth Reprint, 2013
Third Thoroughly Revised Edition, 2019
Reprint, 2021, 2022

ISBN: 978-93-87997-84-4

Published by Sunil Sachdev and printed by Ravi Sachdev at
Allied Publishers Pvt. Ltd., D-5, Sector-2, Noida–201 301

Adorations to the Guru

gururbrahmā gururviṣṇu gurudevaḥ sadā cyutaḥ
na guroradhikaḥ kaścit triṣu lokeṣu vidyate

The Guru is Brahman, the Guru is Viṣnu, the Guru is Lord Achyuta the God;
There is none greater than the Guru in all the three Worlds.

divyajñānopadeṣṭāram deśikam parameśvaram
pujayetparayā bhaktyā tasya jñānaphalam bhavet

The Guru bestows Divine Wisdom; he is the Spiritual Guide and like the Supreme Lord Himself. He who worships the Guru with supreme devotion attains Jñāna.

yathā gurustathaiveśo yathaiveśastathā guruḥ
pūjanīyo mahābhaktyā na bhedo vidyate' nayo

God is like the Guru; the Guru is like God;
There is no difference between the two;
He should be worshipped with great devotion.

nādvaitavādam kurvīta guruṇā saha kutracit
advaitam bhavayedbhaktyā gurordevasya cātmanaḥ
Yogaśikhopaniṣad

The Guru should be obeyed at all times;
With single-minded devotion.
He should be contemplated upon as God and Atman.

"The debt to a Mother can never be repaid."

Dedicated to My Mother

At the lotus feet of Ammā,
who dwells in the abode of Viṣṇu,
who was my Guru,
who gave me the freedom and the moral
courage to follow the path of Yoga.

This book is respectfully dedicated
by her devoted daughter.

Foreword

I was in two minds when both the publisher and the author insisted that only I should write the foreword to this book. The author, Miss Geeta S. Iyengar, is first my daughter, and secondly my pupil. Her filial piety naturally persuaded her to seek the blessings of her parent and even more of her preceptor. Then, the director of the publishing company is my friend as well as my pupil. I could not but accept and write the foreword so as not to sunder the bond between us. Though I am filled with joy that my daughter has made a maiden attempt to write about the disciplines and practices of Yoga for the benefit of her sisters, I have to assess her work in its true perspective, lest what I say may be misconstrued as an expatiation of my daughter's work rather than a dispassionate review and appraisal of its merits. No doubt Yoga is my very breath. My life and my very Being are soaked in its art, science and philosophy.

Although Geeta observed my practices and my teaching of Yoga, she showed no inclination or desire to make a beginning. Her interest arose when she was struck with nephritis. Her ailment became almost fatal when medical treatment produced no signs of progress. As a hapless parent, I could see no way to pay for the inexhaustible list of medicines with my meagre finances. Then I placed a choice before her: either to embrace Yoga, the only panacea for her, or to live until her disease took its toll. Though young in age—barely ten years—she understood my ultimatum and made up her mind to take to Yoga. She gained confidence in herself and dedicated her life to the practice of Yoga. Since then she has undergone rigorous training and has mastered this difficult art. A devoted student, she diligently practised day and night with attention and has been teaching others since 1961. This book is the outcome of her training and experience.

Yoga has a unique place in the search for Self-realisation and through it, God-realisation. Our body is a repository of the faculties of the mind, the intelligence and the soul. In order to extricate the body from the tangle of diseases, the emotional disturbances of the mind and the ruffled intellect need to be transformed to the level of perfect consciousness devoid of prejudices and dualities. Then only the body of the practitioner becomes a worthy abode for that pure consciousness to dwell in. This is the aim of the book.

Having mastered the subtle techniques of this art, Geeta has presented it, highlighting the importance of Yoga in a woman's life, and giving a variety of āsanas with their physical and curative values, prāṇāyāma with its bandhas, and dhyāna–meditation. Their practice will enable the aspirants to lead a peaceful and contented life. Very few women have obtained proficiency in Yoga. Geeta occupies a unique place and is recognised for her knowledge of the art and for her skilled performance. She is a source of inspiration for others to emulate.

Her contribution in Yoga for girls and women lies in the lucid explanations of the terse movements in a lucid style. The āsanas, involving subtle movements, and prāṇāyāma, regulating the flow of energy, act rhythmically on the anatomical, physiological, psychological, and spiritual functions of the human body. She is able to guide students from her knowledge of Āyurveda blended with her knowledge of Yoga. She has given practical steps for advancing from a purely physical plane to a higher level of consciousness. Even from a material standpoint the book aims to help women who are under physical and mental pressure and working for their living. They may be busy housewives or mothers who have to look after the home when they return from the office or the factory. In this age of economic pressures and rapid social and cultural changes, women have to play a very difficult and arduous role. Exposure to the constant stresses and strains of modern life jeopardises their health and mental peace; this plays a decisive role in determining the quality of their children, as the role of the mother is so important. This peace and health can be achieved without the aid of drugs and tonics but through Yoga. It is the answer to health, calmness of nerves, alertness of mind, and ultimately of spiritual repose.

The author has divided the āsanas into various sections dealing with simple standing positions, forward bends, lateral movements, backward extension of the spine, correct breathing techniques during the performance of the āsanas, and giving the effects of the āsanas on the body, the nerves and the mind. This guides the reader step by step in the practice of Yoga. Almost all the illustrations in the book are her own.

The author has also explained how Yoga can be practised in the absence of a teacher. In the section on 'Yoga Kurunta' (Yoga Self-Taught) she has explained with illustrations the various techniques for correct practice in order to help women who cannot attend classes. The devices are very simple: a rope, the support of a wall, and a low-level stool or bench.

It is also interesting to see that she has introduced about twenty illustrations of her sister, Mrs. Vanita Sridharan.

They were taken during advanced pregnancy in order to instil confidence among women to practise Yoga even while pregnant. She has also included illustrations of a few complicated āsanas to show that the women can do them without suffering any adverse effects.

The general notion is that Yoga is not intended for women. It is fallacious and it underrates the moral, intellectual and spiritual legacies to which women are entitled as much as men. The author has shown that Yoga can be taken up by women, in the manner in which other subjects, such as law, history, philosophy, science, engineering, medicine, etc., are offered by Universities. Multitudes of women are seen nowadays who equal and excel men in every faculty. More women can now come forward and strive to attain new heights to enrich Yoga, which is one of our ancient heritages.

I shall feel amply rewarded if this book is well received by all and particularly by women for whom it is written.

B.K.S. Iyengar

Preface

When Mr. P.H. Patwardhan of Orient Longman published *Yoga Dīpikā,* the Marāthī edition of my father, Sri B.K.S. Iyengar's book *Light on Yoga,* he strongly urged me to write in Marāthī a book on Yoga for Women.

For a long time I hesitated, but he continued to insist. I felt I had neither the intellectual ability nor the moral courage to write a book, particularly on Yoga with special reference to the needs of women; but here a pat of encouragement came from my mother—Ammā as I used to call her: 'You must write the book,' she said, 'but not to parade your intellectual attainments. God has given Yoga as a priceless gift for women, and this you must reveal to the world.'

Her remarks, borne out of her experiences in life, were of more value to me than my knowledge obtained from books.

My mother was a saintly woman and led a life of high moral ideals. She did not lecture us on what we should do, but Jñāna (Knowledge), Bhakti (Devotion), Karma (Sense of Duty), and Yoga were expressed in her everyday life and actions. She was an example to us all, the embodiment of pure womanhood.

This book is the outcome of my mother's encouragement. With humility, I wrote a few chapters and gave them to Mr. Patwardhan for his comments. He approved the language as well as the presentation and encouraged me to continue.

It took me a few years to complete the book. When it was ready, he suggested that I give an English version of the Marāthī original, so that its benefits could be shared by women all over the world. His suggestion was too novel for me to say 'yes' immediately, as I had my limitations in the English language and had to borrow the services of an interpreter to convey my thoughts and experiences accurately in that language.

I approached my friend Mr. P.R. Shinde to translate my book, but he was hesitant. I tried others, but no-one else was able to undertake the work. Finally, Mr. Shinde allowed himself to be persuaded and translated the book. He has done so creditably, retaining all the original cadences, and I am grateful to him. I am also thankful to Mr. Patwardhan, but for whose insistence this book might not have seen light.

Before venturing to write this book, I pondered over the present-day economic and social conditions of women contrasted with those of centuries ago. The social and political environment, status, and economic conditions of women years ago led them to a simple life; they were not subjected to the same pressures that burden the women in all walks of life today. Now every item of need has become an indispensable factor of life which is often beyond one's capacity of acquisition. The economic situation has compelled women to contribute an equal share in order to stabilise living conditions and to avoid present as well as future anxieties. She now has to do the double work of having to meet financial pressures and maintaining harmony in the family. It is necessary for her to keep perfect health and harmony to withstand the stresses and strains of life. Yoga is capable of giving this needed relief if she devotes a little of her time daily to its practice.

Rarely does a pupil find the Guru and the Father in one person. I consider myself doubly fortunate in this respect. Annā—my father—is my Guru. Never did he inflict his opinions or thoughts on me, nor did he try to impose the Yoga Sādhanā on me. There was no compulsion or duress. Yoga was my free choice. Verily, I learnt Yoga from him. While teaching me Yoga, he treated me not as his daughter, but as a pupil. I know that he is very exacting as a teacher. He is a stickler for discipline and a taskmaster; but his ways are gentle persuasion and not stern reprimand. He expects discipline and keen attention from his pupils. Is not Yoga Sādhāna the greatest of disciplines?

The fact that life is an admixture of happiness and sorrow cannot become untrue. It should be so, as otherwise life has no meaning and becomes a dead matter. Yoga makes one face both happiness and sorrow with equanimity. So, I am overjoyed in presenting my book *Yoga—A Gem for Women* before my readers, yet my joy is tinged with an imprint of sorrow as my mother is no longer in this world to share in my joy, for it was she who ferried me to a higher shore by example and precept. It is impossible for me to repay the debt of gratitude of my father and mother who became my Gurus, except to follow forever and sincerely the path of Yoga taught by them.

This book is written with my many years of experience and observation but with one objective—to meet the specific needs of women. It does not however, preclude men, as Yoga is useful for both women and men. The book describes simple techniques of Yoga for women and I am happy to be able to share my experiences with my sisters through this presentation.

I am grateful to Mr. Mohan Welling, who took great pains in taking all the photographs and placing his studio at my disposal.

I am thankful to Miss Ramanben Moti for drawing the anatomical charts for the book.

My brother Prashant and sister Mrs. Vanita Sridharan gave me immense help. Besides helping with the script, Vanita willingly agreed to be photographed for the book depicting Yogāsanas during her period of pregnancy. These are valuable photographs and will encourage women to practise Yoga even while pregnant.

I am indebted to Mrs. Silva Mehta for helping me in re-editing the script and Miss Srimathi Rao for typing the final script.

My thanks are due to my father, Sri B.K.S. Iyengar, and to Harper Collins Publishers, U.K., for allowing me to make use of a number of references from the book *Light on Yoga* and *Light on Prāṇāyāma.*

I am indebted to Messrs. Allied Publishers Pvt. Ltd., New Delhi, for publishing this illustrated book and presenting it to the world-wide public, particularly to my sisters in the East and the West.

Geeta S. Iyengar

Contents

Adorations to the Guru .... *vii*
Foreword .... *ix*
Preface .... *xiii*
List of Figures .... *xxiv*
List of Abbreviations .... *xxxii*

Part–I: Theory

Chapter 1: First Steps in Yoga 3

Chapter 2: Four Paths to Liberation 5

Chapter 3: The Path of Yoga 9

Definition of Yoga 9
Patañjali's Definition 11
What is Citta? 11
Aṣṭāṅga Yoga—Eight Branches of Yoga 14
Ṣadāṅga Yoga—Six-Sided Yoga 16
Yama—Social Discipline 20
Niyama—Individual Discipline 24
Āsana—Postures 27
Prāṇāyāma—Breath Control 29
Pratyāhāra—Discipline of the Senses 31
Dhārṇā—Concentration 32
Dhyāna—Meditation 32
Samādhi—Self-Realisation 33

Chapter 4: Are Women Eligible for Yoga? 35

Chapter 5: The Nature of Health 39

Importance of Health 39

Chapter 6: Is Yoga Ideal for Women? 44

Chapter 7: Three Milestones in a Woman's Life 50

Part–II: Practice

Chapter 8: Know Your Body 63

Chapter 9: Yoga Sādhanā—Method of Practice and Prerequisites 74

Mental Attitude 74
Buddhi—Intelligence 76
Ahaṃkāra—Ego 76
Brain 77
Manas—Mind 77
Śarīra—Body 78

Chapter 10: Hints and Suggestions for the Practice of Āsanas 82

Part I: General Hints 82

Part II: Special Hints 90

Chapter 11: Classification, Table and Course of Study 100

Table of Illustrations of Āsanas 103
First Year—Elementary Course 111
Second Year—Intermediate Course 112
Third Year—Advanced Course 113
First Three Months—Introductory Course 115
Weekly Schedules 115
First Year—Elementary Course 115
Second Year—Intermediate Course 118
Third Year—Advanced Course 120
Intensive Course 123

Chapter 12: Yogāsanas—Technique and Effects 125

Section–I: Āsanas: Standing 125

1. *Tādāsana or Samasthiti* 126
2. *Vṛkṣāsana* 127
3. *Utthita Trikoṇāsana* 128
4. *Utthita Pārśvakoṇāsana* 130
5. *Vīrabhadrāsana I* 132
6. *Vīrabhadrāsana II* 134
7. *Vīrabhadrāsana III* 136
8. *Ardha Candrāsana* 138
9. *Parivṛtta Trikoṇāsana* 140
10. *Pārśvottānāsana* 142
11. *Prasārita Pādottānāsana* 145
12. *Pādānguṣṭhāsana* 147
13. *Uttānāsana* 149
14. *Adho Mukha Śvānāsana* 151

Section–II: Āsanas: Forward Bends 154

15. *Daṇḍāsana* 154
16. *Jānu Śīrṣāsana* 156
17. *Ardha Baddha Padma Paścimottānāsana* 159
18. *Triaṅg Mukhaikapāda Paścimottanāsana* 161
19. *Marīcyāsana I* 163
20. *Paścimottānāsana* 165
21. *Parivṛtta Jānu Śīrṣāsana* 169
22. *Parivṛtta Paścimottānāsana* 171
23. *Baddha Koṇāsana* 173
24. *Supta Baddha Koṇāsana* 176
25. *Upaviṣṭa Koṇāsana* 178
26. *Kūrmāsana* 180
27. *Supta Kūrmāsana* 182
28. *Mālāsana* 184

Section–III: Āsanas: Sitting and Supine 187
29. *Siddhāsana* 188
30. *Vīrāsana* 190
31. *Padmāsana* 192
32. *Vīrāsana Cycle* 195
33. *Supta Vīrāsana* 198
Padmāsana Cycle 201
34. *Parvatāsana* 201
35. *Baddha Padmāsana* 203
36. *Yoga Mudrāsana* 205
37. *Matsyāsana* 206

Section–IV: Āsanas: Inverted 208
38. *Sālamba Śīrṣāsana* 208
39. *Pārśva Śīrṣāsana* 220
40. *Parivṛttaikapāda Śīrṣāsana* 221
41. *Ekapāda Śīrṣāsana* 222
42. *Pārśvaikapāda Śīrṣāsana* 224
43. *Upaviṣṭa Koṇāsana in Śīrṣāsana* 226
44. *Baddha Koṇāsana in Śīrṣāsana* 227
45. *Ūrdhva Padmāsana in Śīrṣāsana* 229
46. *Piṇḍāsana in Śīrsāsana* 230
47. *Sālamba Sarvāṅgāsana* 232
48. *Halāsana* 239
49. *Karṇapīḍāsana* 243
50. *Supta Koṇāsana* 244
51. *Pārśva Halāsana* 245
52. *Eka Pāda Sarvāṅgāsana* 247
53. *Pārśvaika Pāda Sarvāṅgāsana* 249
54. *Setu Bandha Sarvāṅgāsana* 251
55. *Ūrdhva Padmāsana in Sarvāṅgāsana* 256
56. *Piṇḍāsana in Sarvāṅgāsana* 257
57. *Pārśva Piṇḍāsana* 259

Section–V: Āsanas: Abdominal and Lumbar 262
58. *Ūrdhva Prasārita Pādāsana* 262
59. *Paripūrṇa Nāvāsana* 267
60. *Jaṭhara Parivartanāsana* 269
61. *Ūrdhva Mukha Paścimottānāsana II* 272
62. *Supta Pādānguṣṭhāsana* 273
63. *Utthita Hasta Pādānguṣṭhāsana* 277

Section–VI: Āsanas: Twists 283
64. *Bhāradvājāsana I* 283
65. *Bhāradvājāsana II* 286
66. *Marīcyāsana III* 287
67. *Ardha Matsyendrāsana* 290
68. *Pāśāsana* 294

Section–VII: Āsanas: Backbends 297
69. *Uṣṭrāsana* 298
70. *Ūrdhva Mukha Śvānāsana* 300
71. *Dhanurāsana* 302
72. *Ūrdhva Dhanurāsana* 304
73. *Dvi Pāda Viparīta Daṇḍāsana* 309

Section–VIII: Āsana: Yoga Kuruṇṭa 315
Arrangement of the Rope 315
74. Variation I: *Bhujaṅgāsana* 317
75. Variation II: *Bhujaṅgāsana and Ūrdhva Mukha Paścimottānāsana II* 320
76. Variation III: *Pūrvottānāsana* 323
77. Variation IV: *Ūrdhva Hasta Dhanurāsana* 324
78. Variation V: *Uṣṭrāsana* 326
79. Variation VI: *Sālamba Sarvāṅgāsana, Halāsana and Variations* 327
80. Variation VII: *Ūrdhva Mukha Paścimottānāsana I* 332

Section–IX: Āsanas and Prāṇāyāma during PREGNANCY 334

Āsanas from Section I

3. *Utthita Trikoṇāsana* 336
4. *Utthita Pārśvakoṇāsana* 337
5. *Vīrabhadrāsana I* 338
6. *Vīrabhadrāsana II* 339
8. *Ardha Candrāsana* 339
10. *Pārśvottānāsana* 340
11. *Prasārita Pādottānāsana* 341

Āsanas from Section II

16. *Jānu Śīrṣāsana* 343
23. *Baddha Koṇāsana* 344
24. *Supta Baddha Koṇāsana* 345
25. *Upaviṣṭa Koṇāsana* 345

Āsanas from Section III

30. *Vīrāsana* 347
32. *Vīrāsana Cycle* 347
33. *Supta Vīrāsana* 348
34. *Parvatāsana* 349

Āsanas from Section IV

38. *Sālamba Śīrṣāsana* 350
39. *Pārśva Śīrṣāsana* 352
40. *Parivṛttaikapāda Śīrṣāsana* 353
47. *Sālamba Sarvāṅgāsana* 354
48. *Halāsana* 356
52. *Eka Pāda Sarvāṅgāsana* 358
55. *Ūrdhva Padmāsana in Sarvāṅgāsana* 359

Āsanas from Section VI

64. *Bhāradvājāsana I* 360

Āsanas from Sections XI and XII

Mudrā, Śavāsana, Prāṇāyāma and *Dhyāna* 361

Order of Practice during Pregnancy 363

Section–X: Āsanas: Advanced 366
81. *Yoganidrāsana* 366
82. *Ūrdhva Kukkuṭāsana* 367
83. *Pārśva Kukkuṭāsana* 368
84. *Pīñcha Mayūrāsana* 368
85. *Kapotāsana* 369
86. *Eka Pāda Rājakapotāsana* 369
87. *Vṛścikāsana* 370
88. *Naṭarājāsana* 370

Part–III: Experience

Chapter 13: On the Threshold of Peace 373
Section–XI: Mudrā and Śavāsana 373
89. *Mahā Mudrā* 374
90. *Ṣaṇmukhī Mudrā* 377
91. *Śavāsana* 380
Chapter 14: Hints and Suggestions for the Practice of Prāṇāyāma 387
Chapter 15: Prāṇāyāma—Techniques and Effects 403
Section–XII 403
I. Preparation for Deep Breathing 404
II. *Ujjāyī Prāṇāyāma I* 406
III. *Viloma Prāṇāyāma* 410
IV. *Ujjāyī Prāṇāyāma II* 413
V. *Sūrya Bhedana Prāṇāyāma* 415
VI. *Nāḍdī Śodhana Prāṇāyāma* 418
Chapter 16: Dhyāna (Meditation) 421
The Nature of Meditation 421
Technique 423

List of Figures

Fig. I: External Organs 65
Fig. II: The System of Bones 67
Fig. III: Skull and Spine 67
Fig. IV: The Muscular System 68
Fig. V: Internal Organs 73
Fig. 1: *Tāḍāsana* (Final Stage) 126
Fig. 2: *Vṛkṣāsana* (Final Stage) 127
Fig. 3: *Utthita Trikoṇāsana* (Intermediate Stage) 128
Fig. 4: *Utthita Trikoṇāsana* (Final Stage) 128
Fig. 5: *Utthita Pārśvakoṇāsana* (Final Stage) 130
Fig. 6: *Vīrabhadrāsana I* (Intermediate Stage) 132
Fig. 7: *Vīrabhadrāsana I* (Final Stage) 132
Fig. 8: *Vīrabhadrāsana II* (Final Stage) 134
Fig. 9: *Vīrabhadrāsana III* (Final Stage) 136
Fig. 10: *Ardha Candrāsana* (Final Stage) 138
Fig. 11: *Parivṛtta Trikoṇāsana* (Final Stage) 140
Fig. 12: *Pārśvottānāsana* (Intermediate Stage) 142
Fig. 13: *Pārśvottānāsana* (Final Stage) 142
Fig. 14: *Pārśvottānāsana* (Intermediate Stage) 143
Fig. 15: *Pārśvottānāsana* (Final Stage) 143
Fig. 16: *Prasārita Pādottānāsana* (Intermediate Stage) 145
Fig. 17: *Prasārita Pādottānāsana* (Intermediate Stage) 145
Fig. 18: *Prasārita Pādottānāsana* (Final Stage) 146
Fig. 19: *Pādānguṣṭhāsana* (Intermediate Stage) 147
Fig. 20: *Pādānguṣṭhāsana* (Final Stage) 148
Fig. 21(a): *Uttānāsana* (Intermediate Stage) 149
Fig. 21: *Uttānāsana* (Final Stage) 150
Fig. 22: *Adho Mukha Śvānāsana* (Final Stage) 151
Fig. 23: *Daṇḍāsana* (Final Stage) 155
Fig. 24: *Jānu Śīrṣāsana* (Intermediate Stage) 156

Fig. 25: *Jānu Śīrṣāsana* (Intermediate Stage) 156
Fig. 26: *Jānu Śīrṣāsana* (Final Stage) 157
Fig. 27: *Ardha Baddha Padma Paścimottānāsana* (Final Stage) 159
Fig. 28: *Triaṅg Mukhaikapāda Paścimottanāsana* (Final Stage) 161
Fig. 29: *Marīcyāsana I* (Final Stage) 163
Fig. 30: *Paścimottānāsana* (Final Stage) 166
Fig. 31: *Paścimottānāsana* (Final Stage) 167
Fig. 32: *Parivṛtta Janu Śīrṣāsana* (Intermediate Stage) 169
Fig. 33: *Parivṛtta Jānu Śīrṣāsana* (Final Stage) 170
Fig. 34: *Parivṛtta Paścimottānāsana* (Final Stage) 171
Fig. 35: *Baddha Koṇāsana* (Final Stage) 173
Fig. 36: *Baddha Koṇāsana* (Final Stage) 174
Fig. 37: *Baddha Koṇāsana* (Final Stage) 174
Fig. 38: *Supta Baddha Koṇāsana* (Final Stage) 176
Fig. 39: *Supta Baddha Koṇāsana* (Final Stage) 177
Fig. 40: *Upaviṣṭha Koṇāsana* (Intermediate Stage) 178
Fig. 41: *Upaviṣṭha Koṇāsana* (Final Stage) 179
Fig. 42: *Kūrmāsana* (Intermediate Stage) 180
Fig. 43: *Kūrmāsana* (Final Stage) 181
Fig. 44: *Supta Kūrmāsana* (Final Stage) 183
Fig. 45: *Mālāsana* (Intermediate Stage) 184
Fig. 46: *Mālāsana* (Easy Stage) 185
Fig. 47: *Mālāsana* (Final Stage) 185
Fig. 48: *Siddhāsana* (Final Stage) 189
Fig. 49: *Vīrāsana* (Final Stage) 190
Fig. 50: *Vīrāsana* (Final Stage) 191
Fig. 51: *Vīrāsana* (Easy Stage) 191
Fig. 52: *Padmāsana* (Final Stage) 192
Fig. 53: *Padmāsana* (Easy Stage) 193
Fig. 54: *Vīrāsana Cycle* (Final Stage) 195
Fig. 55: *Vīrāsana Cycle* (Final Stage) 196
Fig. 56: *Supta Vīrāsana* (Intermediate Stage) 198

Fig. 57: *Supta Vīrāsana* (Intermediate Stage) 199
Fig. 58: *Supta Vīrāsana* (Final Stage) 200
Fig. 59: *Parvatāsana* (Final Stage) 201
Fig. 60: *Baddha Padmāsana* (Final Stage) 203
Fig. 61: *Yoga Mudrāsana* (Final Stage) 205
Fig. 62: *Matsyāsana* (Final Stage) 206
Fig. 63: *Sālamba Śīrṣāsana* (Intermediate Stage) 210
Fig. 64: *Sālamba Śīrṣāsana* (Intermediate Stage) 211
Fig. 64(a): *Sālamba Śīrṣāsana* (Intermediate Stage) 211
Fig. 65: *Sālamba Śīrṣāsana* (Easy Stage) 212
Fig. 66: *Sālamba Śīrṣāsana* (Intermediate Stage) 214
Fig. 67: *Sālamba Śīrṣāsana* (Intermediate Stage) 215
Fig. 68: *Sālamba Śīrṣāsana* (Intermediate Stage) 215
Fig. 69: *Sālamba Śīrṣāsana* (Final Stage) 216
Fig. 70: *Sālamba Śīrṣāsana* (Final Stage) 216
Fig. 70(a): *Sālamba Śīrṣāsana* (Final Stage) 218
Fig. 71: *Pārśva Śīrṣāsana* (Final Stage) 220
Fig. 72: *Parivṛttaikapāda Śīrṣāsana* (Final Stage) 221
Fig. 73: *Eka Pāda Sīrṣāsana* (Final Stage) 222
Fig. 74: *Pārśvaika Pāda Śīrṣāsana* (Final Stage) 224
Fig. 75: *Upaviṣṭha Koṇāsana in Śīrṣāsana* (Final Stage) 226
Fig. 76: *Baddha Koṇāsana in Śīrṣāsana* (Final Stage) 227
Fig. 77: *Ūrdhva Padmāsana in Śīrṣāsana* (Final Stage) 229
Fig. 78: *Piṇḍāsana in Śīrṣāsana* (Easy Stage) 230
Fig. 79: *Piṇḍāsana in Śīrṣāsana* (Final Stage) 230
Fig. 80: *Sālamba Sarvāṅgāsana* (Intermediate Stage) 232
Fig. 81: *Sālamba Sarvāṅgāsana* (Intermediate Stage) 232
Fig. 82: *Sālamba Sarvāṅgāsana* (Intermediate Stage) 233
Fig. 83: *Sālamba Sarvāṅgāsana* (Intermediate Stage) 233
Fig. 84: *Sālamba Sarvāṅgāsana* (Final Stage) 234
Fig. 85: *Sālamba Sarvāṅgāsana* (Final Stage) 234
Fig. 86: *Sālamba Sarvāṅgāsana* (Final Stage) 235
Fig. 87: *Sālamba Sarvāṅgāsana* (Final Stage) 237
Fig. 88: *Halāsana* (Final Stage) 239

Fig. 89: *Halāsana* (Easy Stage) 241
Fig. 90: *Halāsana* (Easy Stage) 241
Fig. 91: *Halāsana* (Final Stage) 242
Fig. 92: *Karṇapīḍāsana* (Final Stage) 243
Fig. 93: *Supta Koṇāsana* (Final Stage) 244
Fig. 94: *Pārśva Halāsana* (Final Stage) 246
Fig. 95: *Eka Pāda Sarvāṅgāsana* (Final Stage) 247
Fig. 96: *Pārśvaika Pāda Sarvāṇgāsana* (Final Stage) 249
Fig. 97: *Setu Bandha Sarvāṅgāsana* (Intermediate Stage) 251
Fig. 98: *Setu Bandha Sarvāṅgāsana* (Easy Stage) 252
Fig. 99: *Setu Bandha Sarvāṅgāsana* (Easy Stage) 252
Fig. 100: *Setu Bandha Sarvāṅgāsana* (Intermediate Stage) 253
Fig. 101: *Setu Bandha Sarvāṅgāsana* (Final Stage) 253
Fig. 102: *Setu Bandha Sarvāṅgāsana* (Intermediate Stage) 255
Fig. 103: *Ūrdhva Padmāsana in Sarvāṅgāsana* (Final Stage) ... 256
Fig. 104: *Piṇḍāsana in Sarvāṅgāsana* (Final Stage) 258
Fig. 105: *Pārśva Piṇḍāsana in Sarvāṅgāsana* (Final Stage) 259
Fig. 106: *Ūrdhva Prasārita Pādāsana* (Intermediate Stage) 263
Fig. 107: *Ūrdhva Prasārita Pādāsana* (Final Stage) 263
Fig. 108: *Ūrdhva Prasārita Pādāsana* (Final Stage) 263
Fig. 109: *Ūrdhva Prasārita Pādāsana* (Final Stage) 264
Fig. 110: *Ūrdhva Prasārita Pādāsana* (Intermediate Stage) 265
Fig. 111: *Paripūrṇa Nāvāsana* (Final Stage) 267
Fig. 112: *Jaṭhara Parivartanāsana* (Intermediate Stage) 269
Fig. 113: *Jaṭhara Parivartanāsana* (Final Stage) 270
Fig. 114: *Jaṭhara Parivartanāsana* (Final Stage) 271
Fig. 115: *Ūrdhva Mukha Paścimottānāsana II* (Final Stage) 272
Fig. 116: *Supta Pādānguṣṭhāsana* (Intermediate Stage) 274
Fig. 117: *Supta Pādānguṣṭhāsana* (Final Stage) 274
Fig. 118: *Supta Pādānguṣṭhāsana* (Final Stage) 275
Fig. 119: *Supta Pādānguṣṭhāsana* (Final Stage) 276
Fig. 120: *Utthita Hasta Pādānguṣṭhāsana* (Intermediate Stage).. 277
Fig. 121: *Utthita Hasta Pādānguṣṭhāsana* (Final Stage) 278
Fig. 122: *Utthita Hasta Pādānguṣṭhāsana* (Intermediate Stage) 279

Fig. 123: *Utthita Hasta Pādānguṣṭhāsana* (Final Stage) 279
Fig. 124: *Utthita Hasta Pādānguṣṭhāsana* (Final Stage) 280
Fig. 125: *Bhāradvājāsana I* (Final Stage) 284
Fig. 126: *Bhāradvājāsana II* (Final Stage) 286
Fig. 127: *Marīcyāsana III* (Final Stage) 288
Fig. 128: *Ardha Matsyendrāsana* (Final Stage) 291
Fig. 129: *Ardha Matsyendrāsana* (Easy Stage) 292
Fig. 130: *Ardha Matsyendrāsana* (Easy Stage) 293
Fig. 131: *Pāśāsana* (Final Stage) 294
Fig. 132: *Pāśāsana* (Easy Stage) 295
Fig. 133: *Uṣṭrāsana* (Final Stage) 298
Fig. 134: *Ūrdhva Mukha Śvānāsana* (Intermediate Stage) 300
Fig. 135: *Ūrdhva Mukha Śvānāsana* (Final Stage) 301
Fig. 136: *Dhanurāsana* (Final Stage) 302
Fig. 137: *Urdhva Dhanurāsana* (Intermediate Stage) 304
Fig. 138: *Urdhva Dhanurāsana* (Intermediate Stage) 305
Fig. 139: *Urdhva Dhanurāsana* (Final Stage) 305
Fig. 140: *Urdhva Dhanurāsana* (Final Stage) 305
Fig. 141: *Urdhva Dhanurāsana* (Intermediate Stage) 307
Fig. 141(a): *Urdhva Dhanurāsana* (Intermediate Stage) 307
Fig. 142: *Urdhva Dhanurāsana* (Intermediate Stage) 307
Fig. 142(a): *Urdhva Dhanurāsana* (Intermediate Stage) 308
Fig. 143: *Urdhva Dhanurāsana* (Easy Stage) 308
Fig. 144: *Dvi Pāda Viparīta Daṇḍāsana* (Intermediate Stage) 309
Fig. 145: *Dvi Pāda Viparīta Daṇḍāsana* (Intermediate Stage) . 310
Fig. 146: *Dvi Pāda Viparīta Daṇḍāsana* (Final Stage) 310
Fig. 147: *Dvi Pāda Viparīta Daṇḍāsana* (Easy Stage) 312
Fig. 148: *Dvi Pāda Viparīta Daṇḍāsana* (Easy Stage) 313
Fig. 149: *Dvi Pāda Viparīta Daṇḍāsana* (Easy Stage) 313
Fig. 150: Rope Arrangement 316
Fig. 151: Variation I: *Bhujaṅgāsana* (Intermediate Stage) 317
Fig. 152(a): Variation I: *Bhujaṅgāsana* (Intermediate Stage).. 318
Fig. 152(b): Variation I: *Bhujaṅgāsana* 318
(Intermediate Stage)

Fig. 153: Variation I: *Bhujaṅgāsana* (Final Stage) 319
Fig. 154: Variation II: *Bhujaṅgāsana, Ūrdhva Mukha Paścimottānāsana I* (Intermediate Stage) 320
Fig. 155: Variation II: *Ūrdhva Mukha Paścimottānāsana* (Final Stage) 321
Fig. 156: Variation II: *Bhujaṅgāsana* (Final Stage) 321
Fig. 157: Variation II: *Ūrdhva Mukha Paścimottānāsana* (Final Stage) 322
Fig. 158: Variation III: *Pūrvottānāsana* (Final Stage) 323
Fig. 159: Variation III: *Pūrvottānāsana* (Intermediate Stage) 324
Fig. 160: Variation IV: *Ūrdhva Hasta Dhanurāsana* (Final Stage) 325
Fig. 161: Variation V: *Uṣṭrāsana* (Final Stage) 326
Fig. 162: Variation VI: *Sālamba Sarvāṅgāsana* (Intermediate Stage) 328
Fig. 162(a): Variation VI: *Sālamba Sarvāṅgāsana* (Intermediate Stage) 328
Fig. 163: Variation VI: *Sālamba Sarvāṅgāsana* (Intermediate Stage) 328
Fig. 164: Variation VI: *Sālamba Sarvāṅgāsana* (Final Stage) 328
Fig. 164(a): Variation VI: *Sālamba Sarvāṅgāsana* (Final Stage) 328
Fig. 165: Variation VI: *Halāsana* (Intermediate Stage) 329
Fig. 166: Variation VI: *Halāsana* (Intermediate Stage) 329
Fig. 167: Variation VI: *Halāsana* (Final Stage) 329
Fig. 168: Variation VI: *Karṇapīḍāsana* (Final Stage) 330
Fig. 169: Variation VI: *Supta Koṇāsana* (Final Stage) 330
Fig. 170: Variation VI: *Pārśva Halāsana* (Final Stage) 331
Fig. 171: Variation VI: *Eka Pāda Sarvāṅgāsana* (Final Stage) 331
Fig. 172: Variation VI: *Pārśvaika Pāda Sarvāṅgāsana* (Final Stage) 331
Fig. 173: Variation VII: *Ūrdhva Mukha Paścimottānāsana* (Final Stage) 332
Fig. 174: *Utthita Trikoṇāsana* (Final Stage) 336

Fig. 175: *Utthita Pārśvakoṇāsana* (Final Stage) 337
Fig. 176: *Vīrabhadrāsana I* (Final Stage) 338
Fig. 177: *Ardha Candrāsana* (Final Stage) 339
Fig. 178: *Pārśvottānāsana* (Intermediate Stage) 340
Fig. 179: *Pārśvottānāsana* (Final Stage) 340
Fig. 180: *Prasārita Pādottānāsana* (Intermediate Stage) 341
Fig. 181: *Prasārita Pādottānāsana* (Easy Stage) 342
Fig. 182: *Jānu Śīrṣāsana* (Intermediate Stage) 343
Fig. 183: *Baddha Koṇāsana* (Final Stage) 344
Fig. 184: *Upaviṣṭha Koṇāsana* (Easy Stage) 346
Fig. 185: *Vīrāsana Cycle* (Final Stage) 347
Fig. 186: *Supta Vīrāsana* (Final Stage) 348
Fig. 187: *Parvatāsana* (Final Stage) 349
Fig. 188: *Sālamba Śīrsāsana* (Final Stage) 350
Fig. 189: *Sālamba Śīrsāsana* (Final Stage) 351
Fig. 190: *Pārśva Śīrṣāsana* (Final Stage) 352
Fig. 191: *Parivṛttaikapāda Śīrṣāsana* (Final Stage) 353
Fig. 192: *Sālamba Sarvāṅgāsana* (Final Stage) 354
Fig. 193: *Sālamba Sarvāṅgāsana* (Easy Stage) 355
Fig. 194: *Halāsana* (Easy Stage) 356
Fig. 195: *Halāsana* (Easy Stage) 356
Fig. 194(a): *Halāsana* (Easy Stage) 357
Fig. 195(a): *Halāsana* (Easy Stage) 357
Fig. 196: *Halāsana* (Easy Stage) 358
Fig. 197: *Ūrdhva Padmāsana in Sarvāṅgāsanaa* (Final Stage) .. 359
Fig. 198: *Bhāradvājāsana I* (Intermediate Stage) 360
Fig. 199: *Śavāsana* (Final Stage) 361
Fig. 200: *Ujjāyī Prāṇāyāma I; Viloma Prāṇāyāma I & II*; 361
Preparation for Deep Breathing I & II (Final Stage)
Fig. 201: *Sūrya Bhedana Prāṇāyāma,* 362
Nāḍi Śodhana Prāṇāyāma (Final Stage)
Fig. 202: *Yoganidrāsana* (Final Stage) 367
Fig. 203: *Ūrdhva Kukkutnsana* (Final Stage) 367
Fig. 204: *Pārśva Kukkuṭāsana* (Final Stage) 368

Fig. 205: *Pīṇcha Mayūrāsana* (Final Stage) 368
Fig. 206: *Kapotāsana* (Final Stage) 369
Fig. 207: *Eka Pāda Rājakapotāsana* (Final Stage) 369
Fig. 208: *Vṛścikāsana* (Final Stage) 370
Fig. 209: *Naṭarājāsana* (Final Stage) 370
Fig. 210: *Mahā Mudrā* (Final Stage) 374
Fig. 211: *Ṣaṇmukhi Mudrā* (Final Stage) 377
Fig. 212: *Savāsana* (Final Stage) 380
Fig. 213: *Ujjayi Prāṇāyāma II* (Final Sage) 392
Fig. 214: *Nāḍī Śodhana Prāṇāyāma,* 395
Sūrya Bhedana Prāṇāyāma (Final Sage)
Fig. 215: *Dhyāna* (Meditation) 425

List of Abbreviations

B.G.	Bhagavad Gītā
C.S.	Caraka Samhitā
H.P.	Haṭhayoga Pradīpikā
I. Ūp.	Iso Upanishad
K. Ūp.	Kaṭhopaniṣad
M.S.	Manu Smṛṭi
Mu. Ūp.	Mundakopaniṣaḍ
P.Y.S.	Patañjāli Yoga Sūtras
R.	Raghuvaṃśa
S.S.	Śiva Samhitā
V.A.H.	Vāgbhatta Aṣṭanga Hṛdaya
Y. Ūp.	Yogapanisad

PART–I

Theory

CHAPTER I

First Steps in Yoga

Poets write sonnets about carefree and joyous childhood; but, for me childhood was a nightmare. At an age when children go plucking raw mangoes or tamarind on the sly, the sickbed was my companion. I was in turn afflicted with chronic fever, headache, cold, cough and stomach-ache. As if this were not enough, I was laid up with typhoid, jaundice and diphtheria. To top it all, I suffered from nephritis (acute inflammation of the kidneys) when I was ten years old. Needless to say, my attendance at school was irregular. I became so weak that climbing even a step was an impossibility for me.

During a severe attack of nephritis, I was unconscious for four days in a nursing home. The doctors did not hold out much hope for my survival and they informed my parents accordingly. By the grace of God I survived and was discharged after three weeks. I heaved a sigh of relief at the thought of being spared so many injections a day! However, I was given a long list of medicines. The return home was like a release from prison. Little did I know then that after this release I was to witness a great upheaval in my life.

On my returning home my father kept the list of medicines aside and said sternly, 'From tomorrow onwards no more medicines. Either you practise Yoga or get prepared to die.'

From the next day I started to practise *Yoga-āsanas*, though not very regularly. Gradually my health showed signs of improvement. Once a week I used to go to the doctors for a checkup. 'Condition improving, continue the medicines,' the doctors would say and I continued my Yoga practice at home! I must, however, admit that I was not very regular.

Later, when foreign students came to study Yoga from my father I felt ashamed. I thought, if foreigners spend a lot of money to derive benefits from Yoga at the hands of my father, surely the least I could do was to be sincere and regular. I resolved that I would learn all about Yoga and one day become a teacher of Yoga as my father. Since 1961 that dream has been fulfilled. This book is the result of my experience as a Yoga teacher. During these years I have given many Yoga demonstrations as well.

An Indian woman's life is a veritable tight-rope walk. Her status in society, the problems she has to face due to social and economic pressures, the burdens nature has imposed on her—all these result in stress and tell upon her health. The more I thought about my sisters—women and their particular problems the more I was convinced that Yoga was the answer.

This book considers how women can achieve fulfilment in their lives through the practice of Yoga.

Chapter II

Four Paths to Liberation

In our scientific age man has reached new heights. With faster and faster modes of travel the world has shrunk. Within hours continents can be reached. With the coming of the space age, man has landed on the moon and now is ambitious to reach other planets. In the field of medicine daring experiments such as heart transplants have been undertaken; with test-tube babies man is now competing with the Creator.

Thanks to the advance in laboursaving devices, man's toil has been reduced to the minimum. With all the technological advances at his doorstep, he has lost his natural birthright—sleep. Insomnia is the curse of our civilisation. Consider the number of patent drugs—sleeping pills and tranquilisers—available in the market. Sleep induced by tranquilisers is not like natural sleep. Natural sleep occurs in a tranquil body and mind and makes one well equipped to face the problems of the day. How important sleep is, has been well described by Vāgbhata in the following stanzas:

nidrāyattam sukham duḥkham
puṣṭiḥ kārśyam balābalam
vṛṣatā klībatā jnānam
ajnānam jīvitam na ca

V.A.H. I, 7.53

[On sleep depend happiness and grief, fatness and leanness, strength and weakness, potency and impotency, knowledge and ignorance, life and death.]

Sound, undisturbed sleep is a life-giver. The conscious mind ceases to function for some hours, recharging batteries for the next day. The nervous system is at rest and one wakes up refreshed the next morning. Can life be happy and progressive if we lose this natural function—sleep?

Sages and philosophers have compared life to a chariot drawn by two horses—the material and the spiritual—both running in unison. Any imbalance in their speed results in unhappiness. The trouble with our age is that the material steed of the chariot is running faster than the other—the spiritual.

A verse from Īśopaniṣaḍ puts this thought aptly:

> *vidyām cāvidyām ca yastad vedobhayam saha*
> *avidyayā mṛtyum tīrtvā vidyayāmṛtamaśnute*
>
> I. Ūp. 11

[Spiritual knowledge and material knowledge—both are necessary. Pursuit of one at the cost of the other leads to downfall. Material knowledge enables one to face life's problems, whereas spiritual knowledge helps one to realise oneself.]

Is there then a way to balance material and spiritual knowledge in order to create harmony in our lives?

There are four paths to Self-realisation: (i) the path of knowledge, (ii) the path of action, (iii) the path of devotion, and (iv) the path of Yoga. Though the paths are different, they lead to the same goal.

The path of knowledge enables one to discriminate between good and evil, to follow right conduct, to discriminate between Prakṛti (Nature) and Puruṣa (Individual Soul), to attain Self-realisation, and finally to be one with God.

The follower of the path of action considers service to humanity as service to God. Good actions and fulfilment of one's duty lead to liberation.

The pursuer of devotion sees the presence of God in every animate and inanimate object. A devotee (Bhakta) is full of love for every living thing and attains liberation with God's name ever on the lips.

The follower of the path of Yoga learns to control the fluctuations of the mind, to stabilise it in order to perceive the Inner Self and through this Self, which is crystal clear, the Supreme is realised.

In the Bhagavad Gītā, Kṛṣṇa advises Arjuna thus:

tapasvibhyodhiko yogī
jnānibhyo'pi matodhikah
karmibhyaścādhiko yogī
tasmād yogī bhavārjuna

B.G VI. 46

[The Yogi is greater than the ascetic, the learned, or the man of action; therefore be a Yogi, Oh Arjuna.]

The fact that the path of Yoga has been highly praised does not mean that the other three paths are inferior, but that Yoga has attained a fullness by absorbing the other three paths of knowledge, devotion and action.

For any attainment, unity is indispensable. Without devotion and love, advaita, non-duality of the Individual Soul with the Universal Spirit, is impossible. Advaita is not attainable through knowledge alone. Knowledge, devotion, and action are so interwoven that without them nothing is attainable. There is no devotion without knowledge, no action without devotion, and Yoga is not possible without the combination of the three paths. In this way Yoga is unique.

In the science of Āyurveda the human body has been divided into six main parts: the head, the chest, the two arms, and the two legs.

The head is the seat of knowledge, the heart that of devotion, the arms and the legs are for action. The path of Yoga combines these three—body, mind and soul—which act in unison. Therefore, Yoga is the foundation for all the other paths.

Explaining the excellence of the art and science of Yoga in Yogabīja, Lord Śiva says to Pārvatī:

jñāna niṣṭo viraktopi dharmajnopi jitendriyaḥ
vinā yogena devopi na mokśam labhate priye

[Oh Pārvati, the learned, the recluse, the righteous, and the one who has controlled the senses, even God Himself, cannot attain liberation without the pursuit of Yoga.]

Lord Śiva again says:

ālokya sarvaśāstrāṇi vicārya ca punaḥ punaḥ
idamekam suniṣpannam yogaśāstram parammatam

S.S. I, 17

[Having studied all the scriptures and sciences, and thought them over again and again, one comes to the conclusion that the art and science of Yoga is the only true and firm doctrine.]

A verse from Atrisamhitā upholds the importance of the path of Yoga:

Yoga helps to attain knowledge; Yoga teaches what one's duty is; Yoga is a penance; hence it is essential to study Yoga.

In Kaṭhopaniṣaḍ, Yama instructed Naciketa to acquire this knowledge from the discipline of Yoga.

mṛtyuproktām naciketo'tha labdhva
vidyāmetām yogavidhim ca kṛtsnam
brahmaprāpto virajo'bhūt vimṛtyuḥ
anyopyevam yo vidadhyātmamevam

K. Ūp. VI, 18

[Naciketa, having acquired this knowledge and the discipline of Yoga from the God of Death, realised the 'Self'; he was purged of all impurities and became immortal. Others also may emulate him and become so.]

Let us now proceed to find out what Yoga is.

Chapter III

The Path of Yoga

The word Yoga evokes all sorts of images in the popular mind. Some associate it with recluses, saffron-robed, body smeared with ashes, with begging bowl in hand, and wandering from town to town; or sitting crosslegged atop a mountain or on the banks of a sacred river. Cartoons depict a Yogi sitting on a bed of nails, performing the rope trick, and walking on water. In others he is a sort of magician drinking acid or swallowing pieces of glass. Thus a confused notion exists in people's minds about Yoga. Now let us examine what Yoga in fact is.

DEFINITION OF YOGA

The word Yoga has its root in the Sanskrit word 'yuj' which means to merge, join, or unite. Yoga is the union of the soul with the eternal truth, a state of unalloyed bliss, arising from conquest of dualities. The study of Yoga discipline sharpens the power of discernment and leads towards understanding the true nature of the soul which cannot be fully comprehended by the senses or the intellect alone. The study of Yoga enables one to attain the pure state of consciousness and to realise the Inner Self.

Yoga frees one from life's sorrows and from the diseases and fluctuations of the mind. It gives serenity and composure, an inward unity amidst the diverse struggles of life. It is the art of knowing oneself and knowing the eternal truth. Yoga is the study of the functioning of the body, the mind and the intellect in the process of attaining freedom. It is the experience of one's self-acquired knowledge, and not the result of book-learning, of battling with logic, or of theoretical argumentation. Yoga is a philosophy, a way of life, wherein art and science meet.

As Lord Kṛṣṇa explains to Arjuna:

buddhiyukto jahātīha
ubhe sukṛtaduṣkrte
tasmād yogāya yujyasva
yogaḥ karmasu kauśalam

B.G. II, 50

[It is the knowledge of Yoga alone that enables an intellectual whose mind is at peace to discriminate between good and evil and to steer the course of his life skillfully.]

Yoga teaches one to do one's duty without thought of reward; to be involved in life's turmoils and yet to remain aloof; to act rightly and to liberate oneself from this life.

Is Yoga an Art?

Living is an art. Yoga enhances the quality of one's life. Hence it is an art. It lifts up one's thoughts and enables one to face life's difficult situations happily and with equanimity; it teaches one to strive to achieve a goal in life; to cultivate friendliness, concentration, piety, contentment, joy, and to discard what is non-essential; to cultivate good habits and to lead a righteous life. Yoga is disciplined action to achieve and attain final emancipation.

Is Yoga a Science?

The science of Yoga consists of acquiring knowledge through observation and experimentation. It is a science which deals with the body and the mind, whereby the rhythm of the mind is conquered by controlling the body. Through the practice of Yoga the health and strength of the body and the mind are acquired. Only when a state of equilibrium is reached between the body and the mind, does one become fit for Self-realisation. The science of Yoga teaches one to attain this harmony in a skillful and systematic way.

Is Yoga a Philosophy?

The human being is swayed by emotions. The mind and, in turn, the body are afflicted by sorrow and happiness, shame and glory, defeat and success. A sādhaka is unaffected by these dualities, learning to become indifferent to conflicting emotions. Yoga is a philosophy that equips one to attain poise and to face all the vicissitudes of life as well as its joys with equanimity. It is a philosophy which turns one away from the material world to the spiritual world in search of truth—to investigate the nature of Being.

PATAÑJALI'S DEFINITION

The great sage Patañjali has defined Yoga as 'yogaḥcittavṛtti nirodhaḥ', which means the control of the fluctuations of the mind, the intellect, and the ego. Just as the moon is not reflected clearly in the turbid waters of a river, so also the Soul is not properly reflected in an oscillating mind. A clear mind alone reflects the Soul. For Self-realisation the fluctuations of the mind have to be removed, enabling one to attain an unruffled mind.

WHAT IS CITTA?

To indicate the mind, the term 'citta' is used in the field of Yoga in a comprehensive sense. Citta is thus composed of mind, intellect and ego. The mind is the bridge connecting the physical entity with the spiritual entity. When it is directed towards the physical, it gets lost in the pursuit of pleasures. When it is directed towards the spiritual, it is reaching its final goal. There is a perpetual tug-of-war between the two, the mind being pulled either way, according to the guṇa or quality which predominates, whether it be sattva, rajas, or tamas.

The sattva state illumines the mind, giving calmness, composure, and serenity.

A rājasic state makes a person active, energetic, tense, and willful. The qualities of ambition, sternness, audacity, and pride will be profuse.

A tāmasic state plunges a person into torpor, inertia, and ignorance.

Five-Faceted Mind

Citta or mindstuff is composed of the three basic qualities of sattva, rajas, and tamas, as explained above. According to the predominant quality, the mental states or modifications are formed. The modifications are fivefold, as follows:

- Pramāṇa is proof as experienced by the five senses and the mind; it is obtained in three ways: pratyakṣa or direct perception, anumāna or inference, and āgama or scriptural testimony.
- Viparyaya is a mistaken view or wrong knowledge, such as mistaking the rope for a snake in the dark.
- Vikalpa is fancy or imagination based on verbal expression without any factual basis; for instance, a barren woman imagining that she has a child.
- Nidrā is sleep.
- Smṛti is memory.

These five modifications or vṛttis of the mind make us extroverts and confine us to the material world; in other words, rajas and tamas qualities dominate. When sattva prevails, the mind turns inwards, and goodness and purity abound. Yoga teaches us to restrain the five vṛttis and to lead a spiritual life.

Control of the Fluctuations of the Mind

Patañjali gives a twofold remedy for controlling the fluctuations of the mind:

abhyāsa-vairāgyābhyām tannirodhaḥ

P.Y.S. I, 12

These are (i) study or practice, and (ii) absence of worldly desires.

(i) *Abhyāsa—Study or Practice*

The poet *Vyāsa* has said:

sukhārtinah kuto vidyā
kuta vidyārthinasukham

[Knowledge cannot be attained by those who are given to pleasures, and pleasures are denied to those who study.]

Without rigorous practice nothing is gained. Without practice, purity of the body and the mind cannot be achieved, fluctuations of the mind cannot be controlled. The fruits of the material world cannot be obtained without sustained effort; this sustained effort has to be multiplied a thousand times to gain Self-knowledge. This rigorous practice is fourfold: moral, physical, mental and spiritual. Patañjali has said:

sa tu dīrghakāla nairantarya
satkārāsevito dṛḍha bhūmiḥ

P.Y.S. I, 14

[This rigorous practice has to be long-lasting, uninterrupted, and performed with dedication and respect; then alone the foundation or the ground is prepared].

(ii) *Vairāgya—Absence of Worldly Desires*

na veṣa dhāraṇam siddheḥ kāraṇam na cu tatkathā
kriyaiva kāraṇam siddheh satyametanna samśayah

H.P. I, 69

[Accomplishment is attained neither by wearing saffron robes nor by discussion; but undoubtedly it can be attained by action and by constant practice.]

The key to success is in effort. Vairāgya or absence of worldly desires can be achieved by controlling the senses, by carrying out one's duties without thought of reward and by acting with goodness and purity. Constant practice and absence of worldly pursuits are interdependent on each other—they are like the wings of an eagle. But successful flight can be achieved only with coordination between both the wings.

AṢṬĀṄGA YOGA— EIGHT BRANCHES OF YOGA

The proper functioning of the body depends on the several limbs. The absence or the sickness of any one limb affects the health of the whole body. The same principle applies to the study of Yoga and its branches. Any inadequacy in the study and the perfection of any of the eight steps of Yoga will not lead to Self-realisation.

yamaniyamāsanaprāṇāyāmapratyāhāra
dhāraṇādhyānasamādhayo'ṣṭāvaṅgāni

P.Y.S. II, 29

The following are the eight steps as formulated by Patañjali:

1. Yama is conduct towards others or social discipline.
2. Niyama is conduct towards oneself or individual discipline.

3. Āsana is practice of the postures for physical discipline.
4. Prāṇāyāma is breath-control for mental discipline.
5. Pratyāhāra is withdrawal or discipline of the senses.
6. Dhāraṇā is concentration.
7. Dhyāna is meditation.
8. Samādhi is Self-realisation.

All the eight steps are interpenetrating and interdependent. They may appear to be different, but all lead to the same goal. As the rays of the sun are refracted to form the spectrum, so has Yoga been divided into eight components which are all interwoven.

As ordinary people, those who are not inclined towards the spiritual aspect can take to Yoga for its physical benefits. Health of the body and the mind is important to all, whether they wish to succeed in their worldly pursuits or in Self-realisation. Yoga gives equal fulfilment to the believer and to the atheist or the agnostic alike. Indeed, through Yoga many an atheist or agnostic has become a believer, and it is one of the beauties of Yoga that it keeps its doors open to all. Even sanyasins, who have renounced the world, can derive benefit from the practice of Yoga, as the health and the mental poise that it gives are necessary to all. On all those who seek physical well-being, mental peace, or concentration of mind, Yoga bestows whatever they demand and satisfies them all.

yogāṅgānuṣṭhānātaśuddhikśaye
jnānadīptiḥāvivekakhyāteḥ

P.Y.S. II, 28

Lord Patañjali says:

> "The study of the eight limbs of Yoga leads to the purification of the body, the mind, and the intellect; the flame of knowledge is kept burning and discrimination is aroused."

ṢADĀṄGA YOGA—SIX-SIDED YOGA

In the Yoga Sūtra of Patañjali, Yoga has been described as eight-limbed. However, some of the Yoga Upaniṣads consider that it has six limbs. In the Amṛtanādopaniṣad the following stanza occurs:

pratyāhārastathā dhyānam prāṇayāmo'tha dhāraṇā
tarkaścaioa samādhiśca ṣadāngo yoga ucyate

Y. Ūp. 6

[Discipline of the senses, meditation, breath control, concentration, logic and Self-realisation are the six branches of Yoga.]

In Yogacūḍāmaṇi Upaniṣad the six limbs of Yoga have been enumerated thus:

āsanam prāṇa saṃrodhaḥ pratyāhāraśca dhāraṇā
dhyānam samādhiretāni yogāṇgāṅi bhavanti ṣaṭ

Y. Ūp. 2

[Postures, breath control, discipline of the senses, concentration, meditation, Self-realisation are the six Yogāṅgas.]

However, these texts also specify that in order to attain samādhi the stages of yama and niyama (social and individual disciplines) are considered as prerequisites, as well as the āsanas like padmakam and svastikam. Therefore, even though they speak of ṣadāṅga Yoga or the Yoga of six limbs, the two additional stages or limbs are understood to be part of the subject and there is thus little difference between aṣṭāṅga and ṣadāṅga Yoga.

The main difference between the two systems is:

Ṣadāṅga Yoga is aimed at small groups, members of particular schools or monasteries, who have to obey their institutional rules and therefore do not need the special injunctions of yama and niyama. Patañjali, on the other hand, lays down a complete philosophical system for everyone and is not confined to any group. He therefore gives elaborate instructions on how to lead one's life and how to attain physical and mental poise through certain rules of conduct in order to gain spiritual bliss.

According to Patañjali, for Self-realisation the soul, the intellect, the mind, and the organs of sense must act in unison. The seeker has to undertake the threefold quest of bahiraṅga sādhanā (external quest), antaraṅga sādhanā (inner quest), and antarātma sādhanā (spiritual quest). The following chart will enable the reader to understand the threefold quest better:

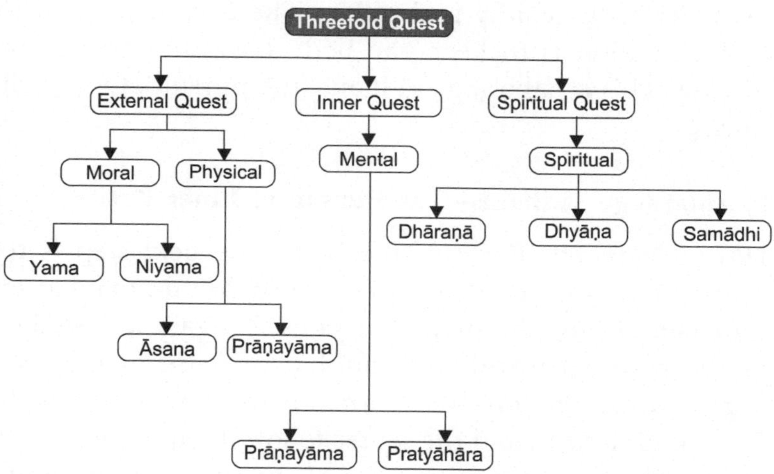

Before we examine the eight facets of Yoga, let us examine the threefold quest:

1. Bahiraṅga Sādhanā—The Pursuit of External Purity

The body is the temple of the Soul. Just as a clean temple evokes pure thoughts, a clean body leads to a pure mind and is thus a fit abode for the Self.

In Yogaśikhopaniṣad the importance of a clean body has been explained thus:

deho devalayah proktaḥ sa jīvaḥ kevalaḥ śivaḥ
tyajedājnānanirmālyam sohaṃ bhāvena pūjayet

Y. Ūp. 1, 168

[The body is a temple and the Soul therein is like Śiva. Therefore shed ignorance and worship the body, considering it as the abode of God.]

God has given us the body as capital to be used for Self-realisation. As a shrewd businessman utilises his capital to obtain gains, so also the body has to be diligently trained by yama, niyama, āsana and prāṇāyāma. It has to be kept perfectly healthy and stable. The first step towards Self-realisation is to keep the body pure and free from disease. This is bahiraṅga sādhanā, the pursuit of external purity.

2. Antaraṅga Sādhanā—The Pursuit of Inner Purity

Having attained purity of the body, the next step is to achieve purity of the mind. In order to do this, one has to understand how the mind functions. To gain knowledge of the external world, the mind makes use of the five organs of perception—nose, tongue, eyes, ears and skin. The mind desires, and the senses follow the mind for their gratification; thus the mind is caught up in the gratification of desires. In controlling the mind and the senses, the purification process is of great help.

The mind has six proclaimed enemies: lust, anger, greed, temptation, pride and jealousy.

In order to conquer these enemies, which come in the way of Self-realisation, prāṇāyāma (breath control) and pratyāhāra (discipline of the senses) are very essential.

In the Haṭhayoga Pradipikā the importance of breath is stressed as follows:

cale vāte calam cittam niścale niścalam bhavet
yogī sthāṇutvamāpnoti tato vāyum nirodhayet

H.P. II, 2

[A disturbed breath leads to a disturbed mind; a steady breath leads to a steady mind. The two go together. Hence, cultivate a steady and quiet breath; thereby the mind is controlled and the life of a Yogi is prolonged.]

It is further stated:

indriyāṇām mana nātho manonāthastu mārutaḥ
mārutasya layo nāthaḥ sa layo nādamāśritaḥ

H.P. IV, 29

[The Lord of the senses is the mind, the Lord of the mind is the breath; the master of breath is the nervous system; quietness of the nerves and concentration depend solely on the steady, smooth and rhythmic sound of inhalation and exhalation.]

Inner purity is therefore achieved by controlling the senses and the mind, which results in self-control. After this the disciple is ready for the next step.

3. Antarātma Sādhanā—The Pursuit of the Soul

In this stage the mind achieves poise and concentration and thus points towards the Soul. Here the last three steps of Aṣṭāṅga Yoga—dhāraṇā (concentration), dhyāna (meditation), and samādhi (self-realisation)—are cultivated.

The seeker lives in the Soul, is active, but devoid of ego and lower self. Indeed, at this time there is no awareness of one's existence because one has reached beyond sensual pleasures and knowledge. Eternal bliss has been found.

The Kaṭhopaniṣad aptly says:

ātmānam rathinam viddhi śarīram rathameva tu
buddhim to sarathim viddhi manaḥ pragrahameva ca
indriyāṇi hayanahuh viṣayamsteṣu gocaṛan
ātmendriyamanoyuktam bhoktetyāhur maniṣiṇaḥ
vijnānasārathiryastu manaḥ pragrahavān naraḥ
so'dhvanaḥ pāramāpnoti tadviṣṇoḥ paramam padam

K.Ūp. III, 3, 4, 9

[In the chariot called the body, the soul is the occupant; the intellect, the rider; and the mind, the reins. To traverse this existence by conquering the senses, the goal of Self-realisation has to be reached. Hence the chariot (body) should be healthy; then alone can the rider (intellect), by using the reins (mind), control the horses (senses).]

Now let us discuss each of the eight facets of Yoga.

YAMA—SOCIAL DISCIPLINE

Yama means restraint or abstention. These are the "do not's" of Yoga, parallel to the Biblical "Thou shalt not".

Man has been a member of society from ancient times. He cannot survive in isolation. As a member of society he has certain obligations and privileges. He has to abide by certain rules in order to make himself and other members of society happy.

āhimsa-satyāsteya-brahmacarya-aparigrahāḥ yamāh
jātideśakāla-samayanavacchinnāḥ sārvābhaumā mahāvratam

P.Y.S. II, 30, 31

Patañjali thus defines social conduct towards others:

Non-violence, truthfulness, non-covetousness, moderation in sex, and non-acquisitiveness. These are the great universal moral commandments which are not limited by birth, place, time, and occasion, i.e., they are applicable at all times. All these qualities result in purity.

Yoga texts have enumerated several such rules which are considered fundamental.

The Yogopaniṣaḍs describe yama as non-violence, truthfulness, non-covetousness, moderation in sex, forgiveness, steady intellect, piety, compassion, moderation in diet and cleanliness. These are ten in number.

The Haṭhayoga Pradīpikā accepts the same ethical principles that are enumerated in the Yoga scriptures.

1. Ahimsā—Non-Violence

Violence is lack of love—without enmity no act of violence can occur. Only love can unite society and make it cohesive. A Yogi has no hatred in the heart, but only love for all. Violence is the outcome of fear, selfishness, anger, and lack of confidence. Non-violence is respect for others; it is a state of mind.

Patañjali says that anyone coming into contact with a Yogi who is devoid of thoughts of violence is bound to cast off feelings of enmity.

2. Satya—Truthfulness

Speak the truth, speak that which is pleasing, but speak not the truth which is unpleasing, nor falsehood which is pleasing; this is traditional religion, says the Mahābhārata.

According to the Darśanopaniṣad, truth is proof obtained by using the five senses.

The Yoga Śāstra says, "When the mind and intellect concur in their judgement, that is the truth, that is the real knowledge."

A student of Yoga ought to be a follower of truth in thought, speech and action.

One who tells a lie is more poisonous than a serpent. The tongue has no bones, hence it can twist as it pleases, and it requires control. Otherwise one does not know at what time it will swerve from the truth.

3. Asteya—Non-Stealing or Non-Covetousness

Like the Old Testament commandment "Thou shalt not steal", asteya is the acceptance of only that which is essential for one's maintenance. Everything else is greed.

To covet other's possessions even mentally is a sin akin to stealing.

A serious student of Yoga who practises asteya has no need for riches; but if riches come, he uses them for the benefit of others.

4. Brahmacarya—Moderation in Sex

Brahmacarya does not mean lifelong celibacy, but moderation in sex between married couples. *Kālidāsa* describes the ideal king in Raghuvamśa:

tyāgāya sambhṛtārthānām prajārtham gṛhamedhinām

R. I, 7

[These kings, who were the descendants of the sun, collected wealth for charity and indulged in sex only with the object of begetting a son.]

Kāma or sex is undoubtedly one of the puruṣārthas or aims of life as well as a driving force in a human being, but it has to be channelled in the right direction. Partners in marriage should be loyal to each other, fulfilling mutual obligations in moderation. Unbridled sex leads to ruin.

The senses should not be distracted from being focused on Brahman, the Supreme, otherwise one is deviating from the path of Yoga.

manasthairye sthirovāyuḥ tato binduḥ sthiro bhavet
bindusthairyāt sadā sattvam piṇḍasthairyam prajāyate

H.P. IV, 28

[The body remains strong and healthy only when manas (mind) and prāṇa (breath) are firm within. When the mind is steady the breath and the vital energy also become steady. By steadying the vital energy, one acquires strength and steadiness of the body.]

5. Aparigraha—Non-Acquisitiveness or Non-Receiving of Gifts

Parigraha is acquisitiveness, or amassing wealth out of personal greed. Once the disease of acquisitiveness sets in, it is impossible to give it up. It is true that a certain amount of money is needed to meet the basic needs, in a monetised economy such as ours; food, shelter, clothes have to be paid for in money. But the physical need is not acquisitiveness. Psychological greed is acquisitiveness: it is a disease. Even while praying to God, we ask for many things out of selfishness. That is not prayer out of gratitude. One who is free from hankering after unnecessary objects and undue sensual pleasures is free from the mental disease of acquisitiveness.

Patañjali has said that "one who has rid oneself of 'I' and 'mine' is able to see things in their proper perspective".

6. Kṣama—Forgiveness

To forgive the enemies who may have tormented him physically or mentally is one of the qualities of a Yogi, reminiscent of the Christ's precept to his disciples to turn the other cheek when some one has slapped them on one cheek.

7. Dhṛti—Steady Intellect

Steadiness of intellect leads to the knowledge that "I am the Self".

8. Dayā—Compassion

Being compassionate to all and practising it in thought, word, and deed is the attribute of a Yogi.

9. Ārjava—Straightforwardness

To be simple, straightforward, and upright is ārjava.

10. Mitahāra—Moderation in Diet

To control one's palate and to eat only for the upkeep of the body, and not for the gratification of the palate, is moderation.

11. Sauca—Cleanliness

Sauca is inner and outer cleanliness of the body.

NIYAMA—INDIVIDUAL DISCIPLINE

Rules of conduct towards oneself consist of certain disciplines which are both physical and mental.

śauca-santoṣa-tapasvādhyāyeśvara-praṇidhānāni niyamāḥ

P.Y.S. II, 32

Cleanliness, contentment, austerity, self-study, and devotion to God are the five rules given by Patañjali.

In addition, seven rules are specified by other texts. These are: faith, charity, modesty, sound mind, repetition of divine names, belief in the scriptures, and observance of vows.

1. Sauca—Cleanliness

Cleanliness has two facets: inner cleanliness and outer cleanliness. This includes cleanliness of the five organs of sense, and personal hygiene. Wearing one's own clothes, thus avoiding contagious diseases, is personal hygiene. Eating simple and nutritious food rather than food which titillates the palate is also a simple factor of external purity without which inner cleanliness or cleanliness of the mind cannot he achieved.

2. Santoṣa—Contentment

Contentment is a state of mind which is essential for the well-being and development of the body and the mind. Discontent leads to greed and envy which are insatiable. Contentment gives a poised mind which results in pure happiness.

3. Tapas—Austerity

Austerity or penance is the conquest of all desires or sensual pleasures by practising purity in thought, speech and action.

To fast on auspicious days, to have brotherly feeling and humility towards all, and to control the senses is the austerity of body or action; not to harbour ill thoughts or feelings towards others is the austerity of thought; to utilise one's speech in the praise of God is the austerity of speech. Austerity removes the impurities of the body and the mind and leads to mastery over the senses. Yogic postures and breath control lead to purity.

4. Svādhyāya—Self-Study

Self-study means performing ordained duties and concentrating all the forces of the body, the mind, and the intellect on Self-realisation. Whether one is awake, in a dream state, or asleep, one should concentrate on uniting the Self with the Supreme.

5. Īśvarapraṇidhāna—Devotion or Surrender to God

To remain aloof and to perform all actions as an offering to God is pure devotion. Devoid of desire, the sādhaka becomes one with God.

In addition to the above, the Haṭhayoga Pradipikā and the Yogopaniṣads list the following Niyamas.

6. Āstikya—Belief

Belief in the existence of God and in the tenets of the Vedas, the Śāstras, and the Purāṇas is Āstikya. Belief is objective, faith is subjective. Faith is potent, hence belief has to be supported by faith.

7. Dānam—Charity

To acquire wealth by legitimate means and to distribute it to the deserving, with compassion, is true charity.

8. Siddhānta Vākya Śravaṇam—Listening to Established Doctrines

To listen to the doctrines that establish the existence of God as Real, Supreme and Limitless is one of the duties of a Yogi.

9. Hrī—Modesty

To cultivate humility while performing good deeds prescribed by the scriptures and feeling modest on their accomplishment is hrī.

10. Mati—Intellectual Faith, Devotion

Confirmed belief in the knowledge gained from the Vedas and from all the scriptures and rejecting the doctrines that are contrary to this is mati.

11. Japa—Recitation of Mantras

Continuous recital of mantras orally and mentally is japa. Mantras are uttered in order to focus attention towards one thought. This brings ekāgratā or pin-pointedness.

12. Vrata—Religious Observances

To perform acts of religious penance is discipline of the mind and the body by the observance of vrata.

The rules of conduct described above are applicable to all, whether or not they follow the path of Yoga. They are enjoined by all religions. The step that follows is found only in Yoga.

ĀSANA—POSTURES

Āsanas are a distinguishing feature of Yoga. They take one from the physical to the spiritual plane. They are the beginning as well as the foundation of Yoga Vidyā, the Science of Yoga.

It is a common belief that Patañjali's Yoga Sutras do not deal with the physical aspect of Yoga but treat exclusively of spiritual sādhanā, mentioning āsana only as coincidental. It is likewise believed that the Haṭhayoga Pradīpikā is concerned only with the physical aspect, mentioning spiritual aims only in passing. Both these views are erroneous interpretations of the Yoga Philosophy.

In the Haṭhayoga Pradīpikā the first discourse describes Yama and Niyama, as enumerated in the several Yoga scriptures, in very general terms, without going into detail because their universal applicability is taken for granted. The treatise therefore commences with the third stage of Yoga, namely, āsana, which is given in great detail, and proceeds gradually towards the Samādhi stage, thus describing all the steps that take one from bondage to liberation.

Āsana means holding the body in a particular posture with the bhavana or the thought that God is within. The āsana has to be held firm or 'sthira' so as not to shake that Divinity. Āsana-Jaya or the conquest of āsana comes when effort ceases and stability sets in. The stability brings about a state of 'sukhatā' or bliss. An āsana held in that state is no longer performed by the physical or the physiological body but by the Inner Self. In this state the body has been conquered, dualities have disappeared, and the union of the body, the mind, and the soul is achieved.

Sage Patañjali describes āsana thus:

sthirasukham āsanam

P.Y.S. II, 46

Posture brings stability of the body and poise of the mind. The Haṭhayoga Pradīpikā, while discussing āsana, affirms:

kuryāttadāsanam sthairyamārogyam cāngalāghavam

H.P. I, 17

[The practice of āsana brings the body to a state of stability, gives freedom from disease, and brings lightness to one's very being.]

While commenting on this śloka, Brahmānanda states that the practice of āsana brings firmness to the body, eliminates the rajoguṇa or the oscillating character of the mind, and makes the mind steady, thus corroborating Patañjali's description of 'sthiratā' and 'sukhatā'. Sthiratā stands for the firmness of the body, while sukhatā stands for a quality of the mind and not of the body: we do not say that the body is happy, but that the mind is contented. Thus 'sukhatā' is not comfort, as it is sometimes translated, but poise of the mind. The two ślokas therefore convey the same meaning.

One may say that the Haṭhayoga Pradīpikā elaborates āsana and takes one step-by-step towards Samādhi, whereas Patañjali's Yoga Sūtras describe āsanas, aptly and exactly, in the context of Samādhi. Both say that one has to start with the physical and then proceed step-by-step to the spiritual.

The body and the mind are interwoven and interdependent.

If there is any disturbance in the body the mind is disturbed and vice versa. In Yoga the body, and the mind are cultivated by a steady process of āsana practice to prevent any impediment in their functioning. This practice gives health, poise, mobility, and immunity from disease.

In mastering the yogic posture lies the secret of the conquest of the body: by this essential step the sādhaka is carried to a spiritual plane and towards Self-realisation.

PRĀṆĀYĀMA—BREATH CONTROL

Prāṇāyāma is breath control, the end product being mental calm and tranquility of the nervous system. The body and the mind become tolerant. The gains of prāṇāyāma have been described thus:

prāṇāyāmena yuktena sarvaroga-kṣayo bhavet

H.P. II, 16

[Breath-control, done in the proper manner, eradicates all diseases.]

With proper breath-control the pulse becomes steady and regular, the body achieves suppleness, and the complexion becomes radiant.

Patañjali describes the effects of prāṇāyāma thus:

tatah kṣīyate prakāśāvaraṇam
dhāraṇāsu ca yogyatā manasaḥ

P.Y.S. II, 52, 53

Practice of breath control leads to a pure mind. It dissolves the covering that hides the effulgence within. Such a mind is fit for concentration.

Prāṇa is air, breath, the very life force; āyāma means expansion of its length and breadth and volume. Thus the systematic lengthening of inhalation and exhalation and the pause in between is breath control.

After gaining mastery of the yogic postures, making the breath deeper and more subtle as well as rhythmic and controlling it systematically to the fullest possible extent is prāṇāyāma.

There are three important functions of breath control: exhalation, inhalation and retention.

1. *Recaka - Exhalation:* Prāṇa-vāyu or the vital force is centred in the region of the navel. It surges upwards into the heart and, traversing the lungs, seeks its outlet through the nostrils. This is recaka or exhalation.
2. *Pūraka - Inhalation:* The pure air from outside, on entering the nostrils, travels through the lungs and the heart and then to the navel region as the vital force. This is pūraka or inhalation.
3. *Kumbhaka - Retention:* Kumbha means a vessel. Like a vessel which can be filled or kept empty, retention is also of two kinds—antara kumbhaka or retention following inhalation and bāhya kumbhaka or retention following exhalation. Antara kumbhaka is the pause after full inhalation when one can fill the lungs no more. Bāhya kumbhaka is the pause after complete exhalation, i.e., after fully emptying the lungs.

   Kevala Kumbhaka: There is yet another stage of retention, more advanced than the foregoing two, where the breath is held by itself without the awareness of inhalation and exhalation. It is beyond inhalation, exhalation, time and space. This is kevala kumbhaka. It is a state which is experienced only in Dhyāna.

The practice of prāṇāyāma confers upon the sādhaka a twofold benefit, namely, Japa Sādhanā and Bhakti Sādhanā, Japa Sādhanā is the practice of the repetition of the mantra or the sacred syllable 'Hamsah'. 'Ham' stands for 'aham' or '1'; 'Sah' means 'He'. Together they mean, 'I am He.' The individual Soul constantly repeats this mantra in the form of the outgoing vital breath which has the sound 'Hum' and with the sound 'Sah' of the incoming breath. This repetitive prayer goes on unconsciously throughout one's life. It is called 'Ajapahamsa Vidyā' or knowledge of unconscious prayer.

In Bhakti Sādhanā, the sādhaka absorbs the Cosmic Energy by inhalation, brings the union of the Cosmic Energy with the Individual Self by inhalation-retention and by exhalation surrenders the self and merges it with the Universal Self.

PRATYĀHĀRA—DISCIPLINE OF THE SENSES

The five organs of sense come in contact with the external world at the instance of the mind. This extroversion of the sense organs due to their hankering after worldly objects has to be restrained and directed inwards towards the Source of all existence. This process of drawing the senses inwards is pratyāhāra or putting the senses under restraint.

The process of acquiring Self-knowledge or cognition is as follows: Object, sense organ, mind, and soul—all these combine to form knowledge. Any disturbance in this combination is like breaking a chain. If a link is broken, an interruption is created. It is a common experience that if the mind is engrossed elsewhere, things happening in front of our eyes do not make any impression; this is called absentmindedness or a dreamy state; such a state is not pratyāhāra, however. In a dreamy state the mind is engrossed in some thought and the sense organs are disconnected from their sense objects, whereas in pratyāhāra the mind is purposefully withdrawn from the sense organs so that they lose contact with the sense objects. This mastery over the mind, which prevents it from becoming dispersed in the external world, is called pratyāhāra. When the dispersed mind (citta) is brought under complete control, the organs of sense are also under control. Having a command over the sense organs and turning them inwards is pratyāhāra.

DHĀRṆĀ—CONCENTRATION

deśabandhaścittasya dhāraṇā

P.Y.S. III, 1

Patañjali has defined concentration as the focusing of all the senses on the Individual Soul. The Śaṅḍilyopaniṣad describes five ways of achieving concentration: focusing the mind on the Individual Self; developing inward vision; controlling the properties of the five elements in one's body; constant remembrance of Brahman; and thought of Iṣṭa Devatā—one's personal deity.

The mind wanders in different directions due to the influences of the five subtle qualities (pañcha tanmātra) of smell, taste, vision, touch and sound. These subtle qualities are felt through the sense organs of nose, tongue, eye, skin and ear. The sādhaka has to learn to restrain the mind from wandering and to turn it inwards towards the Self. When the mind, the intellect, and the ego are totally focused on the Self, that is dhāraṇā. When the sādhaka obtains mastery over this practice, the way is open for the next stage, dhyāna or meditation.

DHYĀNA—MEDITATION

When the sādhaka sustains and maintains the focus of attention throughout the above concentration, unbounded by time and space, it becomes dhyāna or meditation. In such a state of deep concentration and steady undisturbed flow of meditation, the body, the breath, the mind, the intellect, and the ego, all lose their individual existence and merge into one single state of Being. The merging of the Individual Soul with the Universal Soul is meditation.

The deeper the waters of a river, the more quietly it flows.

Similarly, the deeper the focusing of the citta, the more tranquil is the state. Śāṅḍilyopaniṣaḍ describes two states of meditation: Saguṇa and Nirguṇa. Saguṇa means with support, nirguṇa without support. In saguṇa meditation the devotee concentrates on a personal deity with qualities or attributes, while in nirguṇa meditation concentration has no frontier and the sādhaka does not take the support of any particular deity; here there is no pinpointing of thought but name, form, shape, colour and quality are all transcended.

SAMĀDHI—SELF-REALISATION

The eighth and final stage of Yoga is Samādhi. As a river merges into the ocean, losing its identity, so the Individual Soul merges with the Supreme. At this stage, the identity of the sādhaka becomes both externally and internally immersed in meditation. The meditator, the act of meditation, and the object meditated upon, all three shed their individual characteristics and merge into one single vision of the entire cosmos. Supreme happiness, free from pleasure, pain or misery, is experienced.

brahmārpaṇam brahmahaviḥ brahmāgnau brahmaṇā hutam
brahmaiva tena gantavyam brahmakarma samādhinā

B.G. IV, 24

[In Samādhi one offers one's Self, pours it into the pyre of Brahman; it is sublimated and transformed into the Supreme Self, becoming one with It.]

The archer (sādhaka) with the bow of dhyāna (meditation) in hand, with the arrow citta (mind) fixed, aims—with vision centred on the target Self—and attentively hits with a single unfailing stroke (realisation). At that time no differentiation is experienced.

This is the culmination of Yogāngāṇuṣṭhāna, or the practice of all the limbs of Yoga, beginning with Bahiraṇga Sādhanā (external pursuits), proceeding towards Antaraṇga Sādhanā (internal pursuits), and ending with Antarātma Sādhanā (innermost pursuits).

The Path of Devotion (Bhakti Yoga) and the Path of Action (Karma Yoga), like the rivers Gangā and Yamunā, meet and flow together towards the Path of Knowledge (Jñāna Yoga), at the confluence of the invisible river Sarasvati, where Bhakti, Karma and Jñāna become one. This is final beatitude.

Chapter IV

Are Women Eligible for Yoga?

God created man and woman as equal partners to share life, its rewards and burdens, joys and sorrows. If life can be compared to a chariot, then man and woman are its two wheels. The material and spiritual burdens of life fall equally on the shoulders of man and woman. Both desire good health, mental peace and poise in life.

Yoga is beneficial to both men and women. Women need Yoga even more than men as the responsibilities thrust upon them by Nature are greater than men's.

The art of Yoga is as old as the Vedas. When we read of the conditions that prevailed in those days we get the impression that women were pre-eminent in many fields. It was the Goddess Pārvatī who first gained knowledge of Yoga by importuning Lord Śiva to teach her.

Maitreyī, the wife of the great Yogi and philosopher Yājñavalkya, attained liberation through the practice of Yoga. She was instructed in this art by her husband, whose teachings are contained in his book Yogayāgñavalkya.

A well-known episode from the Rāmāyana describes the farewell of Rāma when he was banished for 14 years and sent to live in the forest. His mother Kauśalyā was overcome with grief and knew that any blessings she gave with tears in her eyes would be inauspicious. She practised āsanas and prāṇāyāma to gain composure and only when she had recovered from the shock and earned a composed state did she come before Rāma to give him her blessings.

In the Mahābhārata there is a reference to Sulabhā, a recluse, daughter of King Pradhān, she studied and became proficient in the knowledge of Yoga. Janaka, the King of

Mithilā, was vanquished at her hands during a debate on Yoga.

The legend of Madālasā from our epics gives a good example of women Yoginis. Madālasā was the faithful and devoted wife of King Ṛtudhvaja. She burned herself in 'sati' thinking that her husband was dead, but was brought back to life by Aśvatara Nāgarāja, since Ṛtudhvaja was alive. At first Madālasā did not recognise her husband, as she had lost knowledge of her former existence. However, she was initiated into the art of Yoga and she regained her knowledge. She now recognised the King. She became a great adept in Yoga.

In the Vedic period women were held in high esteem. They enjoyed equal rights and opportunities. Manusmṛti describes them as goddesses.

yatra nāruastu pūjyante ramante tarra devatāh
yatretāstu na pūjyante sarvāstatrāphalāḥ kriyāh

M.S. III. 55

[Where women are respected, there gods dwell. Where they are disregarded, there all deeds go in vain.]

In the Vedic period there were also instances of women undergoing the sacred thread ceremony; they studied the Vedas in the Gurukula and received training in various arts such as wrestling, archery, Yoga, music and drama. Gradually woman's position became a subsidiary one and her freedom was minimised, even though she was regarded as the mother and had to shoulder social responsibilities. She was considered the weaker sex and consequently held no social status. She lost the privileges she had enjoyed during the Vedic times. The Gurukula and thread ceremony were denied to her. In education she lagged far behind. The doors to the study of philosophy, science, arts, and Yoga were shut to her with the result that her position deteriorated still further.

Later Indian history is replete with battles against foreign invaders from the northwest. There was widespread social insecurity and the Indian women suffered because of this. In spite of this, Yoginīs flourished in several parts of the country.

Lallā, a woman saint of the 14th century, flourished in Kāshmir and propagated the Yoga system throughout India. Saint Baḥinābai was an exponent of Yoga and meditation. Sāradā Devī, consort of Sri Rāmakṛṣṇa Paramahamsa, was an adept in āsana and prāṇāyāma.

The path of Yoga is open to all, irrespective of race, caste, creed and sex. Anyone can attain liberation through Yoga.

The status of women today has considerably improved compared to that during the periods of the Smṛti, Purāṇa, and more recent history. Her many facets shine in various fields: her intelligence, acumen, and creativity have wider scope today for fuller expression. On the stage of life she has to perform many roles—daughter, sister, wife, mother and friend. She has to give her best in all these roles.

In Sāṃkhya-Yoga, woman is compared to Prakṛti (nature).

Like nature, she has to remain ever-active. Then her life blossoms and her home is cheerful. That is why Kālidāsa describes woman as the spark of life in a family. This very spark is the uplifter of society.

Apart from her traditional roles mentioned above, a woman has an additional part to play in society. In this age of all-round competition, she has become a doctor, lawyer, politician, professor and has acquitted herself worthily.

Yet, when the struggle exhausts even the upper limits of her patience, her body and mind get fatigued and her natural attention towards her family and children lessens. This results in negligence and frustration.

Her body is biologically created for some specific functions. She has to undergo the four stages of life—childhood, adolescence, middle age and old age. In these four stages physiological changes occur and in each of these she has to face problems and internal conflicts. This affects her physical and physiological organs as well as her mind and much of her energy is lost in coming to terms with life during these periods of change.

Motherhood is woman's ordained duty. This is not merely a physical state, but a divine state. In giving birth new responsibilities begin for her and she has to prove herself. Motherhood adorns her with the sacred qualities of love, sacrifice, faith, tolerance, goodwill and hard work. This is her highest religion—her svadharma. These qualities are ingrained deep into her nature. Sometimes these same qualities make her a little servile when she is overwhelmed by the burdens of her life, because she is not able to free herself from the plethora of duties that nature has thrust upon her. Sometimes she would like to free herself and fly intellectually ahead—but her religion binds her and brings her back to her sense of duty. She has been taught by the Bhagavad Gītā to perform all her duties without expecting any fruits or rewards. The endless struggle of being a woman and a mother, being tied to her work and her duty trains her to face the world and its dualities with equanimity.

For all this, a woman has to pay a high price physically and psychologically in her role of mother, wife, sister and friend. Stabilisation of the physical and mental states is achieved by āsanas and prāṇāyāma. Her salvation lies in practising them.

We shall now examine the nature of health—i.e., the nature of physical and mental well-being.

CHAPTER V

The Nature of Health

IMPORTANCE OF HEALTH

No amount of wealth can equal health. Between the two, the choice is always with health, since wealth cannot be enjoyed without health, whereas wealth can be commanded if one has health. The Upaniṣads say:

> "Health confers longevity, firmness and strength; by this the entire terrestrial sphere will become affluent fully."

All virtuous acts and religious merits are attainable only if there is good health. The Caraka Samhitā, a text of Indian medical science, says:

dharmārtha kāma mokṣāṇām
ārogyam mūlam uttamam

C.S. I, I, 15

> [The fundamental requirement of the body is good health in order to attain the four objectives of human existence, namely, acquisition of religious merits (dharma), wealth for living in comfort and generousness (artha), gratification of permissible pleasures and fulfillment of desires (kāma), and lastly, the endeavour to obtain liberation from the shackles of mundane cycles of births and deaths (mokṣa).]

Without health there is no strength. Strength is preserved only when health is maintained. Health of the body means both physical and mental well-being. It is a sign of a peaceful state of the body and the mind when one is able to follow ethical codes, maintain moral standards, and fulfil social obligations. Therefore, the Upaniṣad says:

nāyamātmā balahīnena labhyaḥ

Mu. Ūp. III, 2.4

[The Self is not realised by a weakling.]

Definition of Health

Life without happiness is mere existence. A concise definition of good health is that it pervades all aspects of our physical, physiological and psychological being. This means freedom from illness, absence of disease, perfect harmony in the functions of the body and the mind. The body is the abode of the citta (a triune of the mental faculty comprising the mind, the intelligence, and the ego). Perfect health is the state in which the functions of the body and the mind are in harmony so that they can turn inward to reach the goal of Self-realisation.

How is Health Achieved?

Good health can neither be bought nor bartered. It cannot be robbed or acquired by force. It is a culture of external and internal cleanliness, dietary control, proper exercise of the limbs and the organs, physical and mental poise, and rest. Just as gold is melted to make it pure, the body and the mind must be purified by careful practice of āsana and prāṇāyāma.

Nature of Disease

Disease may be defined as disturbance in the normal functioning of the body and the mind. Indian medical science (Āyurveda) describes health as the perfect harmony of bodily functions, a well-balanced metabolism and a happy and poised state of the mind and of the senses.

The science of Āyurveda has categorised the physiological functions of the body as falling under three heads, namely, Calana–Movement, Pacana–Digestion or assimilation, and Lepana–Respiration or illumination, which correspond respectively to the three humours of Vāta–Wind, Pitta–Bile and Sleṣma–Phlegm. These humours maintain a harmonious ratio of their own when the body is in a good state of health performing the above three functions. Health is defined as equilibrium among five factors: (i) the doṣās—the humours; (ii) the dhātus—seven juicy secretions from the ingredients of the body; (iii) Agni, i.e., proper functioning of digestion and elimination of waste matter, which is called the metabolism of the body; (iv) clarity or purity of the senses; and (v) tranquility and peace of the mind.

Any deficiency or excess in the normal quantity of the doṣās (humours) or the dhātus (ingredients), or any obstruction in their flow brings about imbalance and results in indisposition causing disease.

According to Āyurveda, the body has thirteen srotas or vessels to carry various substances throughout the body. They are prāṇavaha–breath ducts, trachea, etc.; annavaha–food pipe, oesophagus, etc.; udakavaha–water duct; rasavaha–juice such as bile and pancreatic juice; raktavaha–blood vessels; māṃsavaha–flesh; medovaha–fat; asthivaha–bones; majjāvaha–marrow; śukravaha–seminal duct; śakṛdvaha–waste matter, faeces; etc.; mūtravaha–urinary duct; and svedovaha–sweat pores. When there is imbalance in the three humours of vāta, pitta, and sleṣma, there is an improper flow in the vessels.

In order to ensure good health, the flow in the srotas must be maintained unhindered. In other words, to maintain proper metabolic functioning of the body, the humours (doṣās) must be held in harmony.

As the fluctuations in the physical body are caused by the humours, the mental fluctuations are caused by the rajas and tamo guṇas overshadowing the sattva guṇa. Rajas is one of the constituent qualities causing the activities seen in human beings, in the form of passions and emotions. Tamas is the other constituent quality which causes inertia or inaction which leads one into darkness such as grief sorrow, ignorance, etc. When the rajas and the tamo guṇas dominate or cover the sattva guṇa, the quality of goodness or purity, the mind becomes the abode of disease. Hence the body and the mind both need intelligent care.

Health According to Yoga

Like Āyurveda, Yoga also recognises the threefold afflictions, namely, ādhyātmika, ādhidaivika and ādhibhautika. Ādhyātmika is concerned with both body and mind, i.e., somatic and psychic diseases. Ādhidaivika afflictions are epidemics, unnatural deaths at the hands of beasts, water, burial, accidents and the like. Ādhibhautika are environmental afflictions such as cyclones, tempests, sunstrokes, devastation by floods, caused by nature's fury. Here Yoga adds something more to the definition of health and makes it more comprehensive. According to Yoga, any obstacle that prevents the realisation of the Self is an indication of physical indisposition causing a modification in the mental state—cittavṛtti. The aim of Yoga is to restrain both physical disturbances and mental modifications. The obstacles or impediments are: Sickness, inaction, doubt, delusion, carelessness, non-abstention, erroneous conception; non-attainment, and instability in the Sādhanā, sorrow, dejection, restlessness, and disturbed or unrhythmic breathing. These originate in the body or in the mind. Therefore, health means total freedom from physical and mental afflictions in order to achieve one's goal.

Modern medical science is not at variance with—the above definition and it agrees that the relationship between the body and the mind is intimate.

If life has to be protected, health must be maintained and the functioning of the various organs of the body, especially the central nervous system, should be well taken care of.

Many diseases are due to mental depression, anger, grief, uninhibited sexual indulgence, anxiety, discontent, distrust, and other psychosomatic disturbances. Many people given to mental weakness suffer from diseases of their imagination which in many cases prove fatal. By developing such qualities as good thoughts, enthusiasm, courage, hope, and optimism, even the weak body and mind can turn into a strong and healthy one.

Practice of Yoga brings a perfect balance in body and mind. It makes the body healthy to cooperate with the mind, so that steadiness, composure and firmness are developed. Patañjali explains that the practice of Yoga enables one to avoid the pain which may be in store in the future.

Hence practice of Yoga brings not only physical health, but also mental health. It teaches one how to conquer obstacles so that one can live peacefully and in perfect happiness to achieve the goal of life—Self-realisation.

CHAPTER VI

Is Yoga Ideal for Women?

"Nature meant woman to be her masterpiece" wrote John Ruskin. Her beauty and grace, as well as her soft nature, bear witness to this. She not only possesses external beauty, but her soft and graceful form belies her firmness of character and power of endurance. Woman is soft, tender, and flexible, and this makes her move with ease and grace, contrasted with man whose body is rigid, rough and robust. Yoga demands tremendous elasticity and it seems as if the Creator has favoured woman in making her body fit and suitable for Yoga.

Woman differs greatly from man in her build and stature. Her muscles are soft and light compared to man's which are large, coarse and heavy. Her skeletal structure also is not broad as in man. She has the power to withstand physical strains and mental pressures to a far greater extent than man; this is not due to physical strength or power of endurance, but it is nature's characteristic gift, enabling her to face them.

Nature has, in addition, endowed her with the responsibility of perpetuating mankind. The wealth of a nation and the health of the future generation depend upon her physical and mental well-being. From a careful study of the features distinguishing woman from man, namely, her physical body, her changing physiological functions and emotional states, it follows that, if she chooses to adopt Yogāsana and prāṇāyāma as part of her way of life, they will be even more meaningful and advantageous to her.

Yoga helps woman to fulfil her tasks as well as to maintain her complexion, lustre and femininity. She no longer needs cosmetics, as proper blood circulation makes her skin glow. It is no exaggeration to say that Yogic practices are ideally designed to help her in all conditions and circumstances of her daily life.

Yoga is an ideal form of exercise. The chapters on anatomy in the Caraka and Suśruta Saṃhitās of Āyurveda describe physical exercises as those which are capable of producing beneficial results through actions or movements. Correct performance of them is explained as bringing lightness to the body, ability to work, resistance against disease and discomforts caused by imbalance between the three humours. They stimulate the harmonious functioning of the respiratory, circulatory, digestive, nervous, glandular, genito-urinary and eliminatory systems. The texts have cautioned that incorrect exercise causes sluggishness, exhaustion, vomiting, malfunctioning of the internal organs, dryness, bleeding (internal haemorrhage), cough, fever and other disorders.

Yogāsanas exercise the entire body and revitalise all the physiological systems, resulting in a sound mind in a sound body, as each āsana cultivates the body and the mind evenly. Yogāsanas and prāṇāyāma have stood the test of time for centuries and are helpful for all the needs of men and women in their pursuit of perfect health and supreme happiness.

The body consists of five sheaths or layers. They are:

1. Annamaya—the anatomical body composed of skin, muscles, and bones is the outer sheath.
2. Prāṇamaya—the physiological body composed of the circulatory, respiratory, excretory, digestive, nervous, endocrine or glandular and reproductive systems.
3. Manomaya—the mental or psychological body, composed of mind and emotions.
4. Vijñānamaya—the intellectual body.
5. Ānandamaya—the spiritual body is the innermost sheath encasing the Soul.

All the sheaths are interdependent and interpenetrating, reaching from outer cover to inner core. During the performance of Yogāsanas and prāṇāyāma, total attention is brought to bear on all the sheaths, from the anatomical to the spiritual and vice versa.

All types of exercise have two features—motion and action. Āsanas exercise the anterior, posterior, lateral and interior portions of the body equally, as every posture is a complete entity in which each part of the body has a particular role to play and no part is forgotten. Motion is constant movement from position to position or from place to place. Āsanas, though appearing static externally, are full of dynamic action within. A full range of movements and actions such as horizontal, vertical, diagonal and circumferential extension and expansion are created while performing the postures. This requires skill, intelligence, and application. No portion of the body or the mind is left untouched when an āsana is carefully and correctly performed.

There is a vast difference between Yoga and other physical exercises. Āsanas are psychophysiological, unlike physical exercises which are purely external. Although āsanas develop body consciousness, they also generate internal consciousness and stabilise the mind. Yoga is a culture of the body, the mind, and the soul. In physical exercise body movements may be done with precision, whereas in Yoga, along with precision, a deeper awareness is cultivated, bringing equipoise of body and mind.

Āsanas develop muscles, as do physical exercises, and they remove stiffness so that body movements become free. However, they are concerned more with the physiological body and the vital organs than with the physical body. They strengthen and revitalise organs such as the liver, spleen, intestines, lungs and kidneys. Each āsana works on the entire system. It is an organic exercise which eradicates toxins.

The digestive system is one of the most important systems on which the health of the entire body depends. Its malfunctioning is the root of many diseases and āsanas are an infallible help in alleviating them.

The practice of āsana and prāṇāyāma makes the respiratory system work to its optimum, ensuring proper supply of oxygen to the blood and improving blood circulation throughout the body.

The endocrine glands in our system are very important. They are ductless glands secreting hormones which are circulated throughout the body. A healthy physical and mental state depends on their secretion. Certain āsanas stimulate these glands to ensure their proper functioning, while other āsanas normalise the over-functioning of the hormones and maintain balance in the system.

Āsanas and prāṇāyāma are a great help for the proper functioning of the brain, the nerves, and the spine. The brain is the seat of thinking, reasoning, memorising, perceiving and directing. It is the controller of voluntary and involuntary movements in our body. The body and the brain are constantly interacting. In facing the turmoils of life, they are under continual stress; a tired brain affects the entire system. This constant strain creates anxiety and worry, leading to psychoneurosis, neurasthenia, hysteria, and a host of psychoneurotic diseases. Āsanas such as *Śirṣāsana, Sarvāṅgāsana, Halāsana* and *Setu Bandha Sarvāṅgāsana* supply fresh blood to the brain and keep it alert, active, and at the same time in a restful state. Yoga thus has the unique quality of being able to soothe the nerves, quieten the brain, and make the mind quiet, fresh and peaceful.

Yoga can be done by all at any age. It is particularly beneficial to those over 40 when the recuperative power of the body is declining and resistance to illness is weakened. Yoga generates energy and does not dissipate it. It makes one energetic and full of vitality. With minimum effort one obtains maximum benefit.

Yoga plays an additional role. It is not only preventive, but curative also. Unlike other systems, its aim is to develop symmetry, coordination and endurance in the body. It activates the internal organs and makes them function harmoniously.

Yoga is a naturopathic process of treatment. The progress is slow but certain. None can deny the advances of modern medical science. Drugs and medicines can be of great help, but Yoga can complement them and speed up the process of recovery where medication is being used. Sometimes drugs and medicines have harmful side-effects and Yoga helps to counteract them. Yoga strengthens the body's natural defenses to fight disease. In cases of chronic disease, the advance and the intensity can be checked by the practice of Yoga. Where a surgical operation has to be undergone, it is advisable to practise Yoga before the operation, as this relaxes the nerves and the inner organs and quietens the mind. Practice is again necessary after the operation to help the wound heal quickly and to regain strength. In cases of accident when other forms of exercise are impossible, the door of Yoga is open.

Āsanas are most helpful in eradicating fatigue, aches and pains. They not only make the unhealthy healthy, but help the healthy to remain healthy.

Yoga has a special gift to offer to athletes and sportswomen. The āsanas can help correct the faulty movement of muscles which cause strains and sprains. They create freedom from pressures and tensions and give speed, elasticity, strength, endurance and coordination to the entire system. When sportsmen and sportswomen suffer from exhaustion, they can easily recover their energy by practising āsanas. Āsanas also increase their range of movement.

Thus the art of Yoga is unique in nature. It has everything to give according to one's need. It is especially well designed for women, who with their family responsibilities should welcome the opportunity of being able to perform these wonderful Yogic exercises in the privacy and comfort of their own home.

The practice of Yoga has a tremendous effect on character and makes one morally and mentally strong. The approach to life becomes more positive and tolerant. Pride and egoism are eradicated and humbleness and humility set in. One becomes more thoughtful and discriminative and acquires intellectual clarity. This leads one towards a contemplative state.

CHAPTER VII

Three Milestones in a Woman's Life

Since this book is intended mainly for women, let us consider the three important stages in a woman's life beginning with youth, passing through middle age, and ending in old age:

1. Menstruation
2. Pregnancy and delivery
3. Menopause

These are the trying periods and milestones of her life. Let us examine how these functions in each stage affect her body and mind and whether the practice of āsana and prāṇāyāma is useful to her.

1. Menstruation

When a girl matures, the physiological functions taking place to develop the body into complete womanhood are at their peak to enable her to fulfill the responsibilities which nature has forced upon her; this is an immutable part of her life. Adolescence is the period of growth during which there is a transition from childhood to maturity. At this period important bodily and mental changes occur.

The ovaries, the main female sex organs, are situated at the sides of the uterus and begin to function by producing ova, female sex cells, one of which matures every month. The maturing process begins between the ages of ten and fifteen and stops between forty-five and fifty. The lining of the uterus becomes soft and swollen to receive an ovum and has excess blood to nourish it. When the ovum is not fertilised and the blood is not needed for its nourishment, the swollen membrane and the excess blood are expelled from the uterus through the vagina in the form of a blood discharge. This discharge takes place once a month and is called menstruation.

Hence, menstruation is a periodic change occurring in a female in which discharge of blood takes place from the cavity of the womb. It is a purely physiological process preparing the female body for reproduction, a biological function.

At the base of the brain are situated the pituitary gland divided into two sections—anterior and posterior. Secretions from the anterior section of the pituitary gland stimulate reproduction in women: the posterior section regulates secretions and feeds the involuntary muscles of the uterus and prepares it to function healthily.

During this period of maturation the female body undergoes a visible change. There is a rapid increase in height and weight. The hips become widened and fat is deposited in this region. The vagina becomes fully developed, along with the breasts; the heart and the lungs attain a fuller size; the muscles in the body become harder; the oil glands under the skin secrete more oil, often resulting in acne or pimples around the cheeks and the forehead, a common cause of anxiety among teenagers. The liberal generation of sex hormones also causes excessive secretion of fatty substances under the skin.

A healthy menstruation depends upon the proper functioning of the ovary and this, in turn, upon a healthy pituitary gland. A regular rhythm or cycle within the ovary also depends upon the hypothalamus which is closely connected with the pituitary.

Yogāsanas and prāṇāyāma offer great help at puberty when the body is changing to womanhood. Āsanas such as inverted postures and backbends are useful for stimulating the pituitary gland. Āsanas such as forward bends are also effective as pure blood is supplied to the pelvic organs. For proper skeletal growth and for improving the shape of the body, the standing āsanas are invaluable.

Along with physiological changes, psychological changes also occur at this age. A girl's emotional life is stimulated and acquires an extra edge.

Just as the somatic changes depend upon the hormonal balance of the endocrine system, so also the mental changes depend upon a healthy environment. It is a period when there is a sudden jump from the simplicity of childhood to a complex emotional state. It is a tug-of-war between two minds. Childhood tries to hold her back while adolescence impels her forward.

Self-consciousness and individuality assert themselves at this period. Her mind becomes extra sensitive and her behaviour and moral conduct acquire razor-sharp keenness. Due to the physiological and psychological changes in her body and mind she is in a perplexed state. Hence readjustment is an essential factor. A healthy atmosphere and proper guidance are necessary at this juncture.

Yogic practice at this age gives courage to approach womanhood without any mental disturbances. It helps control and check impulses and emotions; it gives balance of mind. She conquers fear and nervousness and learns to face her changing life and surroundings with confidence.

The foundation of moral conduct can be laid properly and firmly at this age through Yogic practice which builds her character into a fully matured personality. Her beauty blossoms and she becomes a strong woman of high moral principles.

Yoga develops her physiologically, psychologically, morally and spiritually to grow healthily and to lead a pure life. The ages twelve to fourteen are ideal to begin Yoga. This does not mean that Yoga is to be commenced only at that age and not before. On the contrary, if one begins earlier, around the age of eight, it is good; but little ones should not be forced to be too serious. It is sufficient if the child is introduced to Yoga in a playful manner with the purpose of creating interest so that a foundation is laid.

However, even if one does not start at an early age, this should not prevent one from starting later. Yoga may be started at any time:

> *yuvāvṛddho'ativrddho vā vyādhito durbalo'pi vā*
> *abhyāsāt siddhimāpnoti sarvayogeṣvatandritaḥ*
>
> H.P. 1. 64

> [The young, the aged, the diseased, and the weak—all may take to the practice of Yoga and derive its benefits without hindrance.]

My father began to teach Yoga to the Queen Mother of Belgium when she was 84 years old. She had never practised it before. Her head and the whole body had tremors. With perseverance she did *Śirṣāsana* for the next 8 years.

With my father's experience and mine, I say with confidence that women of all ages can learn Yoga. The rate at which they progress may, however, vary according to individual constitution and ability.

Menstrual Disorders

Menstruation is a natural cyclic function occurring within the uterine system. It is a regular process with only a small degree of irregular periodicity varying from person to person. This small irregularity is considered to be a sign of normal health. Also it should be borne in mind that symptoms such as easy fatigue, sleeplessness, change in psychological mood, tenderness or slight swelling of the breasts are due to the heightened activity of the hormones and should be regarded as normal.

The menstrual cycles must occur at regular intervals. Variations in the length of the interval bring about disorders and cause physical and mental afflictions which tell upon pregnancy and maternity.

Many a time, due to general or local conditions the menstrual process may be absent, excessive, irregular, or may cause discomfort and severe pain. It is then considered to be a disorder in menstruation.

The menstrual disorders are:

1. *Amenorrhoea:* The absence of menstruation or delayed puberty is called amenorrhoea. It is found rarely and is due to the underdevelopment of the pituitary gland hindering sexual growth. Sometimes puberty is delayed due to physical as well as psychological causes. Unhealthy physical conditions, strenuous physical work, malnutrition, severe anaemia, tuberculosis, malaria, weak constitution, underdevelopment of the genital organs such as the ovaries or uterus, may cause failure of or delayed menstruation. Sometimes psychological causes such as sudden fright, grief, a weak mind, separation from dear ones, may cause this serious trouble. In all such cases one can take to Yoga without fear of any harm (see Chapter X).
2. *Dysmenorrhoea:* This is a difficult or painful menstruation which may be caused by anaemia, exhaustion, or chills. It may also be due to organic trouble or defects, such as inflammation of the ovaries, fallopian tubes or womb, or due to spasms in the womb caused by nervous temperament or due to maldevelopment of the uterus. Even psychological factors such as fear, disharmony, anxiety and neurosis are involved in dysmenorrhoea.
3. *Menorrhagia:* Excessive bleeding during menstrual periods is called menorrhagia. In this case, the duration of cycles may remain regular, but excessive loss of blood is found each time.
4. *Metrorrhagia:* This is similar to menorrhagia, but here the bleeding is at odd periods before or after menstruation. Hence the cycles are also changing and irregular. Fibroids, tumours, cysts, displacement of

the uterus, inflammation, or miscarriage are common causes of this trouble.

5. *Hypomenorrhoea:* This is scanty discharge. It is due to either underdevelopment of the uterus or to deficiency in the formation of the ovaries or endocrine glands.
6. *Oligomenorrhoea:* Here the cycles are prolonged.
7. *Polymenorrhoea:* Here the cycles are of short duration.
8. *Leucorrhoea:* Excessive white discharge is a common problem which causes physical weakness as well as mental torture. Constitutional, sexual, hormonal and psychic factors are responsible for its cause. Sometimes it is due to new growth in the genital organs, or to foreign bodies in the vagina. Often it is due to hygienic negligence.
9. *Premenstrual Tension:* Many women suffer from this a week or ten days before their period. Strain on the nervous system is generally the cause, resulting in headache, taut nerves, enlarged breasts, tremors, irritability, loss of temper, heaviness in the pelvic region, or inflammation.

All these symptoms of menstrual disorder are due to a number of factors, such as faulty development of the genital organs, imbalance of hormones in the endocrine glands, weak muscles of the reproductive organs, or a weak constitution. Apart from physiological and organic defects, psychological factors are also involved.

Yogic practice is a great help here. Yogāsanas and prāṇāyāma correct the faults or the malfunctioning of the organs. A proper hormonal balance is effected in the endocrine glands and they are stimulated to function efficiently. The muscles of organs such as the uterus are strengthened. The āsanas help one to relax and rest in a proper manner. They ensure a proper menstrual flow.

Moreover, psychological tensions and pressures are reduced through the practice of āsana and prāṇāyāma and one's mental attitude changes from negative to positive.

2. Pregnancy

The saying "As you sow, so shall you reap" is apt in the case of pregnant women. A woman who has looked after her health will reap the reward by having a healthy pregnancy and producing a healthy child. It is absolutely essential for a pregnant woman to maintain her physical and mental well-being both for her own sake and for the sake of the child within.

There are mistaken notions about Yoga for pregnant women. There is a fear in the minds of some women that if Yoga is done during pregnancy, it may lead to miscarriage. This is, however, nothing but an old wives' tale. In āsanas, the uterus is exercised to become strong and to function more efficiently so that delivery can be normal.

"The time to save an unborn baby's life is before pregnancy begins," is a popular saying. It is full of truth. The proper time to begin Yogāsanas, namely puberty, has already been mentioned, and if started then will help the sādhaka to be strong at the time of pregnancy.

Pregnancy is a natural state, like menstruation. Though it brings a great change throughout the body, this subsides after delivery.

One important point has to be stressed here. Deficiency in the internal secretions of the thyroid gland can result in miscarriage. Women should therefore practise āsanas such as *Śirṣāsana*, *Sarvāṅgāsana*, *Setu Bandha Sarvāṅgāsana*, *Janu-Śirṣāsana* from Sections IV and II before conception takes place. The importance of the proper functioning of the ductless glands for good health cannot be over-emphasised and Yogic practice helps bring about this hormonal balance. Yogāsanas are truly beneficial to safeguard against miscarriage owing to defects or abnormal conditions such as inflammation or displacement of the uterus.

Yogāsanas also prove beneficial as a measure of safeguarding against failure to conceive owing to defects of the ovaries, glands, or fallopian tubes.

Hence it is recommended that every woman should begin to practise Yoga before conception, not only to improve maternal health, but also to ensure sound health for future generations.

Pregnant women are advised to be careful during the first three months. Just as medical science, Yoga advises one to take prenatal care. The mother needs good quality blood rich in haemoglobin during pregnancy and also it is important for her to keep her blood pressure normal. To avoid danger signs such as high blood pressure, rapid addition in weight, or albumin in the urine, āsanas are important for her.

There are chances of miscarriage during this period due to improper formation of the placenta, prolapse, or muscular weakness of the uterus. It is dangerous during this period to lift heavy loads and to jump about. Yogāsanas, however, are non-violent; they strengthen the pelvic muscles and improve blood circulation in the pelvic region; they strengthen the reproductive system, exercise the spine, and make the period of confinement bearable.

During this period āsanas especially beneficial are *Parvatāsana, Supta Vīrāsana, Upaviṣṭha Koṇāsana, Baddha. Koṇāsana, Śīrṣāsana* and *Supta Pādānguṣṭhāsana.* These expand the cavity of the pelvic region creating space inside the uterus, ensuring proper blood circulation and adequate room for the movement of the child. In addition, if prāṇāyāma is practised the nerves are calmed, confidence and courage are gained, and fatigue is conquered. Even inverted postures, performed correctly, are beneficial. My father and I have guided many women to perform them till the ninth month. When breathing becomes heavy, however, they should be stopped. A woman in the state of advanced pregnancy is herself the best judge. She can assess that certain āsanas are not possible due to heaviness in the pelvis and abdomen and consequently in the heart. At such times āsanas like *Śīrṣāsana. Sarvāṅgāsana* and

Halāsana have to be discontinued, but other postures such as sitting ones with concave back and spine strengthening āsanas can be done. Do such āsanas which bring lightness in the abdomen and pelvis and which afford nourishment. However, *Ujjāyi Prāṇāyāma I* and *Viloma Prāṇāyāma I & II* can be done throughout pregnancy.

In the early stages of pregnancy, morning sickness, dullness and weakness may appear. Sometimes there are discharges or pains in the pelvic region, swelling or numbness in the feet, swollen veins and varicose veins, backache, constipation, variation in blood pressure, toxaemia, headache, dizziness, blurred vision and infrequent urination. In all these conditions āsanas are most helpful.

However, it is advisable to seek medical treatment if the foetus is found in an abnormal position (transverse or cross) or if it is dead. Yoga done while the foetus is in breach position does not harm.

A short time after miscarriage, āsanas and prāṇāyāma can safely be restarted without straining the abdominal organs. As steadiness and progress is maintained, the time as well as the number of āsanas can be gradually increased.

Delivery

Birth pangs are natural, a sort of signal to various muscles in the pelvic and surrounding region—the lion's share naturally going to the muscles of the uterus which in a series of spasms produce contractions and relaxation and help the expulsion of the child. However, fear and mental stress aggravate labour pains and delay the child from emerging.

If Yogāsanas are practised during the course of pregnancy, they strengthen the uterine muscles so that they are able to function more efficiently during delivery. *Baddha Koṇāsana* and *Upaviṣṭha Koṇāsana* are extremely beneficial as they help make the pelvic area broad and dilate the neck of the womb. Prāṇāyāma strengthens the nerves to enable the mother to breathe calmly in the periods between spasms, which is essential for easy delivery. It helps to relax the nerves and to avoid mental tensions.

If the delivery is normal, or even if a Caesarian operation has to be performed, it is advisable to restart āsana and prāṇāyāma practice in order to regain health and to strengthen the abdominal organs (see Chapter X).

Lactation

After delivery the mother must be ensured of mental and physical rest. The abdominal muscles become loose after delivery, so *Śavāsana* and *Ujjāyī Prāṇāyāma I* are helpful at this stage.

The child must have pure breast feeding. Medical science has said that for every ounce of mother's milk, 400 ounces of oxygen is required. In *Śavāsana* the abdomen and the internal organs do not protrude and in *Ujjāyī Prāṇāyāma* the chest expands fully. Hence the intake of oxygen is increased, which helps lactation.

From the first month onwards āsanas recommended in Part II of Chapter X can be performed; these stimulate the pituitary gland which secretes prolactin that controls lactation. Also these āsanas relieve heaviness in the breasts and bring firmness to their muscle fibres. After delivery fat generally gathers around the buttocks, hips and breasts and there is a tendency towards flabbiness. The growth of fat must be controlled and abdominal organs strengthened. Two months after delivery āsanas that help contract the abdominal and pelvic muscles to their former shape should be performed (see Chapter X).

There is no harm in doing Yoga if one has undergone a surgical operation such as tubectomy or removal of the uterus. However, it should be started carefully and gradually only after taking complete rest and avoiding strain and overstretching. Therefore, correct practice is essential.

3. Menopause (Climacteric)

At around 40 to 50 years, women experience disturbance in the menstrual cycle. Menstruation either stops suddenly or becomes irregular, or the quantity lessens. All these are natural signs that the reproductory functions are coming to an end. Just as at the beginning of menstruation, physical, physiological and psychological disturbances occur, women again have to face disturbances at the stage of menopause. As the ovaries stop functioning, the other glands, namely, the thyroids and the adrenals, become hyperactive and there is an imbalance of hormones. As a result, women suffer from hot flushes, high blood pressure, heaviness in the breasts, headaches, insomnia, obesity, etc. Due to the changes in physiological and metabolic processes and in psychological and emotional states, women have to learn to face the new problem by improving their physical and mental stability.

There can be emotional disturbance, loss of balance and poise resulting in short temper, jealousy, depression, fear and anxiety—all arising out of a feeling that one has lost one's womanhood. This is a critical period of adjustment. At this juncture, practice of Yogāsanas is extremely beneficial, as it calms the nervous system and brings equipoise.

Yoga is a gift for old age. One who takes to Yoga when old gains not only health and happiness but also freshness of mind, since Yoga gives one a bright outlook on life and one can look forward to a happier future rather than looking back into the past which has already entered into darkness. The loneliness and the nervousness which create sadness and sorrow are destroyed by Yoga as a new life begins. Hence it is never too late to begin. Yoga if started in old age is a rebirth which teaches one to face death happily, peacefully, and courageously.

Hence nobody is exempted from doing Yoga practice and there are no excuses for not doing Yoga. How useful Yoga is can only be understood by practising it.

PART– II

Practice

Chapter VIII

Know Your Body

According to Sāṃkhya Yoga Philosophy, a human being is made up of twenty-five components:

Puruṣa or Jīvātmā – Individual Soul
Prakṛti or Avyakta – Nature or Un-evolved Matter
Buddhi or Mahat – Intellect
Ahamkāra – Ego
5 Tanmātra – 5 Subtle Elements (smell, taste, sight, sound, touch)
5 Mahābhūta – 5 Gross Elements (earth, water, fire, air, ether)
5 Jnānendriya – 5 Organs of Sense (nose, tongue, eyes, ears, skin)
5 Karmendriya – 5 Organs of Action (hands, feet, organs of speech, generation and excretion)
Manas – Mind

All these are permeated by the action of the three guṇas of sattva, rajas and tamas, or the three qualities of light, action and inertia.

Āyurveda, the Indian Science of Medicine (Āyus—life, veda—knowledge or science) also accepts this classification but omits the Puruṣa or Jivātmā as being outside of its scope. It is concerned solely with the treatment of diseases and the individual Soul requires no such treatment. It therefore concerns itself only with the remaining twenty-four components.

Further, Āyurveda believes that the body consists of three fundamental elements: doṣa or humours, dhātu or essential ingredients, and mala or impurities. All these are made up of the five mahābhūtas:

3 Doṣa – 3 humours of the body (wind, bile, phlegm)

7 Dhātu – 7 essential ingredients (juice, blood, flesh, fat, bones, marrow, semen)

3 Mala – 3 impurities (faeces, urine, sweat)

The doṣas perform the physiological and physiochemical activities of the body. The dhātus form certain bodily structures which perform specific actions. The malas are impure substances, parts of which are utilised to perform certain physiological functions and parts excreted.

These three fundamental elements of doṣa, dhātu and mala are said to be in a state of equilibrium in the case of good health. When the equilibrium is disturbed, disease sets in.

The air we breathe, the food we eat, and the liquid we drink as well as the dhātus and the malas pass through thirteen types of tubular channels called srotas. These have been enumerated in Chapter V. The srotas together with the dhātus correspond partly to the systems of modern anatomy.

All ancient Indian systems of thought, whether Sāṃkhya, Yoga, Āyurveda, or any other system, believed that a person is a psychophysical as well as a spiritual entity. This is well demonstrated by the Upaniṣadic doctrine of Kośas or sheaths described in Chapter VI. Modern medicine is also rapidly coming to similar conclusions, though the language used is different. The ancient ways were based on a philosophical and religious viewpoint based on analysis, reason and science.

In modern terms, the human body is a complicated mechanism which consists of millions and millions of different types of cells whose products unite to form the various physical structures such as skin, tissues, muscles, veins and arteries, the vital organs and the bones, etc., of which the entire body is composed.

The gross body consists of the head, trunk, arms or upper extremities, and legs or lower extremities (Figure I).

Externally visible on the head are the eyes, ears, nose, mouth, chin, cheeks, temples, forehead and crown of the head. Inside the head is the brain.

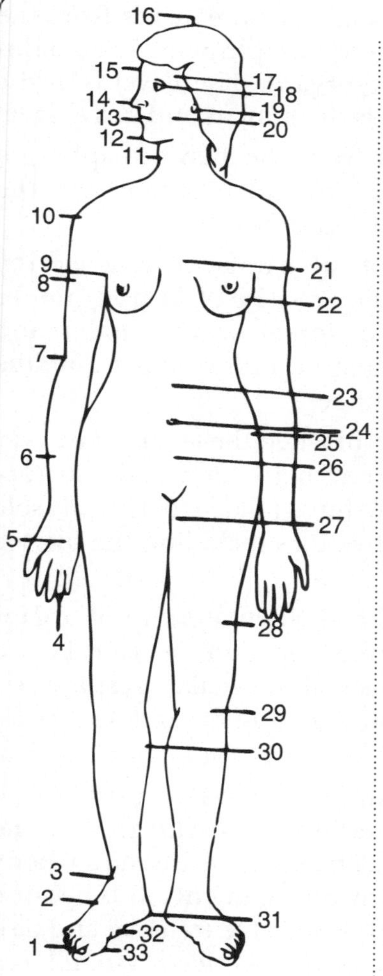

1. Toes
2. Foot
3. Ankle
4. Thumb, index or forefinger, middle, ring, little finger
5. Palm
6. Forearm or lower arm
7. Elbow
8. Upper arm
9. Armpit
10. Shoulder
11. Throat or neck
12. Chin
13. Lips
14. Nose
15. Forehead
16. Crown or top of the head
17. Temple
18. Eye
19. Ear
20. Cheek
21. Chest
22. Breast
23. Stomach
24. Navel
25. Hips
26. Lower Abdomen
27. Groin
28. Thigh
29. Knee
30. Calf
31. Heel
32. Arch of the foot
33. Sole

Fig. I: External Organs

The neck and the throat connect the head to the trunk.

The trunk is divided into three major parts. The upper or the thoracic region extends from the shoulders to the thoracic diaphragm and contains the chest area with the breasts in front and the heart and the lungs within. The back is called the dorsal area.

The middle or the abdominal region extends from the thoracic diaphragm to the pelvic diaphragm. It contains the stomach and the digestive organs. The navel is in the centre. The posterior portion is the lumbar and sacral area.

The lower trunk extends from the pelvic diaphragm to the pubis. It contains the generative organs and the excretory passages. The buttocks are behind.

At the top of either side of the trunk are attached the arms or the upper limbs. They consist of armpit, upper arm, elbow joint, lower arm or forearm, wrist, palm, and five fingers—thumb, forefinger or index finger, middle finger, ring finger, and little finger.

At the base of the trunk are attached the legs or the lower limbs. Each consists of the groin, thigh, knee and kneecap, shin, calf (at the back of the shin), ankle, foot, heel, sole of foot, arch of the foot and five toes including the big toe (Figure I).

The body is highly organised. When a group of organs performs a particular definite function, it is called a system. Thus we have the skeletal, muscular, respiratory, circulatory, digestive, nervous, glandular and excretory systems.

The skeletal system (Figures II & III) consists of all the bones in the body, including the cartilage and the ligaments. There are about 206 bones in the adult body and they are joined together by the ligaments. It is because of these many joints that the body is able to move and also that it is less liable to total injury. The skeletal system has a number of important functions to perform: First, it provides a framework for the body; secondly, it provides levers for

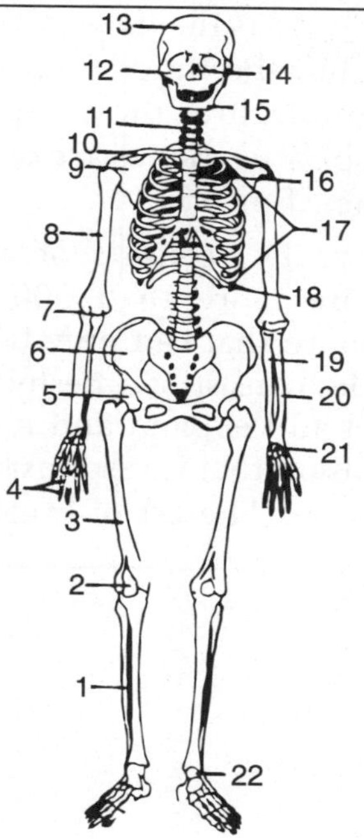

1. Shin bone
2. Kneecap
3. Femur
4. Fingers
5. Pelvic joint or femur
6. Pelvic bone
7. Joint of the elbow
8. Humerus
9. Scapula or shoulder-blade
10. Clavicle
11. Cervical Vertebrae
12. Cheek bone (Zygomatic)
13. Cranium (Skull)
14. Nasal bones
15. Mandible
16. Sternum or breast bone
17. Thorax (Ribs)
18. Floating Ribs
19. Ulna
20. Radius
21. Wrist (Carpal bone)
22. Tarsal (Ankle bone)

Fig. II: The System of Bones

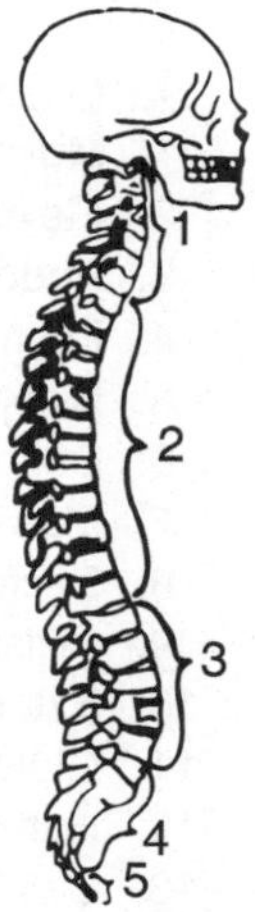

1. Cervical Vertebrae
2. Dorsal Vertebrae
3. Lumbar Vertebrae
4. Sacrum
5. Coccyx

Fig. III: Skull and Spine

the muscles to move; thirdly, it protects the delicate organs of the body such as the brain and the lungs; fourthly, it contains the marrow which manufactures the blood cells; lastly, it stores calcium and phosphorus. Bones are of many shapes and sizes according to their function.

The muscular system (Figure IV) consists of all the muscles of the body. There are more than 500 main muscles, as well as thousands more that can only be seen under a microscope. The muscles consist of a fleshy tissue which has the ability to contract and expand and it is this muscular contraction and expansion that is responsible for all physical movement and motion. The act of breathing,

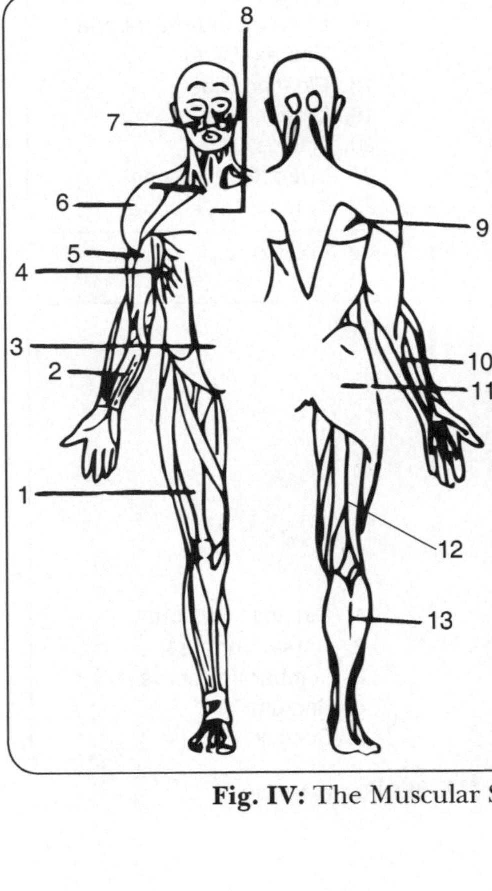

Fig. IV: The Muscular System

the beating of the heart, as well as every other function of our physical organs, is due to muscle action. Indeed, at least half our body is made of muscle, including all our vital organs; muscle makes up for half our body-weight. At all times, whether we are sleeping or resting, innumerable muscles are at work aiding breathing, digestion, etc.

The individual cells of the muscular tissue are long and slim. They shorten and thicken during effort and the whole muscle changes similarly, thus forming a contracted muscle.

There are two types of muscles—voluntary and involuntary. Voluntary muscles are those which are under the control of our will, such as those of the face and the limbs. Involuntary muscles control the working of the inner body over which we have no say, such as are involved in respiratory processes, blood circulation, or digestion. However, those who practise Yoga gradually acquire some degree of control even of the normally involuntary processes.

The respiratory system is made up of all the organs connected with breathing, namely, nose, pharynx or throat, larynx or voice box, windpipe, the bronchii, and the lungs. Its main function is to supply oxygen to the blood and to remove from it waste matter such as carbon dioxide.

Most of the chest area is occupied by the lungs which extend vertically from the thoracic diaphragm to the collar bone and horizontally from side rib to side rib. During inspiration the muscles that line the thoracic cavity raise the sternum and expand the rib-cage horizontally as well as from the back to the front. This increased chest cavity forces the dome of the diaphragm (which is also a muscle) downwards, thereby increasing the cavity vertically also. The diaphragm is contracted and flattened in the manner usual to muscles. The lungs are elastic, they are always inflated, and external air pressure keeps them in contact with the inner rib-cage. When the rib-cage expands air flows into the lungs and when it contracts, air is expelled. Breathing is thus largely the result of the muscular action of the chest and the diaphragm.

The digestive system consists of the mouth, the salivary glands, the food pipe or the oesophagus, the stomach, the intestines, the liver and the pancreas. Food in the form of proteins, carbohydrates, fats, minerals and vitamins gets digested by the chemical action of the various digestive juices that are produced in the digestive tract and gets absorbed into the blood stream and into the lymph vessels. In the liver, much of the digested food is changed for immediate use by the body and some is prepared for storage. The movement of food during the various stages of digestion takes place through muscular action.

There are three processes by which food becomes part of the living body—digestion, absorption and assimilation. In digestion, food is softened and broken down into a form which is soluble in the watery fluids of the body or, in the case of fat, into minute globules. In absorption, the substances formed are carried throughout the body by the blood. In assimilation, these substances deposited from the blood are united with various tissues for their growth and repair. Each of these processes must continue in a regular manner if good health is to be maintained.

Undigested food is excreted as faeces.

The circulatory system is controlled by the heart, a muscular organ which keeps blood in motion by a pumping action. Through large arteries which divide into smaller and smaller ones and through tiny blood vessels called capillaries the heart sends oxygenated blood to nourish every part of the body. The capillaries have extremely thin walls which enable the neighbouring cells to absorb nourishment from them, as well as to use them for sending out the waste matter. The blood then returns to the heart through veins which unite into larger and larger veins. From the heart it is again sent to the lungs to obtain oxygen and to throw off carbon dioxide, after which it returns to the heart. The blood also carries valuable substances such as hormones and minerals to various parts of the body.

The kidneys, the large intestines, the skin, the lungs, and the liver form the excretory system. They rid the body of materials it cannot digest. The lungs remove carbon dioxide and water, the kidneys remove urea and various mineral salts, and the large intestine removes undigested food. The waste matter is excreted in the form of perspiration, urine and faeces.

The nervous system has two major aspects: the central nervous system consisting of the brain which is encased by the skull and the spinal cord, running through the vertebral column. The nerves which emerge from both these radiate to every part of the body and are called the peripheral nervous system. They are connected with the central nervous system but are capable of independent action. In addition to this there is a division of the nervous system which is concerned with the maintenance of functions that are necessary for life, such as breathing or digestion; this is called the visceral or the autonomic system. Another part is concerned with adapting the body to external conditions and this is termed the somatic system. The nervous system controls all the various functions of the body and is responsible for all coordination and smooth working of the entire psychosomatic mechanism.

The nervous system is made up of large number of nerve cells or neurons which are specially adapted to carry messages or impulses very quickly all over the body. Each nerve cell has a body and one or more branches. Groups of nerve cells are called ganglia. Long nerve cells are called nerve fibres or axons. A bundle of such fibres is called a nerve or a nerve trunk.

There are different types of nerves concerning themselves with different aspects of the physical mechanism. Trophic nerves are concerned with growth, nourishment and repair of tissues. Motor nerves stimulate muscular contraction in the uterus and regulate urinary bladder by regulating water level and help the body adjust to external conditions. Autonomic nerves are concerned with the work of the vital organs.

The brain and the spinal cord are made up of masses of nerve cells and intercommunicating fibres. The nerve cell masses are called grey matter and the fibre masses white matter. In the brain, the grey matter is in the outer layer, whereas it is at the centre of the spinal cord.

The endocrine system consists of glands which do not have any ducts but which discharge hormones directly into the blood stream. The following are the principal endocrine glands: the pituitary, which consists of two parts, namely, the posterior lobe which stimulates muscular contraction in the uterus and regulates water balance: and the anterior lobe, which stimulates growth, development of sex organs, secretion of milk, and controls the other endocrine glands. The thyroid regulates general nutrition in the body. The parathyroid controls absorption of limesalt by bones and other tissues. The pancreas adapts sugary foods for incorporation in muscles and other tissues that require sugars. The ovaries and the testicles produce reproductive cells, but also secrete substances which have a general effect upon other tissues. The supra-renal glands or the adrenal bodies secrete adrenaline which diminishes muscle fatigue and raises the metabolic rate.

The reproductive system is responsible for the propagation of the species. Reproductive organs differ in the male and the female. Here we are concerned only with the female reproductive organs, which consist externally of the vagina and breasts and internally, within the pelvic cavity, the uterus (womb), fallopian tubes and ovaries. The ovary is a gland of the size and shape of an almond. In it is found the ovum which when united with the male sperm forms the embryo.

(For the benefit of the student Figures V are given to show the location of some of the main internal organs.)

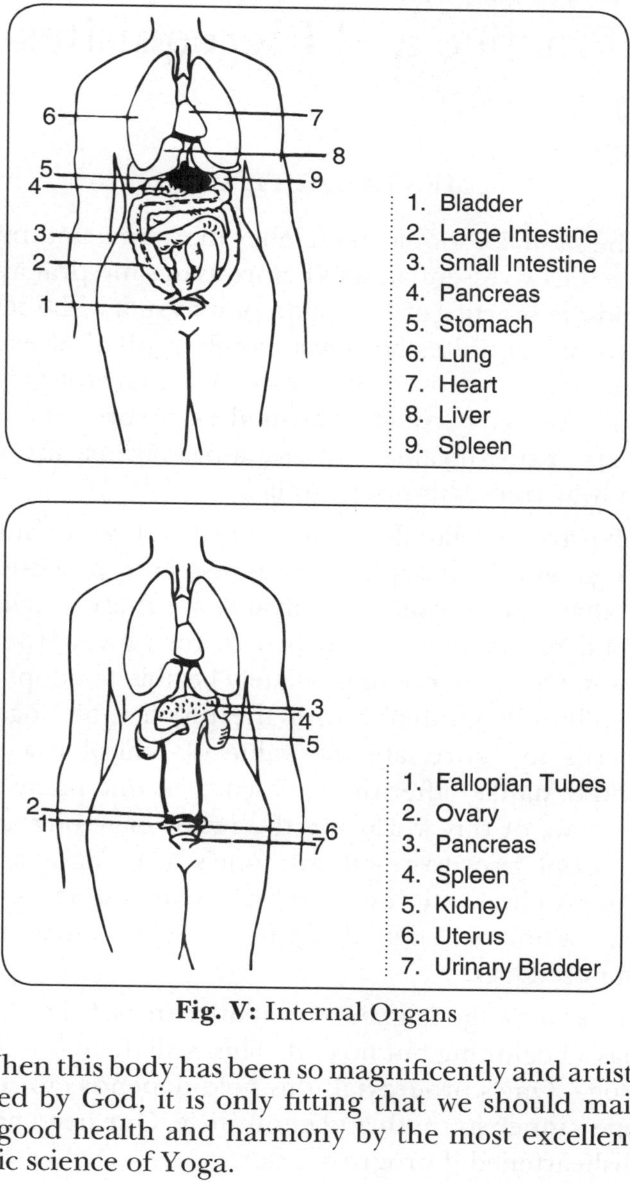

Fig. V: Internal Organs

When this body has been so magnificently and artistically created by God, it is only fitting that we should maintain it in good health and harmony by the most excellent and artistic science of Yoga.

CHAPTER IX

Yoga Sādhanā—Method of Practice and Prerequisites

MENTAL ATTITUDE

1. The sādhaka should remember that yama and niyama are the two essential steps before āsana and prāṇāyāma, and the practice of āsana and prāṇāyāma without these two prerequisites becomes merely a physical exercise and not a psychosomatic subject. Without ethical discipline practice becomes meaningless, according to Yoga texts. Yama-niyama and āsana-prāṇāyāma are like a railway track, running parallel.
2. The average family woman need not be afraid that Yoga with its discipline is impossible to practise. The Mahāvratas of yama and niyama are there to cultivate good habits and to help people turn away from bad ones. One may not immediately be able to adopt them totally, but gradually with the practice of Yoga one learns to appreciate the value of ethical disciplines and to hanker after them. One learns that many of the sorrows of this world are the result of wrong actions and one tries to re-educate one's own conduct to be more in line with the universal commandments which one admires. Yoga discipline then becomes a self-imposed task.
3. No knowledge is gained instantly. In fact, knowledge has a beginning but no end. This is all the more true of Yoga. One's progress in this field depends entirely on one's inner strength and endurance. One need not feel disheartened if progress is slow.

4. Yoga should not be taken lightly, as if it were a hobby. It is not an entertainment. It should be approached seriously, with faith, enthusiasm, determination, keenness, courage, will and dedication.
5. Patañjali has spoken of three types of pupils:

   tīvrasaṁvegānāmāsannaḥ
   mṛdu madhyādhimātratvāttatopi viśeṣaḥ

   P.Y.S. I, 21.22

   The practice of a sādhaka falls into three categories, namely, mild, middling, and intense, according to physical and mental capacity and inclination; each category is likewise divided into three, for example, as mild-mild, middle-mild, intense-mild, and so on. This is further categorised into even subtler degrees of practice. The achievement of spiritual absorption is close to the extremely courageous sādhaka whose practice is highly intense. A warning, however, is to be given that severity of practice by itself is not the yardstick for measuring the nearness to success, as the qualities of Tamas, Rajas and Sattva are also involved in the method of concentration and practice. A pure mind and a right intention are necessary. Hence Yoga must be done gradually whilst watching one's own progress so that it brings inner purification.
6. Quite often a flair for Yoga prompts sādhakas to begin in earnestness. Being beginners, the subtleties of Yoga cannot be imbibed by their body, mind, or intelligence. So they jog along. Yoga practice may become tedious during such times, but they should persevere with a firm will. They should remember the adage that "Rome was not built in a day". With constant practice, perseverance and faith they will begin to understand the subtlety and the beauty of Yoga.

BUDDHI—INTELLIGENCE

7. In the performance of āsana and prāṇāyāma, intelligence plays the main role. In this context, Chapter VI on *Is Yoga Ideal for Women?* may be re-read which describes how movements should be done for maximum effect. A movement during āsana practice is not mere twisting of the body. It has a bearing not only on the physical aspect, but on the physiological and the psychological as well. Āsanas and prāṇāyāma have to be done with care, skill and attention.

8. Often a sādhaka will grasp the āsana and the method of its performance by her intelligence, but finds it hard to translate the same into practice. Mere academic knowledge of the āsanas remains illusory. Theoretical knowledge and its application in practice alone leads to an understanding of its reality. When theoretical knowledge and experienced knowledge meet, harmony, clarity and wisdom set in. This is called Prajnā.

AHAṂKĀRA—EGO

9. After gaining some proficiency in the practice of Yoga, one should not abandon it, saying that it is merely the pursuit of the external. Likewise, one should never feel complacent that one has fully mastered the art and that nothing more remains to be learned. Equally, it is wrong to claim that one has already subdued one's senses and that the discipline of Yoga is no longer necessary. This would be the beginning of an inflated ego and one's downfall in Yoga.

10. No doubt, Yoga brings about a transformation in one's physical, mental and moral well-being. This should not be mistaken for mastery of the subject. Ego, which

manifests itself grossly, penetrates the personality in a subtle form and permeates it totally. It is the greatest enemy in the practice of Yoga. Hence the sādhaka should take care not to be caught in such a web and should cultivate humility. Whatever attainments are gained should be considered as having been bestowed by the Grace of God and one should surrender to Him. This is humbleness.

11. Śankarāchārya and Jñāneśvar, having attained the highest knowledge of the Formless Eternal Truth, composed all their hymns and prayers in praise of God with Form and Attributes. The Self, though formless, has a form in the shape of the body. The sādhaka should bear in mind that one must start with the body, which is the external covering of the Self. This gradually leads to the pursuit of the internal—the mind and the innermost Self.

BRAIN

12. The brain should be cool, alert, and watchful, examining the movements of the body and the fluctuations of the mind during every moment of practice. By adopting this habit of self-observation, one's mistakes will become apparent quickly and can be corrected. The body should be the performer and the brain the observer.

MANAS—MIND

13. Āsanas are performed according to the pliability of the body. This gives one the idea that this is my capacity. Here mental mobility is required and such an attitude has to be replaced by will-power, so that the mind can be extended beyond its limited operation. The will-power has to be followed by action so that the barriers of both body and mind are broken in order to proceed

further. Everyday practice has to be accompanied by a spirit of research so that the intellect can penetrate deeper and deeper.

14. Always there is a tug-of-war between the body and the mind while performing an āsana. Sometimes the body is elastic but the mind rigid and at other times the mind is more elastic but the body remains stiff and unenthusiastic. Whichever is the dull one should be activated with concentration and attention. Laziness and lethargy are arch-enemies of Yoga while cheerfulness and enthusiasm are the friends that elevate the practitioner.

ŚARĪRA—BODY

15. If you experience restlessness of the body or mind, be assured that the sādhanā has some serious faults. At this stage it is wise to seek the Guru's guidance.

16. The beginner will experience aches in the limbs after beginning the sādhanā. It is so in all walks of life. With regular practice the aches gradually becomes less and less and ultimately disappears. If, however, the ache persists, stop the āsanas which cause pain and do simpler ones from the same Section. After a few days again try those which caused you trouble cautiously and carefully.

17. Find out the causes of pain in the postures by repeating the movements on either side and observing the reactions. Suppose the right side pains and not the left; see how you performed on the left. Imitate the same movement on the right and vice versa if the pain is on the opposite side. By trial and experience you will learn to perform correct āsanas and get relief from wrong pains.

18. However, during the continuance of sādhanā minor aches and pains do come, but they can be endured. Pains may occur even while walking or running, if one is not accustomed to walk or run long distances. Such pains disappear with continued practice; in the same way pains through Yoga also vanish soon.

19. One should learn to distinguish between healthy and unhealthy pain. A healthy pain is a natural pain which occurs when the range of action is increased. It does not hinder us in our everyday life; hence we know that it is not harmful and we can continue to practise.

    Unhealthy pains continue for a long time; they hinder practice as well as our normal life. Sometimes they disturb the organic functions and even the nervous system, thereby causing mental instability, nervousness and depression. These are danger signals in one's practice and in this case the intensity of practice should be lessened and, if necessary, guidance should be sought.

20. Most sādhakas will feel a peculiar sensation that either the right or the left portion of the body is more elastic than the other. In such cases the easier side must act as a guide to the less efficient or stiffer side. Here the body needs an intellectual adjustment.

21. Certain bodies are stiff and others elastic by nature. Some sādhakas will notice that their body bends forward easily while for others backward movement is easy. This is quite natural, depending on the elasticity of the spine. Do not despair if a posture eludes you: continue the practice and elasticity will be achieved in due course. A challenge and response interaction takes place between the intelligence and the body. If one challenges, the other has to respond with equal vigour and vice versa.

22. Sometimes the sādhaka feels that the practice is ineffective or faulty due to lack of alertness. Here one must again apply one's mind and intelligence to watch the challenges and the responses taking place in the mind and the body. Such care and attention will enliven not only one's practice but one's very Being.
23. In order to reach the final posture, do not move with an aggressive mind or by hardening the muscles. You should be passive and attentive. When once the final posture is reached, remain firm in it and observe its accuracy; adjust and extend further to perfect it.
24. Beginners should try to grasp the subtleties of movements involved in each āsana. This will enable them to perform the āsana easily and with poise.
25. In doing āsana and prāṇāyāma an inward vision is necessary to analyse oneself.
26. Aim at the quality of the āsanas and not the quantity. Quality means doing the postures accurately, steadily and whole-heartedly.
27. Be alert and watchful in every limb, as the entire body should be responsive to the āsanas.
28. Āsanas should be done with the discipline of the senses—the roots of sādhanā should come from the innermost Self. Therefore, convert and transform all the āsanas from the external to the internal and turn your attention inward whenever you practise.
29. Faultless sādhanā leads to radical changes in one's personality: One becomes moderate in habits, food, sleep and sex. As the mind and the body become pure, spiritual awakening dawns.
30. Sādhanā has three stages, namely, śravaṇa—listening, manana—thinking, and nididhyāsana—putting into practice and experiencing. Patañjali explains these three aspects using a different terminology, namely,

japa—repetition, artha—understanding the meaning, and bhāvanā—realisation.

In Yoga-sādhanā all the three processes have to be followed for one's practice to bear fruit. For example, āsana has to be repeated again and again, day after day, year after year; this is śravaṇa or japa. It is Karma Mārga.

This repetition leads one to the mental process of thinking, where one penetrates deeper and deeper from Annamaya Kośa to Ānandamaya Kośa. This is called manana, which gives meaning and understanding of the action which is being performed by the sādhaka. This is Jnāna Mārga in sādhanā.

This repeated (japa) and well-thought-over (artha) action gives a new experience to the sādhakā. It is a form of worship in which one offers every āsana as a flower to God. The sādhaka becomes one with the action and remains absorbed in it (bhāvanā). This enlightened state of Self-realisation is Bhakti Mārga. Then Karma, Jñāna and Bhakti all merge into one. This is Nididhyāsana.

This type of sādhanā alone brings completion to the practice.

CHAPTER X

Hints and Suggestions for the Practice of Āsanas

PART I: GENERAL HINTS

Time

1. For any study or practice, early morning is the ideal time. For beginners, however, morning is not the best as their muscles are rigid at that time of the day. It is better for them to commence practice in the afternoon or in the evening when the muscles are elastic. Later, as they progress and their muscles loosen they can switch over to the early hours of the morning.

   However, āsanas may be practised at other times of the day so long as the period between meal-times and Yoga study is observed.

2. Women may find it difficult to adhere to a fixed time for practice. Even then, it is not harmful to practise at any hour, but for discipline it is ideal to stick to a definite time.

3. Generally, the mind and the body are fresh and relaxed in the morning. This is therefore the most beneficial time for difficult āsanas to be practised. After the day's toil, evening is ideal for āsanas such as *Sālamba Śīrṣāsana* (Figure 69), *Sālamba Sarvāṅgāsana* (Figure 84), *Halāsana* (Figure 88), *Setu Bandha Sarvāṅgāsana* (Figures 99, 101), and *Paścimottānāsana* (Figure 30). These āsanas relieve fatigue and help obtain sound sleep and peace of mind.

Duration of each Āsana

4. Suggestions have been given about the duration of āsanas while explaining the techniques.

Age

5. Āsanas can be practised at any age. It is ideal to begin at the age of seven or eight but this does not mean that one cannot begin later. It is, however, essential to choose āsanas according to one's capacity. Postures selected in this book are suitable for everyone irrespective of age. The sādhakā should use her discretion to master the particular āsanas which are most useful to her. I have introduced special methods of performing āsanas correctly using the wall as a guide.

Hygienic Habits

6. It is essential to finish one's morning hygienic chores before practising āsanas.
7. If one is suffering from acute or chronic constipation, the following āsanas should be practised: *Sālamba Śīrṣāsana* (Figure 69), *Pārśva Śīrṣāsana* (Figure 71), *Parivṛttaikapāda Śīrṣāsana* (Figure 72), *Sālamba Sarvāṅgāsana* (Figure 84), *Halāsana* (Figures 88, 91), *Pārśva Halāsana* (Figure 94), *Piṇḍāsana* (Figure 104), and *Pārśva Piṇḍāsana* (Figure 105). These āsanas relieve constipation. Motion or stools should not be obstructed during the process of doing the postures; one should relieve oneself and continue one's practice afterwards.
8. It is easier to do āsanas after a bath. But if one is accustomed to hot water, then the āsanas should not be practised immediately afterwards as the dilated blood vessels tend to make one dizzy. A period of 15 to 20 minutes should elapse before starting to practise.

9. There is no rule that a cold bath should be taken, nor that one should bathe in the early morning before dawn. The habits to which one is accustomed should be followed.
10. If you wish to take a bath again after practice due to sweating, by all means do so. In that case, however, it is best to wait for 15 or 20 minutes after *Śavāsana*.

Food

11. Āsanas should preferably be practised on an empty stomach. A cup of tea, coffee, or milk preceding the practice is not harmful. However, an hour should elapse if one has had a light meal and four hours after a full meal before practice. Light beverages may be taken after āsanas, but one hour should elapse before solid foods are eaten. Solid food taken immediately after practice may harm digestion.
12. However, there are a few āsanas which can be done after a meal if so desired. They do not harm digestion and, on the contrary, may help it. These are *Siddhāsana* (Figure 48). *Vīrāsana* (Figures 49, 50), *Padmāsana* (Figure 52). *Supta Vīrāsana* (Figure 58), *Baddha Koṇāsana* (Figure 5), *Supta Baddha Koṇāsana* (Figures 38, 39) and *Matsyāsana* (Figure 62). These āsanas relieve one from a heavy feeling in the stomach after meals.
13. A balanced diet, in moderation, is the best. Āyurveda says that the stomach should be filled with two parts of solid food and one part of water, and that one part of the stomach should be kept free for the movement of air. Food which is not congenial to the system should be avoided. Too oily, dry, spicy and sour foodstuff are not good for the system. A diet which is balanced, light, varied, and well cooked is ideal for health.

Those who suffer from stomach and heart troubles, diabetes, obesity should regulate their diet carefully. It is important to notice the change that the practice of āsanas brings. In the beginning the appetite grows as digestion improves. Later the intake of food is reduced, without affecting energy. Even a little quantity is relished. The system starts rejecting hot and spicy dishes. By regular practice one's own constitution guides one as to what is good and what is to be avoided in food.

Sunshine

14. It is not advisable to practise Yoga immediately after being exposed to the hot Sun, nor to practise directly in the sun. However, if you have to, then first do *Jānu Śīrṣāsana* (Figure 26), *Paścimottānāsana* (Figures 30, 31), *Uttānāsana* (Figure 21), and *Adho Mukha Śvānāsana* (Figure 22) before attempting *Sālamba Śīrṣāsana* (Figure 69), *Sālamba Sarvāṅgāsana* (Figure 84) and *Halāsana* (Figure 88).

Place

15. Select an airy place free from insects and noise. The place should be well ventilated and the floor even.

Mat

16. Spread a mat or blanket on the floor; it should not be too thick nor too thin. The hardness of the floor should not be a discomfort to the head or to the body.

Clothing

17. Do not use tight-fitting clothes for practice. Loosen all tight fittings so that you can breathe freely. The movement of the ribs and the chest should not

be obstructed. I have known cases where tight-fitting clothes have led to breathing through the mouth and burning in the region of the chest. Use a loose blouse and stretch pants. The body should feel free while moving.

Mirror

18. The beginner should avoid the use of a mirror because it is necessary to be inwardly aware of what one is doing. By the use of a mirror one gets confused, especially during the inverted positions.
19. After gaining a certain amount of proficiency, however, a mirror may be used occasionally to observe subtle movements. See that the mirror is properly fixed to the wall, exactly perpendicular and not slanting, so that you are parallel to it.
20. The fixed mirror should touch the floor level for proper observation of such āsanas as *Sālamba Śīrṣāsana* (Figure 69), *Dvi Pāda Viparīta Daṇḍāsana* (Figure 146) and so on.

Śavāsana

21. Do *Śavāsana* only at the end and not between āsanas. To alternate *Śavāsana* with āsanas in quick succession is harmful and disturbs the nervous system. Moreover, neither the other āsanas nor *Śavāsana* will be properly performed if one follows this procedure. During the day *Śavāsana* may be done by itself at any time for relaxation.
22. The minimum duration of *Śavāsana* in normally 5 to 10 minutes; however, it may continue for 20 to 40 minutes, or until the whole body and the mind are relaxed.

23. The pause between two āsanas is largely a matter of personal discretion. Generally it should last for 4 to 5 breaths or 15 to 20 seconds. Those who are prone to breathlessness will need a longer time. It really depends on one's breathing habits. However, this pause should not be increased just because there is pain in the body. The greater the delay, the greater the possibility of the body becoming dull and inactive for another āsana and the mind is given a chance to wander and laziness sets in. The time lag between the difficult āsanas in Sections VI and VII is likely to be increased to 30 or 35 seconds. Do not be impatient while doing the āsanas. Only when you are morose or feeling out of sorts and wish to remove mental sluggishness, then the āsanas from Sections I, II and VII have to be performed in succession rather more briskly and energetically than usual. But do not make a habit of this type of practice. The order which is given in the sections should normally be followed.
24. Do not make the facial muscles taut. Relax the eyes, the ears, and the tongue. Keep the jaws loose and do not clench the teeth. If you are tense, the benefit of the āsana is lost.
25. Do not shut your eyes while practising āsanas as all the movements have to be observed carefully. A beginner will lose all awareness if the eyes are shut.
26. As you gain experience, after mastering an āsana, if you feel that you can observe its subtleties better with the eyes shut, you may do so.
27. For tension in the eyes due to overwork or mental fatigue, the following āsanas may be practised with the eyes shut: *Halāsana* (Figure 90), *Setu Bandha Sarvāṅgāsana* (Figure 99), *Uttanāsāna* (Figure 21), *Paścimottānāsana* (Figures 30, 31).

Breathing

28. In the āsana techniques, whenever a particular instruction for inhalation or exhalation is given it should be followed otherwise it should be taken for granted that breathing is to be kept normal. However, with regular Yoga practice normal breathing automatically becomes deeper.
29. Do not inhale and exhale through the mouth, but only through the nostrils.
30. Do not hold the breath during practice. Only sometimes, while a limb is being stretched or during particular movements, there is a suspension of breath. Normal breathing should be continued after that particular action ceases. For instance in *Ardha Matsyendrāsana* (Figure 128), while the trunk is being turned after exhalation, or in *Sālamba Sarvāṅgāsana* (Figure 84), while it is being lifted up after exhalation, breath is suspended. When the body has reached the desired position, normal breathing is resumed.

Blood Pressure

31. For high blood pressure, dizziness, etc., practice *Paścimottānāsana* (Figure 30), *Uttānāsana* (Figure 21), and *Adho Mukha Śvānāsana* (Figure 22), followed by *Halāsana* (Figure 90), *Setu Bandha Sarvāṅgāsana* (Figure 99), and then *Sālamba Sarvāṅgāsana* (Figure 86). Finish the cycle with the first three āsanas in reverse order, i.e., as in Figures 22, 21 and 30. When the blood pressure comes to normal, āsanas from Section I and *Sālamba Śīrṣāsana* (Figure 65 or 69) may be introduced. *Śavāsana* and *Viloma Prāṇāyāma II* (Figure 212), as well as *Sūrya Bhedana Prāṇāyāma* (Figure 214) should also be regularly practised.
32. For low blood pressure first practise *Sālamba Śīrṣāsana* (Figures 69, 70) and *Sālamba Sarvāṅgāsana* (Figure 84),

then do *Jānu Śīrṣāsana* on both sides (Figure 26) for one minute or longer. Then practise the other postures according to your capacity.

Heart Disease and other Serious Conditions

33. It is wise to seek the advice of a guru if one is suffering from serious illnesses such as heart trouble or coronary diseases as they need direct attention and guidance, Nevertheless, from my teaching experience I can say that the following may safely be practised by heart patients without fear of aggravating their condition: *Setu Bandha Sarvāṅgāsana* (Figures 98, 99), *Sālamba Sarvāṅgāsana* (Figures 85, 87), *Halāsana* (Figures 89, 90), *Jānu Śīrṣāsana* (Figure 26), *Supta Vīrāsana* (Figures 58, 186), *Matsyāsana*, Lying on a high pillow under the back as in *Supta Vīrāsana* (Figure 186), also *Śavāsana*, *Ujjāyī Prāṇāyāma I*, and *Viloma Prāṇāyāma I* and *II* (Figure 200).

Running Ear or Ear Fungus

34. Inverted postures should be avoided or should be performed under the strict supervision of your guru. *Ardha Halāsana* (Figures 89, 90) is good but should not be done independently as it requires a special adjustment of the inner ear to make sure there is no pressure on it.

Displacement of the Retina

35. Here again, the guidance of an experienced teacher is necessary. Āsanas from Section II are very good as they quieten the eyes. Āsanas from Section I and IV should be avoided, with the exception of *Ardha Halāsana* (Figures 89, 90) which has to be performed in a special way by binding the eyes with a soft cloth to stabilise them so that they are free from tension while the posture is being performed.

PART II: SPECIAL HINTS

Menstruation

36. All the āsanas mentioned in this book are effective. Regular and proper practice of the āsanas and prāṇāyāma is beneficial especially for those suffering from menstrual disorders. However, some practices are more effective than others and are mentioned in the following hints.
37. While doing āsanas from Section I, the abdominal muscles and the organs have to be moved towards the spinal column as well as up towards the chest to avoid undue pressure on the uterus.
38. During the monthly period (48 to 72 hours) complete rest is advisable. Āsanas should not be practised, but if there is some tightness or tension then forward bends from Section II are helpful; over-exertion should be avoided. Normal practice may be resumed after the flow stops completely.
39. *Viloma Prāṇāyāma I* and *II* and *Śavāsana* (Figure 200) are especially helpful during menstruation.
40. The following āsanas should be practised if one suffers from numbness, heaviness and aches.

    Section I : *Utthita Trikoṇāsana* (Figure 4), *Utthita Pārśva Koṇāsana* (Figure 5).

    Section II : *Baddha Koṇāsana* (Figure 35), *Supta Baddha Koṇāsana* (Figure 38), *Upaviṣṭha Koṇāsana* (Figure 40), *Kūrmāsana* (Figure 43), *Mālāsana* (Figure 46).

    Section III : *Vīrāsana* (Figures 49–51), *Supta Vīrāsana* (Figure 58), *Matsyāsana* (Figure 62).

    The duration of these āsanas should be determined by one's physical condition. If you have tremors or are weak, it is better to avoid practice and to rest in *Śavāsana*.

41. During the period if there is pain in the abdomen, profuse discharge, cramp or dysmenorrhoea, practise *Baddha Koṇāsana* (Figure 35), *Supta Baddha Koṇāsana* (Figure 38), *Upaviṣṭha Koṇāsana* (Figure 40), *Vīrāsana Cycle* (Figures 54, 55), and *Supta Vīrāsana* (Figure 58).

42. For profuse discharge or menorrhagia practise āsanas given in No. 41 above and add *Uttānāsana* (Figure 21), *Paścimottānāsana* (Figures 30, 31), *Kūrmāsana* (Figure 43), *Ūrdhva Prasārita Pādāsana* (Figure 109) with feet and legs supported by a wall, *Adho Mukha Śvānāsana* (Figure 22), *Pādānguṣṭhāsana* with concave back (Figure 19), and *Prasārita Pādottānāsana*, concave back only (Figures 16 and 17).

43. During menstruation the following must be avoided:

    All āsanas from Sections IV, V, VII and VIII. Under no circumstances should *Salamba Śīrṣāsana* (Figure 69) and *Sālamba Sarvāṅgāsana* (Figure 84) be performed.

44. Section V must be avoided completely by one who suffers from displaced uterus, serious menstrual disorders and leucorrhoea.

45. *Leucorrhoea:* Regular practice of the following āsanas is helpful:

    Section II : *Baddha Koṇāsana* (Figures 35, 36), *Supta Baddha Koṇāsana* (Figures 38, 39), *Upaviṣṭha Koṇāsana* (Figures 40, 41).

    Section III : *Vīrāsana* (Figures 49, 50), *Vīrāsana* Cycle (Figures 54, 55), *Supta Vīrāsana* (Figure 58), *Matsyāsana* (Figure 62).

    Section IV : *Sālamba Śīrṣāsana* (Figures 69, 70), *Upaviṣṭha Koṇāsana* in *Śīrṣāsana* (Figure 75), *Baddha Koṇāsana* in *Śīrṣāsana* (Figure 76), *Sālamba Sarvāṅgāsana* (Figures 84, 85, 87), *Halāsana* (Figures 89, 90), *Supta Koṇāsana* (Figure 93), *Setu Bandha Sarvāṅgāsana* (Figures 98, 99,101).

Section XI : *Mahā Mudrā* (Figure 210).

Section XII: *Sūrya Bhedana Prāṇāyāma* (Figure 214).

46. *Amenorrhoea:* All āsanas in this book are recommended, especially those from Sections IV, VI, VII and VIII.
47. *Dysmenorrhoea:* Regularly practise āsanas from Sections I, II, III, IV and VI; during menstruation follow the hints given in No. 38 or 41 of this chapter.
48. For complaints such as cramp in the muscles, pain in the stomach, waist, and back, heaviness in the abdomen, and burning sensations practise all āsanas regularly, but during menstruation practise the following: *Baddha Koṇāsana* (Figure 35), *Supta Baddha Koṇāsana* (Figures 38, 39), *Upaviṣṭha Koṇāsana* (Figures 40, 41), *Mālāsana* (Figure 46), *Vīrāsana* (Figure 49), *Supta Vīrāsana* (Figure 58), *Bharadvājāsana I* (Figure 125), *Mahā Mudrā* (Figure 210), *Viloma Prāṇāyāma I & II*, and *Śavāsana* (Figure 212).
49. *Menorrhagia, metrorrhagia:* It is advisable to take complete rest and not to practise any āsanas during the period, but for continued discharge or profuse discharge causing discomfort, practise āsanas given in Nos. 41 and 42.

    However, in order to become free of these complaints, it is important to practise thoroughly the āsanas in Sections II, III and IV when one is not in menses.
50. *Hypomenorrhoea:* Follow the instructions in rules 36 and 37 and practise the āsanas in Sections I, II, IV and *Ūrdhva Dhanurāsana* (Figures 139, 140), and *Dvi Pāda Viparīta Daṇḍāsana* from Section VII (Figure 146).
51. *For oligomenorrhoea:* Sections IV and VII are beneficial. *For polymenorrhoea*: Sections II and III are helpful.
52. During menstruation, if feeling dizzy, do the following:

    Section III : *Virāsana Cycle* (Figure 55), *Supta Vīrāsana* (Figure 58).

Section II : *Jānu Śīrṣāsana* (Figure 26), *Ardha Baddha Padma Paścimottānāsana* (Figure 27), *Triang Mukhaikapāda Paścimottānāsana* (Figure 28), *Maricyāsana I* (Figure 29), *Paścimottānāsana* (Figure 30, 31).

Section XI : *Śanmukhī Mudrā* (Figure 211), *Śavāsana* (Figure 212).

Section XII: Preparation for Deep Breathing I and II (Figure 212).

53. During pre-menstrual tension the following are beneficial:

Section II : *Baddha Koṇāsana* (Figures 35, 36, 37), *Supta Baddha Koṇāsana* (Figures 38, 39).

Section III : *Supta Vīrāsana* (Figure 58), *Matsyāsana* (Figure 62).

Section IV : *Sālamba Śīrṣāsana* (Figure 69), *Sālamba Sarvāṅgāsana* (Figure 84), *Halāsana* (Figures 89, 90), *Setu Bandha Sarvāṅgāsana* (Figure 99 on bench).

Section VII: *Dvi Pāda Viparīta Daṇḍāsana* (Figures 148, 149 on bench).

Section XI : *Mahā Mudrā* (Figure 210), *Śavāsana* (Figure 212).

Section XII: *Viloma Prāṇāyāma I* and *II* (Figure 212), *Sūrya Bhedana Prāṇāyāma* (Figure 214).

54. After the menstruation period one has to begin with the following āsanas and prāṇāyāma to make the vagina dry and this practice should be continued for four days to soothe the nerves and to regain the physical strength to enable normal practice to be resumed:

Section I : *Uttānāsana* (Figure 21), *Adho Mukha Śvānāsana* (Figure 22).

Section II : *Jānu Śīrṣāsana* (Figure 26), *Paścimottānāsana* (Figure 30), *Baddha Koṇāsana* (Figures 35,

36, 37), *Supta Baddha Koṇāsana* (Figures 38, 39), *Upaviṣṭha Koṇāsana* (Figure 41).

Section IV : *Sālamba Śīrṣāsana* (Figures 69, 70), *Upaviṣṭha Koṇāsana* in *Śīrṣāsana* (Figure 75), *Baddha Koṇāsana* in *Śīrṣāsana* (Figure 76), *Sālamba Sarvāṅgāsana* (Figures 84, 85, 87), *Setu Bandha Sarvāṅgāsana* (Figures 98, 99, 101).

Section V : *Supta Pādānguṣṭhāsana* (Figure 119).

Section VII: *Dvi Pāda Viparīta Daṇḍāsana* (Figures 147, 148, 149, 146).

Section XII: *Ujjāyī Prāṇāyāma I* and *II* (Figures 200, 213), *Viloma Prāṇāyāma I* and *II* (Figures 212), *Sūrya Bhedana Prāṇāyāma* (Figure 214).

Pregnancy

55. It is advisable for all women after marriage and before pregnancy to build up their health by regular practice of āsanas and prāṇāyāma.
56. Those who have conceived may, for the first three months, practise all the āsanas and prāṇāyāma given in this book except *Ūrdhva Prasārita Pādāsana* (Figures 106 to 110), *Jathara Parivartanāsana* (Figures 112 to 114), *Paṛipurna Nāvāsana* (Figure 111), from Section V and all āsanas from Section VIII.
57. Do all āsanas from Sections I, II, III, IV and VI, especially those which stretch the spinal column and broaden the pelvis.
58. A tendency to repeated miscarriages is observed in cases of hypothyroidism. To remedy this, āsanas from Section IV are helpful.
59. To facilitate easy delivery, the following āsanas should be practised often, until late in pregnancy: *Baddha*

Koṇāsana (Figures 35, 183, 184), *Supta Baddha Koṇāsana* (Figure 38), *Upaviṣṭha Koṇāsana* (Figures 40, 168), and those contained in Section II. In fact, whenever you have some free time you may do these poses.

60. After three months, as the foetus grows in size, Section IX is the guide for practice until the time of delivery.
61. If a miscarriage takes place, practise *Viloma Prāṇāyāma I* and *II* in *Śavāsana* (Figure 212) and *Sūrya Bhedana Prāṇāyāma* (Figure 214) for the first two to four weeks. Thereafter āsanas from Section IV may be begun, starting for some days only with *Sālamba Sarvāṅgāsana* (Figure 86) and *Halāsana* (Figure 90). Later *Sālamba Śīrṣāsana* may be added, and when one's strength is fully recovered āsanas from Sections I and II may gradually be resumed.
62. Those who are prone to miscarriage will find Yogāsana beneficial. During pregnancy they should practise all āsanas in Section IX (Figures 174 to 199) and prāṇāyāma and its variations.
63. Those who are prone to miscarriages due to glandular trouble or muscular weakness and weak constitution should concentrate on the practice of āsanas from Sections II, III and IV. *Mahā Mudrā* (Figure 210) and *Śavāsana* (Figure 212) from Section XI are essential. On no account should āsanas from Section V be attempted. This programme should be followed as a curative measure at all times, whether or not one is pregnant.

Natural Delivery

64. For the *first month* after delivery: After a fortnight of rest do *Śavāsana*, *Ujjāyī* and *Viloma Prāṇāyāma* (total 20 to 30 minutes) every morning or evening or both times. In prāṇāyāma the abdominal organs and the muscles are toned and massaged towards the spinal column

and towards the chest. This strengthens the abdomen and helps the uterus return to normal. It also improves the quality of the mother's breast milk by purifying it and increases the secreting ability of the breasts so that more milk is produced. In addition, with this practice the whole nervous system becomes relaxed.

65. *Second Month:* The following āsanas should be practised, the previous week's āsanas being performed in addition to those shown for the current week:

First Week

Section I : *Vṛkṣāsana* (Figure 2), *Utthita Trikoṇāsana* (Figure 4), *Utthita Pārśvakoṇāsana* (Figure 5).

Section IV : *Sālamba Sarvāṅgāsana* (Figure 86), *Halāsana* (Figure 90).

Second Week

Section I : *Virabhadrāsana II* (Figure 8), *Uttānāsana* (Figure 21).

Third Week

Section II : *Paścimottānāsana* (Figure 30), *Jānu Śīrṣāsana* (Figure 26).

Section IV : *Sālamba Śīrṣāsana* (Figure 65).

Section XI : *Mahā Mudrā* (Figure 210).

Fourth Week

Section III : *Parvatāsana* (Figure 59).

Section V : *Paripurṇa Nāvāsana* (Figure 111).

Section VI : *Setu Bandha Sarvāṅgāsana* (Figure 99).

Section VI : *Bharadvājāsana I* (Figure 125).

Duration: Sālamba Sarvāṅgāsana, Halāsana, Setu Bandha Sarvāṅgāsana on a bench and *Paścimottānāsana* should be done for 3 to 5 minutes each, according to capacity; the rest for 15 to 20 seconds each.

A point needs to be clarified. The above schedule is for the average woman based on my teaching experience. Yoga practice, however, is very personal, so the duration of āsanas and the selection from the above programme should be made to suit the individual. The duration should be increased gradually by judging one's own physical strength; practice of Yoga should not end in fatigue. Prāṇāyāma should be done along with the above course.

66. *Third Month:* By the third month, the mother has regained the original shape and strength of her organs; post-natal fatigue has also vanished by this time. Once normalcy is regained all āsanas from Sections I, V and VI may be restarted. After completion of three months, practice of all āsanas may be resumed.

Effects: Practice of āsanas after delivery strengthens the spinal column; the stomach and the abdomen do not accumulate fat, the waist tends to become slim, and, the buttocks do not become flabby. The muscles of the breast are pulled upwards and the breasts do not drop down. Weakness due to bleeding vanishes and the nervous system is toned.

67. *Caesarean:* In the case of an abnormal delivery or of a Caesarean operation, one has to do *Śavāsana*, *Ujjāyī Prāṇāyāma I* and *Viloma Prāṇāyāma I* (Figure 212) until the wound heals. This normally takes two months. Then the following āsanas should be started:

Section IV : *Sālamba Sarvāṅgāsana* (Figure 84), *Halāsana* (Figures 89, 90), *Setu Bandha Sarvāṅgāsana* (Figure 99 on bench).

Section III : *Parvatāsana* (Figures 59, 187).

Section II : *Jānu Śīrsāsana* (Figure 182).

Section XI : *Mahā Mudrā* and *Śavāsana* (Figures 210, 212).

After six months you can gradually begin with the normal course given in this book.

Menopause

68. The following āsanas give a soothing sensation to the nerves:

    Section I : *Prasārita Pādottānāsana* (Figure 18), *Uttānāsana* (Figure 21), *Adho Mukha Śvānāsana* (Figure 22).

    Section II : *Jānu Śīrṣāsana* (Figure 26), *Paścimottān-āsana* (Figure 30, 31).

    Section III : *Supta Vīrāsana* (Figure 58), *Matsyāsana* (Figure 62).

    Section IV : *Sālamba Śīrṣāsana* (Figures 69, 70), *Sālamba Sarvāṅgāsana* (Figure 86), *Halāsana* (Figures 89, 90), *Setu Bandha Sarvāṅgāsana I* (Figures 98, 99).

    Section V : *Dvi Pāda Viparīta Daṇḍāsana* (Figures 147, 148, 149).

    Section XI : Complete.

    Section XII: *Ujjāyī Prāṇāyāma I* (Figure 212) and *II* (Figure 213), *Viloma Prāṇāyāma* (Figures 200, 212), *Sūrya Bhedana Prāṇāyāma* (Figure 214).

69. To correct the functioning of the endocrine system, the following are extremely helpful:

    All āsanas in Sections IV and VII—especially *Setu-bandha Sarvāṅgāsana* (Figures 98, 99, 101), *Dvi Pāda Viparīta Daṇḍāsana* (Figures 146 to 149); āsanas from Section XI and *Viloma Prāṇāyāma*, *Sūrya Bhedana Prāṇāyāma* and *Ujjāyī Prāṇāyāma I* and *II* (Figures 212, 213, 214) from Section XII.

70. To keep the head cool, relaxing āsanas must be practised, as, for instance, the following:

    Section I : *Pārśvottānāsana* (Figure 15), *Prasārita Pādottānāsana* (Figure 18), *Pādānguṣṭhāsana* (Figure 20), *Uttānāsana* (Figure 21), *Adho Mukha Śvānāsana* (Figure 22).

    Section II : *Jānu Śīrṣāsana* (Figure 26), *Ardha Baddha Padma Paścimottānāsana* (Figure 27), *Triang Mukhaikapāda Paścimottānāsana* (Figure 28), *Marīcyāsana I* (Figure 29), *Paścimottānāsana* (Figures 30, 31).

71. Whenever one's condition is normal during the menopause period, all the āsanas and prāṇāyāma given in this book may be practised.

CHAPTER XI

Classification, Table and Course of Study

The learning and practising of any subject requires a method; so also with Yoga. The physical body, the sense organs, the emotions, the mind, and the consciousness are trained slowly and gradually in Aṣṭāṅga Yoga.

Here a practical method of training oneself in āsana, prāṇāyāma, and dhyāna are given, whereby one learns to discipline the body and the mind and to acquire control over oneself.

The classification of the āsanas is based, first, on the anatomical structure of the body; secondly, on the anatomical range of the movement of the spine as well as of the rest of the body; and, lastly, on the effects they have on the body and the mind.

The practical aspect of the āsanas is divided into twelve Sections. The first ten sections are concerned with āsanas, Section XI deals with mudrās and *Śavāsana*, while the last section contains prāṇāyāma and dhyāna. In each section, as one progresses, one gains physical firmness, the patience to persevere and sustain the practice; one disciplines the mind, develops endurance, will-power, and pin-pointed attention to experience the divinity within. Each section trains the sādhaka in each of these aspects in a definite way. Thus Yoga sādhanā starts with the body and ends with Self-realisation.

The āsanas have been grouped and graded into ten sections to enable one to practise them with ease and attention.

The first section consists of standing poses. Beginners should start with these as they bring elasticity in the joints and the muscles, as well as building up stamina and physical stability. This constitutes the most basic training in the early stages of Yoga sādhanā. The second section consists of forward bending āsanas in which the posterior portion of the body is stretched and extended. These prepare the body to proceed further and bring consistency and evenness in the development of physical and mental pliability.

The third section has sitting, upright and supine extending positions. This section prepares one physically and mentally for prāṇāyāma.

The fourth section deals with the inverted postures which help one recover from the strains and stresses of everyday life. They give vitality, mental balance and emotional stability.

The āsanas from the fifth section tone and massage the abdominal organs and strengthen the pelvic and the lumbar areas.

The sixth section contains lateral stretches and twists of the spine, giving new life to the spine, toning the internal organs, and bringing new horizons of tranquility to the mind.

The seventh section, consisting of backbends, brings physical and mental sharpness and alertness. The postures are the direct opposite of those in Section II and the effects are also opposite. In Section II the posterior spine is extended, bringing consistency and mental peace, whereas in Section VII the anterior spine is stretched and the effect is invigorating and enlivening.

Thus different groups of āsanas help develop firmness, fitness, pliability, strength, poise, balance, alertness and mental peace.

The eighth section deals with 'Yoga Kuruṇṭa' which is a method of performing the āsanas with the help of a rope to enable one to attain accuracy, agility and balance. It is good for stiff people, old people, and for those who have fear complexes or who cannot perform the āsanas independently.

The ninth section is for pregnant women. Here the āsanas and prāṇāyāmas are given to maintain the health of the expectant mother and the foetus.

The tenth section has been included to demonstrate that women can practise complicated and advanced āsanas without fear of losing their femininity. It is intended for serious and intensive students who wish to advance in this sādhanā, However, the techniques are not given here.

The eleventh section gives mudrās and *Śavāsana*.

The last section is devoted to prāṇāyāma and dhyāna, Each section has been sub-titled for the convenience of the reader.

A table of āsanas and prāṇāyāma, which is divided according to sections is given here. It has five columns.

The first column gives the index number of the āsanas and the second column the name. The last three columns refer to the illustrations. The third column gives the Figure numbers, showing the Intermediate Stages of some of the āsanas. The fourth column gives the Figure numbers of the Easy Stages of an āsana. Easy Stages are for those who cannot do an āsana independently and who need the support of a table, a wall, or a piece of furniture. The last column gives the Figure number of the Final Stage of each āsana.

The following Table will enable the reader to find the sections, the āsanas, and the illustrations easily.

Index No. of Āsanas	Name of Āsanas	Figure No. Intermediate Stage	Easy Stage	Final Stage
Section I: Āsanas: Standing				
1.	Tāḍāsana	–	–	1
2.	Vṛkṣāsana	–	–	2
3.	Utthita Trikoṇāsana	3	–	4
4.	Utthita Pārśvakoṇāsana	–	–	5
5.	Vīrabhadrāsana I	6	–	7
6.	Vīrabhadrāsana II	–	–	8
7.	Vīrabhadrāsana III	–	–	9
8.	Ardha Candrāsana	–	–	10
9.	Parivṛtta Trikoṇāsana	–	–	11
10.	Pārśvottānāsana	12, 13, 14	–	15
11.	Prasārita Pādottānāsana	16, 17	–	18
12.	Pādānguṣṭhāsana	19	–	20
13.	Uttānāsana	21a	–	21
14.	Adho Mukha Śvānāsana	–	–	22
Section II: Āsanas: Forward Bends				
15.	Daṇḍāsana	–	–	23
16.	Jānu Śīrṣāsana	24, 25	–	26
17.	Ardha Baddha Padma Paścimottānāsana	–	–	27
18.	Triang Mukhaikapāda Paścimottānāsana	–	–	28
19.	Marīcyāsana I	–	–	29
20.	Paścimottānāsana	–	–	30, 31
21.	Parivṛtta Jānu Śīrṣāsana	32	–	33
22.	Parivṛtta Paścimottānāsana	–	–	34

Index No. of Āsanas	Name of Āsanas	Figure No. Intermediate Stage	Easy Stage	Final Stage
23.	Baddha Koṇāsana	–	–	35,36, 37
24.	Supta Baddha Koṇāsana	–	–	38, 39
25.	Upaviṣṭha Koṇāsana	40	–	41
26.	Kūrmāsana	42	–	43
27.	Supta Kūrmāsana	–	–	44
28.	Mālāsana	45	46	47
Section III: Āsanas: Sitting and Supine				
29.	Siddhāsana	–	–	48
30.	Vīrāsana	–	51	49, 50
31.	Padmāsana	–	53	52
32.	Vīrāsana Cycle	–	–	54, 55
33.	Supta Vīrāsana	56, 57	–	58
34.	Parvatāsana	–	–	59
35.	Baddha Padmāsana	–	–	60
36.	Yoga Mudrāsana	–	–	61
37.	Matsyāsana	–	–	62
Section IV: Āsanas: Inverted				
38.	Sālamba Śīrṣāsana	63, 64, 64a, 66, 67, 68	65	69, 70, 70a
39.	Pārśva Śīrṣāsana	–	–	71
40.	Parivṛttaikapāda Śīrṣāsana	–	–	72
41.	Eka Pāda Śīrṣāsana	–	–	73
42.	Pārśvaika Pāda Śīrṣāsana	–	–	74
43.	Upaviṣṭha Koṇāsana in Śīrṣāsana	–	–	75

Index No. of Āsanas	*Name of Āsanas*	*Figure No.*		
		Inter-mediate Stage	*Easy Stage*	*Final Stage*
44.	Baddha Koṇāsana in Śīrṣāsana	–	–	76
45.	Ūrdhva Padmāsana in Śīrṣāsana	–	–	77
46.	Piṇḍāsana in Śīrṣāsana	–	78	79
47.	Sālamba Sarvāṅgāsana	80, 81, 82, 83	86	84, 85, 87
48.	Halāsana	–	89, 90	88, 91
49.	Karṇapīḍāsana	–	–	92
50.	Supta Koṇāsana	–	–	93
51.	Pārśva Halāsana	–	–	94
52.	Eka Pāda Sarvāṅgāsana	–	–	95
53.	Pārśvaika Pāda Sarvāṅgāsana	–	–	96
54.	Setu Bandha Sarvāṅgāsana	97, 100, 102	98, 99	101
55.	Ūrdhva Padmāsana in Sarvāṅgāsana	–	–	103
56.	Piṇḍāsana in Sarvāṅgāsana	–	–	104
57.	Pārśva Piṇḍāsana in Sarvāṅgāsana	–	–	105
Section V: Āsanas Abdominal and Lumbar				
58.	Ūrdhva Prasārita Pādāsana	106, 110, 107, 108	–	109
59.	Paripūrṇa Nāvāsana	–	–	111
60.	Jaṭhara Parivartanāsana	112	–	113, 114

Index No. of Āsanas	Name of Āsanas	Figure No. Intermediate Stage	Easy Stage	Final Stage
61.	Ūrdhva Mukha Paścimottānāsana II	–	–	115
62.	Supta Pādānguṣṭhāsana	116	–	117, 118, 119
63.	Utthita Hasta Pādānguṣṭhāsana	120, 122	–	121, 123, 124
Section VI: Āsanas: Twists				
64.	Bhāradvājāsana I	–	–	125
65.	Bhāradvājāsana II	–	–	126
66.	Marīcyāsana III	–	–	127
67.	Ardha Matsyendrāsana	–	129, 130	128
68.	Pāśāsana	–	132	131
Section VII: Āsanas: Backbends				
69.	Uṣṭrāsana	–	–	133
70.	Ūrdhva Mukha Śvānāsana	134	–	135
71.	Dhanurāsana	–	–	136
72.	Ūrdhva Dhanurāsana	137, 138, 141, 141a, 142, 142a	143	139, 140
73.	Dvi Pāda Viparīta Daṇḍāsana	144, 145	147, 148, 149	146
Section VIII: Āsanas: Yoga Kuruṇṭa				
74.	Variation I (Bhujaṅgāsana)	151, 152a, 152b	–	153

Index No. of Āsanas	*Name of Āsanas*	*Figure No.*		
		Inter-mediate Stage	*Easy Stage*	*Final Stage*
75.	Variation II (Bhujaṅgāsana, Ūrdhva Mukha Paścimottānāsana I, II)	154, 155	–	156, 157
76.	Variation III (Pūrvottānāsana)	159	–	158
77.	Variation IV (Ūrdhva Hasta Dhanurāsana)	–	–	160
78.	Variation V (Uṣṭrāsana)	–	–	161
79.	Variation VI (Sālamba Sarvāṅgāsana)	162, 162a, 163	–	164, 164a
	(Halāsana)	165	166	167
	Karṇapīḍāsana	–	–	168
	Supta Koṇāsana	–	–	169
	Pārśva Halāsana	–	–	170
	Eka Pāda Sarvāṅgāsana	–	–	171
	Pārśvaika Pāda Sarvāṅgāsana	–	–	172
80.	Variation VII (Ūrdhva Mukha Paścimottānāsana I)	–	–	173
Section IX: Āsanas and Prāṇāyāma: Pregnancy				
3.	Utthita Trikoṇāsana	–	–	174
4.	Utthita Pārśvakoṇāsana	–	–	175
5.	Vīrabhadrāsana I	–	–	176
8.	Ardha Candrāsana	–	–	177
10.	Pārśvottānāsana	178	–	179

Index No. of Āsanas	Name of Āsanas	Figure No.		
		Inter-mediate Stage	Easy Stage	Final Stage
11.	Prasārita Pādottānsana	180	181	–
16.	Jānu Śīrṣāsana	182	–	–
23.	Baddha Koṇāsana	–	–	183
25.	Upaviṣṭha Koṇāsana	–	184	–
32.	Vīrāsana Cycle	–	–	185
33.	Supta Vīrāsana	–	–	186
34.	Parvatāsana	–	–	187
35.	Sālamba Śīrṣāsana	–	–	188, 189
36.	Pārśva Śīrṣāsana	–	–	190
37.	Parivṛttaikapāda Śīrṣāsana	–	–	191
47.	Sālamba Sarvāṅgāsana	–	193	192
48.	Halāsana	–	194, 195, 194a, 195a	–
52.	Eka Pāda Sarvāṅgāsana	–	196	–
55.	Ūrdhva Padmāsana in Sarvāṅgāsana	–	–	197
64.	Bhāradvājāsana I	198	–	–
91.	Śavāsana	–	–	199
Prāṇāyāma				
1.	Preparation for Deep Breathing I, II	–	–	200
2.	Ujjāyī Prāṇāyāma I	–	–	200

Index No. of Āsanas	Name of Āsanas	Figure No. Inter-mediate Stage	Easy Stage	Final Stage
3.	Viloma Prāṇāyāma I, II	–	–	200
5.	Sūrya Bhedana Prāṇāyāma	–	–	201
6.	Nāḍi Śodhana Prāṇāyāma	–	–	201
Section X: Āsana: Advanced				
81.	Yoganidrāsana	–	–	202
82.	Ūrdhva Kukkuṭāsana	–	–	203
83.	Pārśva Kukkuṭāsana	–	–	204
84.	Pīñcha Mayūrāsana	–	–	205
85.	Kapotāsana	–	–	206
86.	Eka Pāda Rājakapotāsana	–	–	207
87.	Vṛścikāsana	–	–	208
88.	Naṭarājāsana	–	–	209
Section XI: Mudrā and Śavāsana				
89.	Mahā Mudrā	–	–	210
90.	Ṣaṇmukhī Mudrā	–	–	211
91.	Śavāsana	–	–	212
Section XII: Prāṇāyāma and Dhyāna				
1.	Preparation for Deep Breathing I, II	–	–	212
2.	Ujjāyī Prāṇāyāma I	–	–	212
3.	Viloma Prāṇāyāma I, II	–	–	212
4.	Ujjāyī Prāṇāyāma II	–	–	213
5.	Sūrya Bhedana Prāṇāyāma	–	–	214
6.	Nāḍi Śodhana Prāṇāyāma	–	–	214
7.	Dhyāna (Meditation)	–	–	215

Each section begins with simple āsanas and advances step-by-step to the highest range of intensity, building up the physical and mental calibre of the practitioner to master the sections gradually.

The course of study given in this book is to last a minimum of three years and has been divided into three parts elementary, intermediate and advanced—each part lasting for one year. These parts have again been subdivided to enable the sādhaka to practise systematically and step-by-step. Some sādhakas may take longer to complete the course. However, Yogasādhanā cannot be bound by time and much depends upon the sādhaka's approach to the subject and on the intensity of her efforts to reach the Highest Goal.

Although the course is divided into three parts each containing a number of āsanas and different types of prāṇāyāma, mastery of all the postures has to be maintained; for this reason the āsanas from one part are incorporated into the subsequent programmes. Each āsana creates its own intelligence in the body and if that āsana is no longer practised, then the body loses that particular intelligence and refinement and fresh efforts have to be made to regain it. Constant practice is necessary to maintain control and one should not assume that one will retain mastery of a posture if one neglects to practise it. It is better not to lose what has been gained by sincere effort and hard work.

Now follow the lists of āsanas and prāṇāyāma divided into Elementary, Intermediate and Advanced Courses:

(The numbers within parentheses after the āsanas denote Figure Numbers.)

I. FIRST YEAR—ELEMENTARY COURSE

Section I

1. Tāḍāsana (1)
2. Vṛkṣāsana (2)
3. Utthita Trikoṇāsana (4)
4. Utthita Pārśvakoṇāsana (5)
5. Vīrabhadrāsana I (7)
6. Vīrabhadrāsana II (8)
9. Parivṛtta Trikoṇāsana (11)
10. Pārśvottānāsana (15)
11. Prasārita Pādottānṡana (18)
13. Uttānāsana (21)
14. Adho Mukha Śvānāsana (22)

Section II

15. Daṇḍāsana (23)
16. Jānu Śīrṣāsana (26)
17. Ardha Baddha Padma Paścimottānāsana (27)
18. Triang Mukhaikapāda Paścimottānāsana (28)
19. Marīcyāsana (29)
20. Paścimottānāsana (30)
23. Baddha Koṇāsana (35, 36, 37)
25. Upaviṣṭha Koṇāsana (41)
28. Mālāsana (46)

Section III

29. Siddhāsana (48)
30. Vīrāsana (49, 50)
31. Padmāsana (52)
32. Vīrāsana Cycle (54, 55)
33. Supta Vīrāsana (58)
34. Parvatāsana (59)
37. Matsyāsana (62)

Section IV

38. Sālamba Śīrṣāsana (65)
47. Sālamba Sarvāṅgāsana (84, 87)
48. Halāsana (89, 90, 88, 91)
49. Karṇapīḍāsana (92)
50. Supta Koṇāsana (93)
52. Eka Pāda Sarvāṅgāsana (95)
53. Pārśvaikapāda Sarvāṅgāsana (96)
54. Setu Bandha Sarvāṅgāsana (98, 99)

Section V

58. Ūrdhva Prasārita Pādāsana (109)
59. Paripūrṇa Nāvāsana (111)
63. Utthita Hasta Pādānguṣṭhāsana (121, 123)

Section VI

64. Bharadvājāsana I (125)
65. Bharadvājāsana II (126)
67. Ardha Matsyendrāsana (129)

Section VII

70. Ūrdhva Mukha Śvānāsana I (135)
73. Dvi Pāda Viparīta Daṇḍāsana (148, 149)

Section VIII

74. Yoga Kuruṇṭa Variation 1(153)
75. Yoga Kuruṇṭa Variation II (156)
80. Yoga Kuruṇṭa Variation VII (173)

Section XI

89. Mahā Mudrā (210)
91. Śavāsana (212)

Section XII

1. Preparation for Deep Breathing - I, II (212)
2. Ujjāyī Prāṇāyāma I (212)
3. Viloma Prāṇāyāma I, II (212)

II. SECOND YEAR—INTERMEDIATE COURSE*

Section I

7. Vīrabhadrāsana III (9)
8. Ardha Candrāsana (10)
12. Pādānguṣṭhāsana (20)

Section II

21. Parivṛtta Jānu Śīrṣāsana (33)
24. Supta Baddha Koṇāsana (38, 39)
26. Kūrmāsana (43)
28. Mālāsana (47)

Section III

35. Baddha Padmāsana (60)
36. Yoga Mudrāsana (61)

Section IV

39. Pārśva Śīrṣāsana (71)
40. Parivṛttaikapāda Śīrṣāsana (72)
41. Eka Pāda Śīrṣāsana (73)
42. Pārśvaikapāda Śīrṣāsana (74)
43. Upaviṣṭha Koṇāsana in Śīrṣāsana (75)
44. Baddha Koṇāsana in Śīrṣāsana (76)
51. Pārśva Halāsana (94)

Section V

58. Ūrdhva Prasārita Pādāsana (107, 108, 109, 110)
60. Jaṭhara Parivartanāsana (113, 114)
62. Supta Pādānguṣṭhāsana (117, 118)

Section VI

66. Marīcyāsana III (127)
67. Ardha Matsyendrāsana (128)

Section VII

69. Uṣṭrāsana (133)
70. Ūrdhva Dhanurāsana (139, 140)

Section VIII

76. Yoga Kuruṇṭa Variation III (158)
78. Yoga Kuruṇṭa Variation V (161)

Section XI

90. Ṣaṇmukhī Mudrā (211)

Section XII

4. Ujjāyī Prāṇāyāma II (213)
5. Sūrya Bhedana Prāṇāyāma (214)

* To be studied in conjunction with the Elementary Course.

III. THIRD YEAR—ADVANCED COURSE**

Section II

22. Parivṛtta Paścimottānāsana (34)
27. Supta Kūrmāsana (44)

Section IV

45. Ūrdhva Padmāsana in Śīrṣāsana (77)
46. Piṇḍāsana in Śīrṣāsana (79)
55. Ūrdhva Padmāsana in Sarvāṅgāsana (103)
56. Piṇḍāsana in Sarvāṅgāsana (104)
57. Pārśva Piṇḍāsana in Sarvāṅgāsana (105)

Section V

61. Ūrdhva Mukha Paśchimottānāsana II (115)
62. Supta Pādānguṣṭhāsana (119)
63. Utthita Hasta Pādānguṣṭhāsana (124)

Section VI

68. Pāśāsana (131)

Section VII

69. Dhanurāsana (136)
73. Dvi Pāda Viparīta Daṇḍāsana (146)

Section VIII

77. Yoga Kuruṇṭa Variation IV (160)

Section XII

6. Nāḍi Śodhana Prāṇāyāma (214)

**To be studied in conjunction with the Elementary and the Intermediate Courses.

To assist the sādhaka, a weekly schedule of āsanas has been given for each course. This does not mean that all the āsanas mentioned for a particular day have to be practised; as these are practice-sheets to be followed throughout the year, one should start with the simpler postures given for a particular day at the beginning of the year and gradually add more difficult ones throughout the year. Regularity in practice throughout the year yields better results than practising all the āsanas with interruptions during the year. Consistency in practice leads to the best results.

In addition, a separate Introductory Course for the first three months is given to familiarise the sādhaka with the way the course has to be progressively followed during the next three years.

By learning in a systematic way from the beginning, as given in the course, a correct habit will be instilled in her to practise methodically, thereby ensuring even and balanced development of her body and mind through Yoga.

FIRST THREE MONTHS—INTRODUCTORY COURSE

Schedule for Daily Practice

Section I

1. Tāḍāsana (1)
2. Vṛikṣāsana (2)
3. Utthita Trikoṇāsana (4)
4. Utthita Pārśvakoṇāsana (5)
5. Vīrabhadrāsana I (7)
6. Vīrabhadrāsana II (8)
10. Pārśvottānāsana (15)
11. Prasārita Pādottānsana (18)

Section IV

47. Sālamba Sarvāṅgāsana (84, 87)
48. Halāsana (89, 90)

Section II

15. Daṇḍāsana (23)
16. Jānu Śīrṣāsana (26)
17. Ardha Baddha Padma Paścimottānāsana (27)
20. Paścimottānāsana (30)

Section III

30. Vīrāsana (49, 50, 51)
32. Vīrāsana Cycle (54, 55)

Section VI

64. Bharadvājāsana I (125)

Section XI

91. Śavāsana (212)

WEEKLY SCHEDULES

I. FIRST YEAR—ELEMENTARY COURSE

To be followed after completing the three month Introductory Course.

First Day

Sālamba Śīrṣāsana (65); *Vṛkṣāsana* (2); *Utthita Trikoṇāsana* (4); *Utthita Pārśvakoṇāsana* (5); *Vīrabhadrāsana I, II* (7, 8); *Parivṛtta Trikoṇāsana* (11); *Pārśvottānāsana* (15); *Prasārita Pādottānsana* (18); *Uttānāsana* (21); *Adho Mukha Śvānāsana* (22); *Vīrāsana*

Cycle (54, 55); *Sālamba Sarvāṅgāsana* (84, 87); *Halāsana* (89, 90); *Baddha Koṇāsana* (35); *Upaviṣṭha Koṇāsana* (40, 41); *Bharadvājāsana I, II* (125, 126); *Ardha Matsyendrāsana* (129); *Yoga Kuruṇṭa Variation I, II* (153, 156); *Dvi Pāda Viparīta Daṇḍāsana* (148, 149); *Setu Bandha Sarvāṅgāsana* (98, 99); *Śavāsana* (212).

Preparation for Deep Breathing I, II (212); *Śavāsana* (212).

Second Day

Sālamba Śīrṣāsana (65); *Sālamba Sarvāṅgāsana* (84, 87); *Halāsana* (89, 90); *Karṇapīḍāsana* (92); *Supta Koṇāsana* (93); *Eka Pāda Sarvāṅgāsana* (95); *Pārśvaika Pāda Sarvāṅgāsana* (96); *Ūrdhva Prasārita Pādāsana* (109); *Paripūrṇa Nāvāsana* (111); *Siddhāsana* (48); *Vīrāsana* (49, 50); *Vīrāsana Cycle* (54, 55); *Supta Vīrāsana* (58); *Padmāsana* (52); *Parvatāsana* (59); *Matsyāsana* (62); *Jānu Śīrṣāsana* (26); *Ardha Baddha Padma Paścimottānāsana* (27); *Triang Mukhaikapāda Paścimottānāsana* (28); *Marīcyāsana I* (29); *Paścimottānāsana* (30); *Baddha Koṇāsana* (35); *Upaviṣṭha Koṇāsana* (40, 41); *Mālāsana* (46); *Bharadvājāsana I, II* (125, 126); *Ardha Matsyendrāsana* (129); *Setubandha Sarvāṅgāsana* (98, 99); *Śavāsana* (212).

Mahā Mudrā (210); *Ujjāyī Prāṇāyāma I* (212); *Śavāsana* (212).

Third Day

Sālamba Śīrṣāsana (65); Āsanas from Section I as on the first day (4, 5, 7, 8, 11, 15, 18, 21, 22); *Utthita Hasta Pādānguṣṭhāsana* (121, 123); *Ūrdhva Mukha Śvānāsana* (135); *Vīrāsana* (49, 50); *Sālamba Sarvāṅgāsana* (84, 87); *Halāsana* (89, 90); *Baddha Koṇāsana* (35); *Bharadvājāsana I, II* (125, 126); *Ardha Matsyendrāsana* (129); *Yoga Kuruṇṭa Variation I, II* (153, 156); *Dvi Pāda Viparīta Daṇḍāsana* (148, 149); *Setu Bandha Sarvāṅgāsana* (98, 99); *Śavāsana* (212).

Preparation for Deep Breathing I, II (212); *Śavāsana* (212).

Fourth Day

Sālamba Śīrṣāsana (65); *Sālamba Sarvāṅgāsana* (84, 87); *Halāsana* (89, 90); *Karṇapīḍāsana* (92); *Supta Koṇāsana* (93); *Eka Pāda Sarvāṅgāsana* (95); *Pārśvaika Pāda Sarvāṅgāsana* (96); *Ūrdhva Prasārita Pādāsana* (109); *Paripūrṇa Nāvāsana* (111); *Jānu Śīrṣāsana* (26); *Ardha Baddha Padma Paścimottānāsana* (27); *Triang Mukhaikapāda Paścimottānāsana* (28); *Marīcyāsana I* (29); *Paścimottānāsana* (30); *Supta Vīrāsana* (58); *Matsyāsana* (62); *Bharadvājāsana I, II* (125, 126); *Ardha Matsyendrāsana* (129); *Setu Bandha Sarvāṅgāsana* (98, 99); *Śavāsana* (212).

Mahā Mudrā (210); *Ujjāyī Prāṇāyāma I* (212); *Śavāsana* (212).

Fifth Day

Follow the programme as on the first day.

Sixth Day

Follow Sections IV and II as on the second day; then, *Yoga Kuruṇṭa Variation VII* (173); *Supta Vīrāsana* (58); *Matsyāsana* (62); *Bharadvājāsana I, II* (125, 126); *Ardha Matsyendrāsana* (129); *Setu Bandha Sarvāṅgāsana* (98, 99); *Śavāsana* (212).

Mahā Mudrā (210); *Ujjāyī Prāṇāyāma I* (212); *Śavāsana* (212).

Seventh Day

Take complete rest;

or

Śavāsana (212); Preparation for Deep Breathing I, II (212); *Ujjāyī Prāṇāyāma I* (212); *Śavāsana* (212);

or

Sālamba Śīrṣāsana (65); *Sālamba Sarvāṅgāsana* (84, 85); *Halāsana* (89, 90); *Setu Bandha Sarvāṅgāsana* (98, 99); *Śavāsana* (212); *Ujjāyī Prāṇāyāma* I (200); *Śavāsana* (212).

II. SECOND YEAR—INTERMEDIATE COURSE

First Day

Sālamba Śīrṣāsana (69, 70); All āsanas from Section I (1, 2, 4, 5, 7, 8, 9, 10, 11, 15, 18, 20, 21, 22); *Vīrāsana* (50); *Vīrāsana Cycle* (54, 55); *Sālamba Sarvāṅgāsana* (84); *Halāsana* (88, 91); *Baddha Koṇāsana* (35, 36); *Supta Baddha Koṇāsana* (38); *Upaviṣṭha Koṇāsana* (41); *Paścimottānāsana* (30); *Yoga Kuruṇṭa Variations I, II, III, V* (153, 156, 157, 158, 161); *Uṣṭrāsana* (133); *Ūrdhva Dhanurāsana* (139); *Dvi Pāda Viparīta Daṇḍāsana* (147, 148, 149); *Bharadvājāsana I, II* (125, 126); *Ardha Matsyendrāsana* (128); *Setu Bandha Sarvāṅgāsana* (101); *Śavāsana* (212).

Ṣaṇmukhī Mudrā (211); *Viloma Prāṇāyāma I, II* (212); *Ujjāyī Prāṇāyāma I* (212); *Śavāsana* (212).

Second Day

Sālamba Śīrṣāsana (69, 70); *Pārśva Śīrṣāsana* (71); *Parivṛttaikapāda Śīrṣāsana* (729; *Eka Pāda Śīrṣāsana* (73); *Pārśvaika Pāda Śīrṣāsana* (74);· *Upaviṣṭha Koṇāsana in Śīrṣāsana* (75); *Baddha Koṇāsana* in *Śīrṣāsana* (76); *Sālamba Sarvāṅgāsana* (84, 85); *Halāsana* (88, 91); *Karṇapīḍāsana* (92); *Supta Koṇāsana* (93); *Pārśva Halāsana* (94); *Eka Pāda Sarvāṅgāsana* (95); *Pārśvaika Pāda Sarvāṅgāsana* (96); *Setubandha Sarvāṅgāsana* (98, 99, 101); *Ūrdhva Prasārita Pādāsana* (107, 108, 109); *Jaṭhara Parivartanāsana* (113, 114); *Paripūrṇa Nāvāsana* (111); *Jānu Śīrṣāsana* (26); *Ardha Baddha Padma Paścimottānāsana* (28); *Marīcyāsana I* (29); *Parivṛtta Jānu Śīrṣāsana* (32); *Baddha Koṇāsana* (35, 36, 37); *Upaviṣṭha Koṇāsana* (41); *Kūrmāsana* (43); *Vīrāsana Cycle* (54, 55); *Yoga Mudrāsana* (61); *Mālāsana* (46, 47); *Marīcyāsana III* (127); *Ardha Matsyendrāsana* (128); *Paścimottānāsana* (30); *Śavāsana* (212).

Sūrya Bhedana Prāṇāyāma, Ujjāyī Prāṇāyāma II, Śavāsana (212).

Third Day

Sālamba Śīrṣāsana (69, 70); All āsanas from Section I (1, 2, 4, 5, 7, 8, 9, 10, 11, 15, 18, 20, 21, 22); *Utthita Hasta Pādānguṣṭhāsana* (121, 123); *Supta Pādānguṣṭhāsana* (117, 119); *Supta Baddha Koṇāsana* (38); *Sālamba Sarvāṅgāsana* (84, 85); *Halāsana* (88, 91), *Setubandha Sarvāṅgāsana* (98, 99); *Yoga Kuruṇṭa Variations I, II, III, V* (153, 156, 157, 158, 161); *Uṣṭrāsana* (133); *Ūrdhva Dhanurāsana* (139); *Dvi Pāda Viparrta Daṇḍāsana* (147, 148, 149); *Vīrāsana Cycle* (54, 55); *Bharadvājāsana I, II* (125, 126); *Marīcyāsana III* (127); *Ardha Matsyendrāsana* (128); *Paścimottānāsana* (30); *Śavāsana* (212).

Viloma Prāṇāyāma I, II; Ujjāyī Prāṇāyāma I; Śavāsana (212).

Fourth Day

Sections IV and V as on the second day (IV 69, 70, 71, 72, 73, 74, 75, 76, 84, 85, 88, 91, 92, 93, 94, 95, 96, 98, 99; V 107, 108, 109, 113, 114; 111) *Jānu Śīrṣāsana* (26); *Ardha Baddha Paścimottānāsana* (27); *Triang Mukhaikapāda Paścimottānāsana* (28); *Marīcyāsana I* (29); *Paścimottānāsana* (30); *Bharadvājāsana I, II* (125, 126); *Marīcyāsana III* (127); *Ardha Matsyendrāsana* (128); *Supta Vīrāsana* (58); *Supta Baddha Koṇāsana* (38); *Matsyāsana* (62); *Śavāsana* (212).

Mahā Mudrā (210); *Ujjāyī Prāṇāyāma II* (213); *Ujjāyī Prāṇāyāma I* (212); *Savāsana* (212).

Fifth Day

All āsanas and prāṇāyāma to be performed as on the first day.

Sixth Day

Section IV as on the second day (69, 70, 71, 72, 73, 74, 75, 76, 84, 85, 88, 91, 92, 93, 94, 95, 96, 98, 99); Section II (26, 27, 28, 29, 30, 33); *Baddha Koṇāsana* (35, 36, 37);

Upaviṣṭha Koṇāsana (41); *Kūrmāsana* (43); *Ūrdhva Mukha Paścimottānāsana I* (173); *Vīrāsana Cycle* (54, 55); *Parvatāsana* (59); *Baddha Padmāsana* (60); *Yoga Mudrāsana* (61); *Matsyāsana* (62); *Bharadvājāsana I, II* (125, 126); *Marīcyāsana III* (127); *Ardha Matsyendrāsana* (128); *Śavāsana* (212).

Sūrya Bhedana Prāṇāyāma (214); *Ujjāyī Prāṇāyāma II* (213); *Śavāsana* (212).

Seventh Day

Take complete rest;

or

Sūrya Bhedana Prāṇāyāma (214); *Śavāsana* (212);

or

Sālamba Śīrṣāsana (69, 70); *Sālamba Sarvāṅgāsana* (84); *Halāsana* (88, 91); *Setubandha Sarvāṅgāsana* (98, 99); *Śavāsana* (212); *Ujjāyī Prāṅāyāma I* and *Śavāsana* (212).

III. THIRD YEAR—ADVANCED COURSE

First Day

Sālamba Śīrṣāsana (69, 70); All āsanas from Section I (1, 2, 4, 5, 7, 8, 9, 10, 11, 15, 18, 20, 21, 22); *Utthita Hasta Pādānguṣṭhāsana* (121, 123, 124); *Yoga Kuruṇṭa Variations I to V* (153, 156, 158, 160, 161): All āsanas from Section VII (133, 135, 136, 139, 140, 146): *Adho Mukha Śvānāsana* (22); *Vīrāsana* and *Cycle* (50, 54, 55); *Sālamba Sarvāṅgāsana* (84); *Halāsana* (88, 91); All āsanas from Section VI (125, 126, 127, 128, 132); *Paścimottānāsana* (30); *Śavāsana* (212).

Viloma Prāṇāyāma I, II; Ujjāyī Prāṇāyāma I; Śavāsana (212).

Second Day

All āsanas from Section IV (69, 70, 71, 72, 73, 74, 75, 76, 77, 79 and 84, 85, 88, 91, 92, 93, 94, 95, 96, 101, 103,

104, 105); Section II (26, 27, 28, 29, 30, 33, 34); *Ūrdhva Mukha Paścimottānāsana I, II* (115, 173); *Baddha Koṇāsana* (35, 36, 37); *Upaviṣṭha Koṇāsana* (41); *Kūrmāsana* (43); *Supta Kūrmāsana* (44); *Mālāsana* (46, 47); *Yoga Mudrāsana* (61); All āsanas from Section VI (125, 126, 127, 128, 132); *Śavāsana* (212).

Sūrya Bhedana Prāṇāyāma (214); *Ujjāyī Prāṇāyāma II* (213); *Śavāsana* (212).

Third Day

Sālamba Śīrṣāsana (69); All āsanas from Section I (1, 2, 4, 5, 7, 8, 9, 10, 11, 15, 18, 20, 21, 22); *Utthita Hasta Pādānguṣṭhāsana* (121, 123, 124); *Yoga Kuruṇṭa Variations I to V* (153, 156, 158, 160, 161); All āsanas from Section VII (133, 135, 136, 139, 140, 146); *Adho Mukha Śvānāsana* (22); *Vīrāsana* and *Cycle* (50, 54, 55); *Supta Pādānguṣṭhāsana* (117, 118, 119); *Supta Vīrāsana* (58); *Matsyāsana* (62); *Supta Baddha Koṇāsana* (38, 39); *Sālamba Sarvāṅgāsana* (84); *Halāsana* (88, 91); All āsanas from Section VI (125, 126, 127, 128, 131); *Paścimottānāsana* (30); *Śavāsana* (212).

Nāḍi Śodhana Prāṇāyāma (214); *Ujjāyī Prāṇāyāma II* (213); *Śavāsana* (212).

Fourth Day

All āsanas from Section IV (69, 70, 71, 72, 73, 74, 75, 76, 77, 79, 84, 85, 88, 91, 92, 93, 94, 95, 96, 101, 103, 104, 105); *Ūrdhva Prasārita Pādāsana* (107, 108, 109); *Vīrāsana Cycle* (54, 55); *Jaṭhara Parivartanāsana* (113, 114); *Paripūrṇa Nāvāsana* (111); *Ūrdhva Mukha Paścimottānāsana I, II* (173, 115); *Mālāsana* (46, 47); *Yoga Mudrāsana* (61); *Kūrmāsana* (43); *Supta Kūrmāsana* (44); *Paścimottānāsana* (30); *Parivṛtta Jānu Śīrṣāsana* (33); *Parivṛtta Paścimottānāsana* (34); all āsanas from Section VI (125, 126, 127, 128, 131); *Supta Vīrāsana* (58); *Matsyāsana* (62); *Supta Baddha Koṇāsana* (38, 39); *Śavāsana* (212).

Sūrya Bhedana Prāṇāyāma (214); *Ujjāyī Prāṇāyāma II* (213) *Śavāsana* (212).

Fifth Day

All āsanas to be followed as on the first day of the week.

Nāḍi Śodhana Prāṇāyāma (214); *Ujjāyī Prāṇāyāma II* (213); *Śavāsana* (212).

Sixth Day

All āsanas from Section IV (69, 70, 71, 72, 73, 74, 75, 76, 77, 79, 84, 85, 88, 91, 92, 93, 94, 95, 96, 101, 103, 104, 105); *Jānu Śīrṣāsana* (26); *Ardha Baddha Padma Paścimottānāsana* (28); *Marīcyāsana I* (29); *Vīrāsana Cycle* (54, 55); *Parvatāsana* (59); *Baddha Padmāsana* (60); *Yoga Mudrāsana* (61); *Supta Vīrāsana* (58); *Matsyāsana* (62); *Supta Baddha Koṇāsana* (38, 39); All āsanas from Section VI (125, 126, 127, 128, 131); *Paścimottānāsana* (30); *Śavāsana* (212).

Sūrya Bhedana Prāṇāyāma (214); *Ujjāyī Prāṇāyāma II* (213); *Śavāsana* (212).

Seventh Day

Take complete rest; or

Nāḍi Śodhana Prāṇāyāma (214); *Śavāsana* (212);

or

Sālamba Śīrṣāsana (69); *Sālamba Sarvāṅgāsana* (84); *Halāsana* (88, 91); *Paścimottānāsana* (30); *Setu Bandha Sarvāṅgāsana* (98, 99); Śavāsana (212).

Nāḍi Śodhana Prāṇāyāma (214); *Śavāsana* (212).

The above courses of study are intended for the average sādhaka whose object is to maintain good physical and mental health. Those who are eager to make Yoga a special study may follow a more rigorous routine, as given in Section IV on next page.

IV. INTENSIVE COURSE

All the āsanas and prāṇāyāma from the respective courses should be performed.

Example: A first year student should perform all the āsanas and prāṇāyāma in the Elementary Course.

1. Early Morning Practice

Dhyāna (Meditation) (215); Prāṇāyāma (212, 213, 214).

2. Morning Practice

(allowing a minimum of half an hour to elapse after the previous practice).

All āsanas from Sections I, II, III, V, VI, VII; Section VIII (153, 156, 157, 158, 160, 161, 173); *Śavāsana* (212).

3. Early Evening Practice

All āsanas from Section IV.

Note: If following the intensive course, simple postures such as *Siddhāsana* (48), *Vīrāsana* (49, 50) and *Padmāsana* (52) may be dropped from everyday practice as they are covered in the courses and in prāṇāyāma practice.

Before proceeding to Chapter XII, I should like to clarify a few points. At first the techniques may appear complicated. Gradually as one re-reads and studies them, they become easier to understand and one learns to incorporate them in one's practice. The technical points have been elaborated to enable the sādhaka to practise thoughtfully and to avoid mistakes. As a teacher with about twenty years of teaching experience, I have noticed that often the same mistakes are committed again and again by many practitioners. Therefore, do not omit even the minutest technical details that have been given in the instructions. One may not be able to carry out all the instructions at once, but gradually the body will become habituated to carry them out naturally.

All the instructions and points of observation that are given have to be performed on the right as well as on the left side, as one of the aims of Yoga practice is to develop both sides of the body evenly, otherwise integration is not possible.

After reaching the final position of an āsana, one has to observe and adjust a number of points to bring stability and poise in that particular āsana. Therefore, certain points are stressed for observation during the final position of each āsana, so that the sādhaka develops a new perspective and vision. This in turn will lead to a concentrated action integrating the body, the mind and the self. Here begins spiritual sādhanā.

Now nothing remains to be said further before coming to the practical aspect which follows, except to pray to Sage Patañjali to bless the sādhaka and to help her succeed in her quest:

ābāhu puruṣākāram śankhacakrāsi dhariṇam
śahasra śirasam śvetam praṇamāmi patañjalim.

Chapter XII

YOGĀSANAS— Technique and Effects

Section-I

Āsanas: Standing

We stand on our legs throughout our waking state; thus, the foundation for movement and action are the legs. The legs have to be trained to make them firm and steady. Without a firm foundation, a building cannot stand. Similarly, without the firm foundation of strong legs and feet, the brain, which is the seat of intelligence, cannot be held in correct alignment with the spine. Hence the standing poses are introduced first.

The āsanas in Section I are mainly standing positions. These are elementary poses. They are designed to bring first flexibility and then to make the body strong and steady. Beginners should start practising with this Section.

Note: Those with weak heart or suffering from high blood pressure should first practise *Sālamba Sarvāṅgāsana* (Figure 84), *Halāsana* (Figures 90, 91), and *Setu Bandha Sarvāṅgāsana* (Figure 99), followed by āsanas in this section such as *Utthita Trikoṇāsana* (Figure 4), *Utthita Pārśvakoṇāsana* (Figure 5), *Pārśvottānāsana* (Figure 15), *Prasārita Pādottānāsana* (Figure 18), *Pādāṅguṣṭhāsana* (Figure 20), *Uttānāsana* (Figure 21), *Adho Mukha Śvānāsana* (Figure 22), followed by *Śavāsana* (Figure 212). Then do *Ujjāyi Prāṇāyāma I* (Figure 212), 6 to 8 cycles. Once you feel strong enough and the blood pressure becomes normal, the following āsanas may be practiced.

1. *TĀḌĀSANA* OR *SAMASTHITI*

This is one of the simplest and the most basic postures for Yogāsana practice. *Tāḍāsana* means steady and erect like a mountain.

Technique

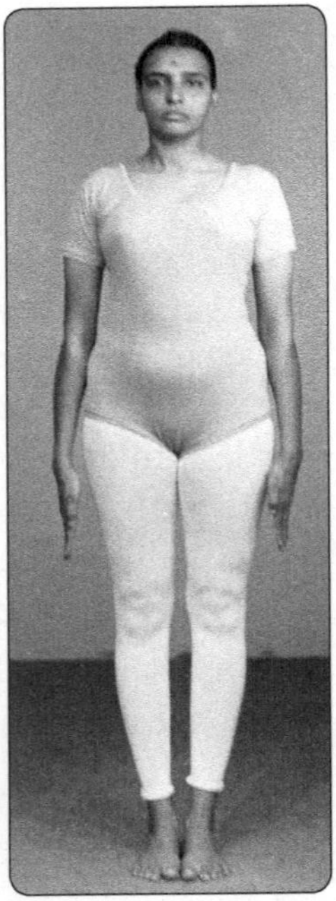

Fig. 1: *Tāḍāsana* (Final Stage)

1. Stand erect with the feet together and the big toes and the heels touching. See that the weight of the body is neither on the heels nor on the toes but in the centre of the arches.
2. Do not tighten the toes, but stretch them from the bottom and keep them relaxed. (This is the position of the toes in all standing postures.)
3. Keep the ankles in line with each other.
4. Tighten the knees, pull the knee-caps upwards and tighten the quadriceps. Keep the shin bones in line with the thigh bones. Breathe normally.
5. Compress the hips and tighten the buttocks.
6. Keep the spine erect, raise the sternum expand the chest. Do not protrude the abdomen but lift it upwards.
7. Keep the neck erect and the head straight; do not tilt forwards or backwards. Look straight ahead.
8. Keep the arms by the sides of the body, extending downwards and keep the palms facing the thighs, in line with them. Do not lift the shoulders. Keep the fingers together (Figure 1).
9. Stand still for 20 to 30 seconds and breathe normally.

Effects: Before attempting to balance on the head, it is essential to stand erect on one's feet. Most people do not know how to stand. Some stand with knees bent, others protrude the abdomen, while others throw the weight of the body on one foot or the other, or have the feet at an angle. All these standing defects tell upon the spinal column which in turn affects the mind. So for an alert body and alert mind and brain, *Tāḍāsana* is very useful.

2. *VṚKṢĀSANA*

Vṛkṣa means a tree. In this posture, the whole body extends upwards like a tree.

Technique

1. Stand erect as in *Tāḍāsana* (Figure 1).
2. Interlock the fingers, turn the wrists and palms outwards, and stretch the arms forward in line with the shoulders.
3. Take the extended arms upwards by the side of the ears. The palms should face the ceiling.
4. Move the back ribs forwards. Lift the chest and take the shoulder-blades deep in.
5. Keep the head erect and look straight forward.
6. Breathing normally, maintain this posture for 10 to 15 seconds.
7. Now lower the arms, first forwards and then down. Release the interlock.

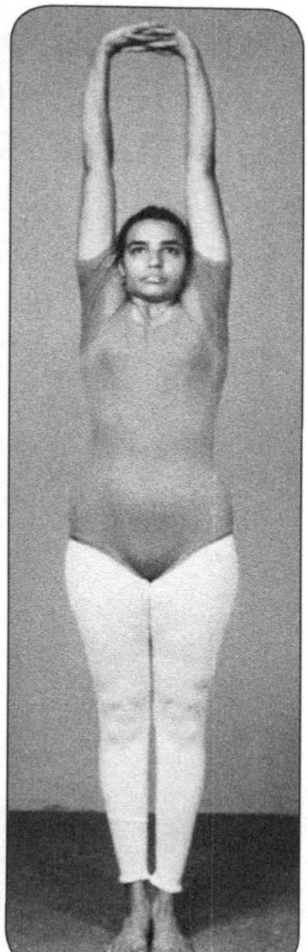

Fig. 2: *Vṛkṣāsana* (Final Stage)

Effects: This posture tones the shoulder muscles and gives one poise and balance.

3. *UTTHITA TRIKOṆĀSANA*

Utthita is extended, trikoṇa is triangle. This is an extended triangle posture.

Technique

1. Stand erect in *Tāḍāsana* (Figure 1).
2. While inhaling, jump with the legs three feet apart and stretch the arms sideways in line with the shoulders (Figure 3). Keep the palms facing the floor.
3. Turn the right leg sideways 90° to the right. Turn the left foot slightly inwards. Tighten the knees and the thighs. Take one or two breaths.
4. While exhaling, bend the trunk sideways to the right. Hold the right ankle with the right hand (Figure 4).
5. Raise the left arm in line with the shoulders and the right arm. Keep the left palm facing forwards. Stretch both the arms, keeping the elbows tight.
6. Turn the neck and gaze at the thumb of the left hand.

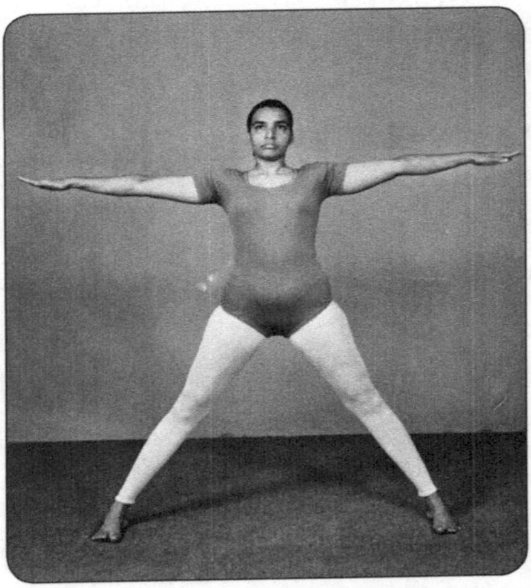

Fig. 3: *Utthita Trikoṇāsana* (Intermediate Stage)

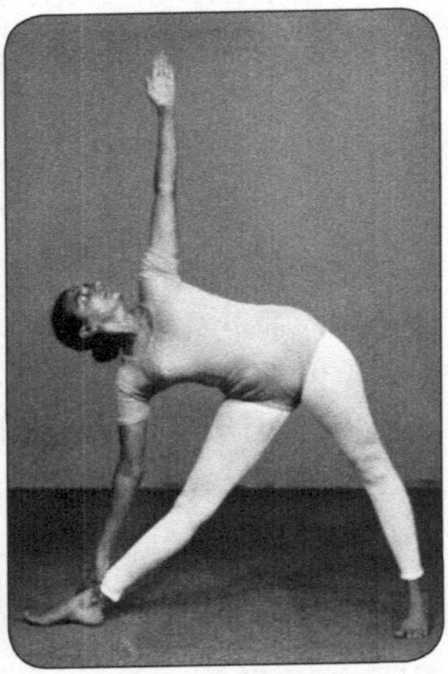

Fig. 4: *Utthita Trikoṇāsana* (Final Stage)

7. This is the final position of the āsana. Breathe normally and remain steady for 20 to 30 seconds, observing the following points:
   (a) keep the thigh muscles tight and the kneecaps pulled in and up;
   (b) the back of the left leg, the hips, and the back of the chest should be in one plane;
   (c) expand the chest by tucking the shoulder-blades in.
8. Now, with an inhalation, lift the right palm from the ankle, raise the trunk, and come back to the position in Technique 3 and then in 2 (Figure 3).
9. Repeat the posture on the left side, following Techniques 3 to 8 and substituting the word right for left and vice versa. Exhale and jump to *Tāḍāsana* (Figure 1).

Special Instructions

1. While in position 2 (Figure 3), keep the feet facing forward and not turned outwards.
2. Extend the toes, do not tighten them.
3. After turning the right leg sideways see that the ankle, the knee, and the middle of the thigh are in one line.
4. In position 3, (a) while turning the right foot, do not bend the left knee; (b) the left hand should remain stable and should neither go up nor drop down; (c) the trunk should not tilt towards the right. The anal mouth and the head should remain in line with each other.
5. Beginners who find it difficult to bend may hold the shin instead of the ankle.

Effects: This āsana corrects deformity in the legs and relieves backache and neckache.

4. UTTHITA PĀRŚVAKOṆĀSANA

This is an extended lateral angle posture.

Technique

1. Stand in *Tāḍāsana* (Figure 1).
2. While inhaling, jump to get the feet 4 to 4½ feet apart. Extend the arms sideways as in Figure 3.
3. Turn the right leg out to 90° and the left foot slightly in. Tighten the knees and the thighs.
4. Bend the right leg at the knee until the thigh and calf form a right angle. The right thigh is parallel and the shin perpendicular to the ground. Take one or two breaths.
5. Exhale and take the trunk sideways to the right. Place the right palm on the floor by the side of the right foot.
6. Stretch the left arm over the ear; turn the neck and look up (Figure 5).
7. This is the final position. Breathe normally and stay for 20 to 30 seconds observing the following points:
   (a) tuck the right buttock in so that it remains in line with the outer right knee;
   (b) tighten the quadriceps and stretch the hamstrings of the left leg;

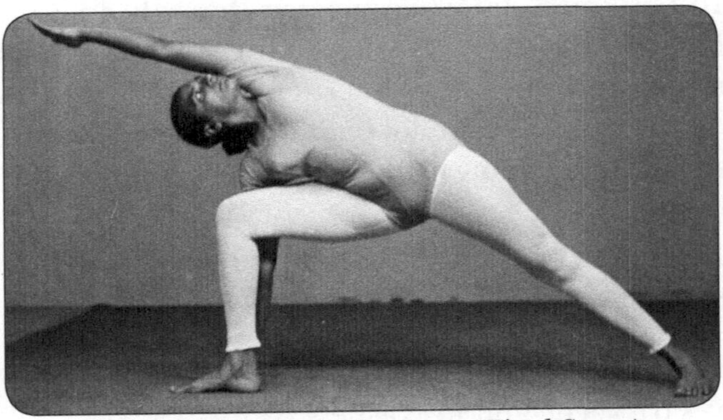

Fig. 5: *Utthita Pārśvakoṇāsana* (Final Stage)

(c) extend the left armpit, the biceps, the wrist and the elbow. From the left ankle to the left wrist there should be one stretch so that the body does not sway;

(d) tuck in the shoulder-blades. Turn the left side of the trunk upwards, and backwards so that the chest is expanded and the posterior side of the body remains in one plane.

8. While inhaling, lift the right palm off the floor and raise the trunk, keeping the right leg at a right angle. Take a breath.
9. Inhale, straighten the right knee and come to position as in Figure 3.
10. Repeat the same posture on the left side, following all Techniques but changing the words right to left. Come back to *Tāḍāsana* (Figure 1).

Special Instructions

1. It is important to adjust the distance between the legs, otherwise the bent leg does not form a right angle. If the distance is too great, an obtuse angle is formed; and if it is too small, it forms an acute angle. The distance should be adjusted according to the height of the person. While adjusting, the left foot should be moved inwards or backwards and not the right foot when doing the pose on the right side and vice versa. The leg which is already bent should not be disturbed.
2. The left palm should remain facing the floor while rotating the left side of the trunk upwards.
3. Beginners can keep the tips of the fingers on the floor if they are stiff.

Effects: This āsana reduces fat around the waist and hips; it relieves sciatic and arthritic pains and helps digestion and elimination.

5. *VĪRABHADRĀSANA I*

This posture is named after Vīrabhadra from Kumārasambhava, a play by Kālidāsa, The āsana has three varieties, each of increasing intensity.

Technique

1. Stand in *Tāḍāsana* (Figure 1).
2. While inhaling, jump with the legs 4 to 4½ feet apart and extend the arms sideways in line with the shoulders.
3. Turn the palms up. Stretch them upwards and join the palms. Keep the elbows straight. Take a breath or two.
4. Exhale and turn the right leg and trunk 90° to the right and the left foot slightly in (Figure 6). Take one breath.
5. While exhaling, bend the right knee to 90°.
6. Take the head back and look up at the thumbs (Figure 7).

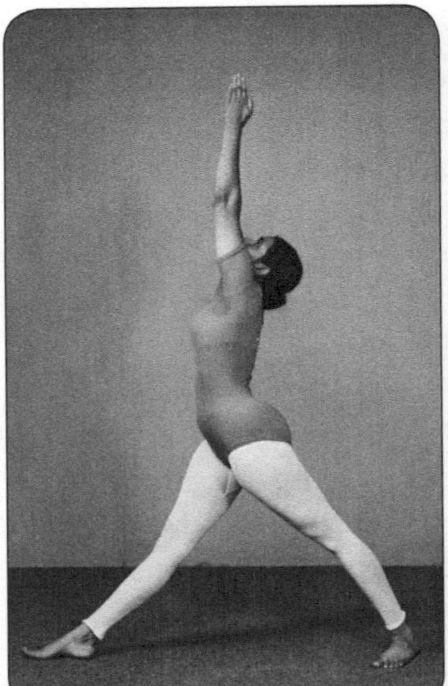

Fig. 6: *Vīrabhadrāsana I* (Intermediate Stage)

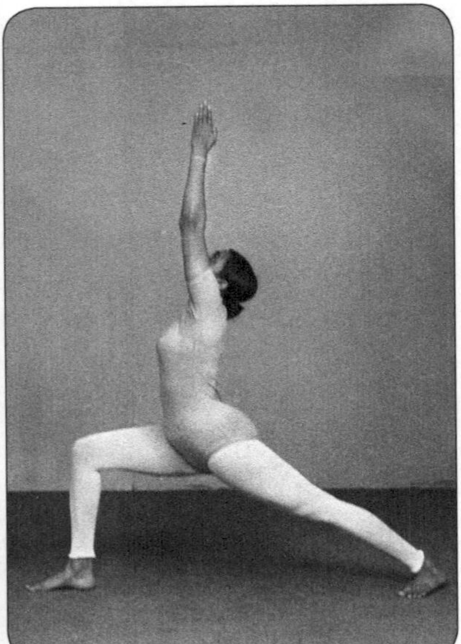

Fig. 7: *Vīrabhadrāsana I* (Final Stage)

7. This is the final position. Breathe normally and stay for 15 to 20 seconds, observing the following points:
   (a) keep the left leg firm and straight while bending the right leg;
   (b) stretch the arms up, keeping the muscles of the chest lifted up. Do not drop this lift;
   (c) keep the palms, the head and the anus in line with each other;
   (d) both the pelvic bones should be parallel to each other, facing forwards and should not tilt to the side;
   (e) tighten the hips.
8. Inhale and come to position as in Figure 6, then turn to the centre.
9. Repeat the posture on the left side following Techniques 3 to 8 and reversing all processes. Return to *Tāḍāsana* (Figure 1).

Special Instructions

1. While bending the right leg to 90° do not bend the left knee. Keep the quadriceps tight.
2. Beginners and those who find it difficult to balance should keep the head straight and facing forward.
3. Women suffering from heart trouble should avoid this āsana and those who are weak should not remain in this position for long.
4. Those who find it difficult to keep the elbows straight while stretching the arms when the palms are together may keep the arms apart so that they remain in line with the armpits.

Effects: The expansion of the chest makes the breathing deep. The posture relieves stiffness in the shoulders and strengthens the legs. By taking the head back, the neck is extended and the thyroid and the parathyroid glands are massaged.

6. *VĪRABHADRĀSANA II*

Technique

1. Stand in *Tāḍāsana* (Figure 1).
2. While inhaling, jump with the feet 4 to 4½ feet apart and stretch the arms sideways in line with the shoulders, palms facing down (Figure 3).
3. Turn the right leg sideways 90° to the right and the left foot slightly in. Keep the legs straight. Take a breath.
4. While exhaling, bend the right leg to 90°.
5. Turn the head to the right and keep the left eye focused on the right palm (Figure 8).
6. This is the final position. Breathe normally and remain steady for 20 to 30 seconds, observing the following points:
   (a) expand the chest; stretch both the arms sideways as though they are being pulled apart in a tug-of-war;
   (b) see that the anal mouth and the crown of the head remain in line with each other;

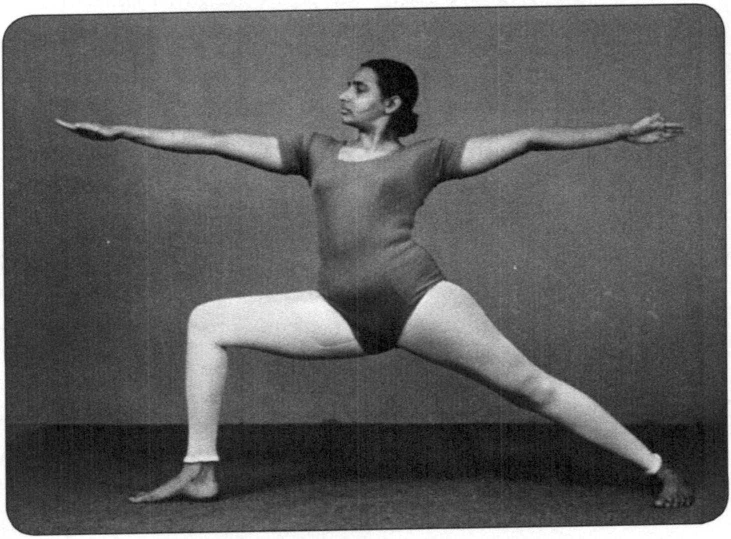

Fig. 8: *Vīrabhadrāsana II* (Final Stage)

(c) tighten the right thigh towards the hip and the left frontal thigh towards the back of the thigh.

7. Inhale and come back to position as in Figure 3.
8. Repeat the same on the left side, following Techniques 3 to 7, reversing all processes from right to left and return to *Tāḍāsana* (Figure 1).

Special Instructions

1. Do not allow the trunk to lean towards the bent leg while bending the right knee and vice versa.
2. Both sides of the trunk should be kept parallel.
3. While turning the head to the right, do not turn the trunk to the right.

Note: For Āsanas 3 to 6.

1. Remember that while doing the posture on the right side, resistance should be created in the left leg and vice versa. If the feet slide, stand sideways to a wall and place the left leg against the wall while doing the posture on the right and vice versa.
2. Those who are on the heavy side may find it difficult to turn the trunk, to stretch the spine, or to balance. In this case use the support of a wall. This can be done in two ways:
   (a) standing at a right angle to the wall and, while doing the posture on the right side, keeping the heel of the left foot against the wall and vice versa;
   (b) standing with the back to the wall and keeping the heels, the hips and the back of the head touching the wall while performing all the āsanas.
3. Those suffering from backache, slipped disc; sciatica, and lumbago should not jump into the standing āsanas but should do them with the support of a wall.
4. Elderly persons who find it difficult to jump should do the postures against a wall, as mentioned in Note 2.

7. *VĪRABHADRĀSANA III*

Technique

1. Stand in *Tāḍāsana* (Figure 1).
2. While inhaling, jump with the legs 4 to 4½ feet apart and raise the arms sideways in line with the shoulders (Figure 3). Take a breath.
3. Exhale, turn to the right, and come to *Vīrabhadrāsana I* (Figure 7) on the right side. Take a breath.
4. Exhale and bend the trunk over the right leg, stretch it forward extending the arms forward and keeping the palms together. Keep the chest close to the right thigh.
5. Move the trunk towards the arms. Raise the left heel up, keeping the left knee tight. Take one or two breaths.
6. Exhale and slowly lift the left leg up until it comes parallel to the ground. Keep the right leg tight and perpendicular to the ground (Figure 9).
7. Gaze at the thumbs.

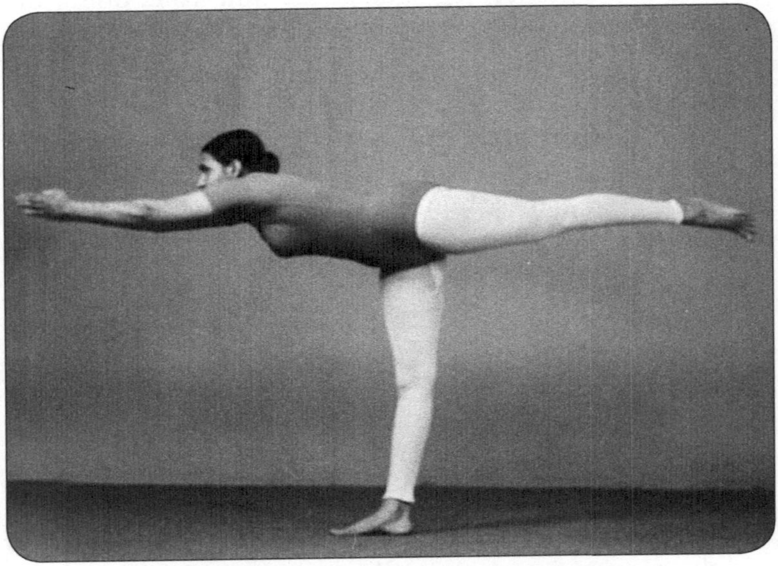

Fig. 9: *Vīrabhadrāsana III* (Final Stage)

8. Breathe normally, and remain in this final position for 10 to 15 seconds observing the following points:
   (a) keep the body parallel to the ground from the fingers to the heel;
   (b) keep the right leg firm and steady;
   (c) stretch the left leg backwards and the trunk forwards as though the trunk were challenging the left leg. This is called challenge and response. The centre of gravity is in the right thigh, which should be firm like a rod;
   (d) extend the sides of the trunk towards the arms.
9. Exhale and slowly take the left foot to the ground by raising the trunk up, like a lever.
10. Come back to *Vīrabhadrāsana I* (Figure 7).
11. Inhale and come to position as in Figure 6; turn to the centre, then repeat the posture on the left side, balancing on the left leg, following Techniques 3 to 10, but reading right for left and vice versa. Return to *Tāḍāsana* (Figure 1).

Special Instructions

1. Those who are weak and find it hard to straighten the arms may keep them apart.
2. Those who are overweight may do the posture directly without performing *Vīrabhadrāsana I* (Figure 7). Or take the support of a wall or a table, stand 3 to 3½ feet away from the wall, place the hands on the wall, and lift the legs up alternately.
3. The raising of the left leg up and the stretching of the right leg back should synchronise.

Effects: This āsana develops poise and balance, makes the legs strong and tones the abdominal organs. It is recommended for runners as it brings agility and vigour.

8. *ARDHA CANDRĀSANA*

Ardha means half; candra means the moon. This pose resembles the half moon.

Technique

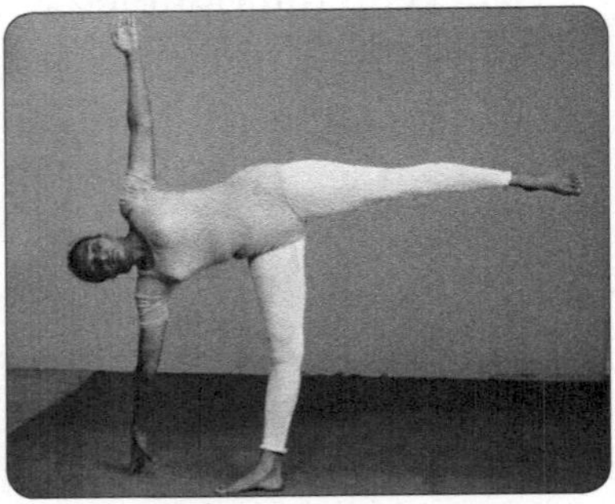

Fig. 10: *Ardha Candrāsana* (Final Stage)

1. Stand in *Tāḍāsana* (Figure 1).
2. While inhaling, jump with the legs 3 to 3½ feet apart and extend the arms horizontally in line with the shoulders.
3. Do *Utṭhita Trikoṇāsana* on the right side (Figure 4). Take one or two breaths.
4. Exhale and bend the right leg slightly. Rest the tips of the fingers of the right hand on the floor, about one foot in front of the right leg.
5. Move the trunk towards the head so that the left heel comes off the floor. Take a breath.
6. Exhale, extend the trunk towards the head, and raise the left leg up until it is parallel to the floor. Straighten the right leg and keep it firm.
7. Raise the left arm up in line with the shoulders (Figure 10).
8. This is the final position. Breathing normally, remain steady for 10 to 15 seconds observing the following points:
   (a) keep the right leg perpendicular and the left leg parallel to the ground;
   (b) extend the toes of the left foot;
   (c) synchronise the action of raising the left leg and straightening the right leg;

(d) tuck the shoulder-blades in and expand the chest;
(e) the back of the left leg, the back of the trunk, and the back of the head should be in line;
(f) the weight of the body remains on the right thigh and hip;
(g) the left side of the trunk should face the ceiling;
(h) widen the pelvis by turning the left pelvic bone up.

9. Exhale, bend the right leg slightly at the knee, and lower the left leg to the ground.
10. Come to the position as in Figure 3 and repeat the posture on the left side, balancing on the left leg, following all the techniques but substituting the word right for left and vice versa. Come back to *Tāḍāsana* (Figure 1).

Special Instructions

1. The left leg should extend in line with the left side of the trunk and should not be raised higher nor be lower down.
2. This posture can also be done by keeping the left palm over the left hip. Here the leg has a tendency to drop down, whereas the body balances more easily when the arm is kept up.
3. Those who find it difficult to balance independently may support the whole body against a wall.
4. Those who are overweight may do the posture without going into the position as in Figure 4. For them, the placing of the fingers on the floor and the raising of the leg should synchronise. Or the fingers may be placed on a block as in Section IX, Figure 177.

Effects: This posture helps damaged legs. It tones the lumbar spine and cures gastric troubles. It is good for backache and dysmenorrhoea.

9. *PARIVṚTTA TRIKOṆĀSANA*

Parivṛtta means revolved or turned around. The pose is a revolving or a reverse triangle.

Technique

1. Stand in *Tāḍāsana* (Figure 1).
2. While inhaling, jump with the legs 3 to 3½ feet apart and raise the arms sideways in line with the shoulders (Figure 3).
3. Turn the right leg sideways to 90° and the left foot slightly inwards. Tighten the knees and the thighs. Take one or two breaths.
4. Exhale, rotate the trunk to the right so that the left arm faces the right leg.

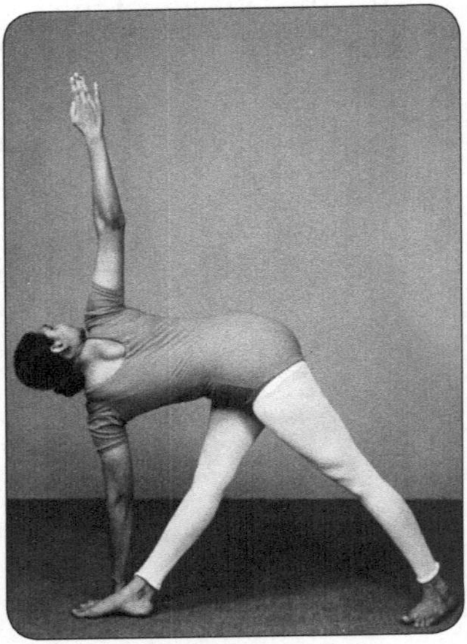

Fig. 11: *Parivṛtta Trikoṇāsana* (Final Stage)

5. Place the fingers of the left palm on the floor near the outer side of the right foot.
6. Raise the right arm up, bringing it in line with the left arm.
7. Turn the head and look at the right hand (Figure 11).
8. This is the final position. Breathing normally, stay for 20 to 30 seconds observing the following points:
   (a) tighten both the legs;
   (b) tuck in the left shoulder-blade and keep the chest expanded;

(c) keep both the edges of the trunk parallel and in line with the right leg;

(d) keep the trunk in line from the hips to the head.

9. Inhale and raise the left hand off the floor and come to position (Figure 3) by turning the right foot in.
10. Repeat on the left side and come to *Tāḍāsana* (Figure 1).

Special Instructions

1. While rotating the trunk, turn the left thigh and knee inwards and also the left hip joint so that the spine revolves more.
2. Keep both legs firm to turn the pelvic region.
3. Extend the trunk towards the head in such a way that the abdominal muscles not only revolve but also move towards the chest.

Effects: This āsana increases the blood supply to the lower part of the trunk and invigorates the abdominal organs.

OVERALL EFFECTS OF ĀSANAS 2 to 9

These āsanas have an overall strengthening effect on the body.

They tone the leg muscles and correct the deformities in the feet, the ankles and the legs.

They help to get rid of constipation, acidity and improve the blood circulation and digestion. They also rectify and correct malfunctioning of the liver, spleen and kidneys. In addition to these, they are good for stiff shoulders, hunch-back, rheumatic pains, lumbago and slipped discs.

They improve the functioning of the reproductive system, malfunctioning of the ovaries, displaced uterus and other such disorders.

They develop stamina, strength, flexibtlity, lightness and balance.

10. *PĀRŚVOTTĀNĀSANA*

Pārśva means side or flank; uttāna means an intense stretch. In this posture the sides of the chest are stretched intensely.

Technique

1. Stand in *Tāḍāsana* (Figure 1).
2. Join the palms behind the back, fingers pointing downwards towards the waist. Turn the wrists and the palms inwards and bring both the palms up above the middle of the back of the chest. Keep the fingers in level with the shoulder-blades and pointing upwards (Figure 12).

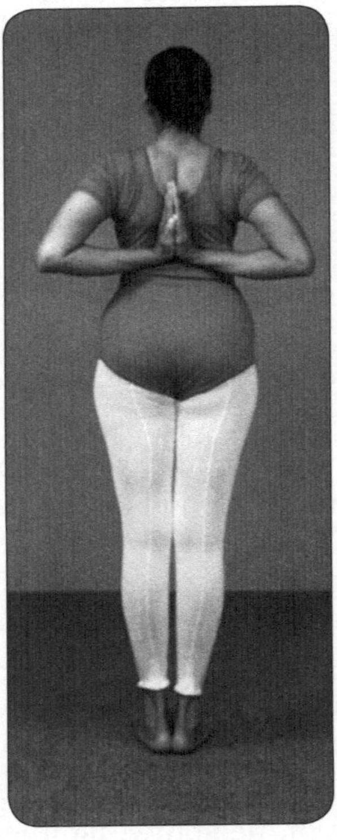

Fig. 12: *Pārśvottānāsana* (Intermediate Stage)

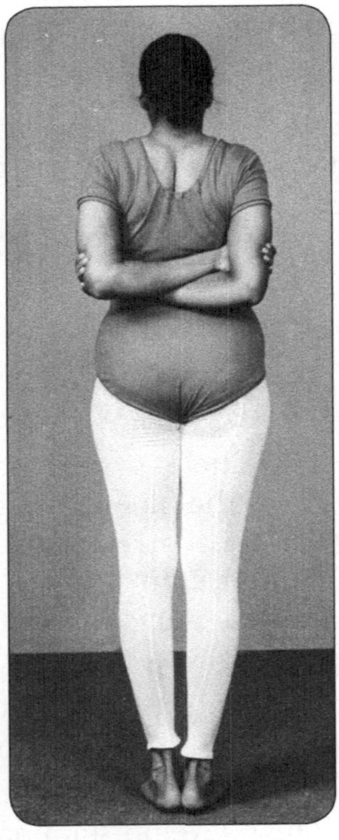

Fig. 13: *Pārśvottānāsana* (Intermediate Stage)

3. Press the palms against each other and take the elbows backwards so that the chest is not constricted. Expand the chest and raise the sternum.
4. While inhaling, jump with the legs 3 to 3½ feet apart. Remain in this position for a while, breathing normally.
5. Turn the right leg sideways 90° out and the left foot inwards. Simultaneously turn the trunk to the right.
6. Extend the head backwards, remain in this position for a while (Figure 14) and take a few breaths.
7. Exhale and lift the head up, extend the spine, bend the trunk forward, and touch the knee with the head (Figure 15). Do not bend the right knee while bending to the right.
8. This is the final posture. Breathing normally, remain for 20 to 30 seconds observing the following points:
   (a) keep the centre of the trunk over the centre of the thigh;
   (b) tighten the legs, extend the spine towards the head;
   (c) keep the chest expanded;
   (d) keep both the pelvic bones parallel;

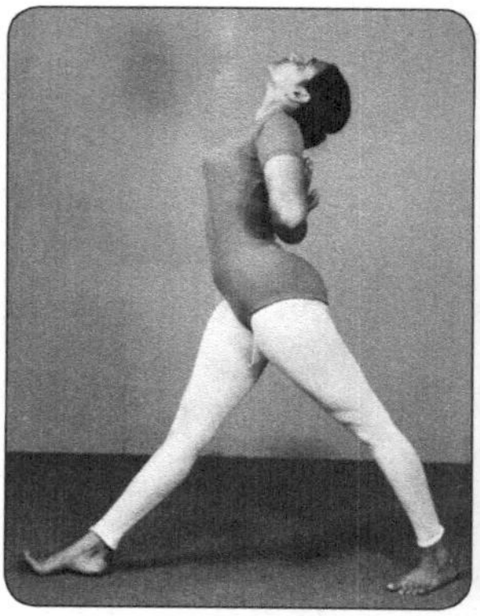

Fig. 14: *Pārśvottānāsana* (Intermediate Stage)

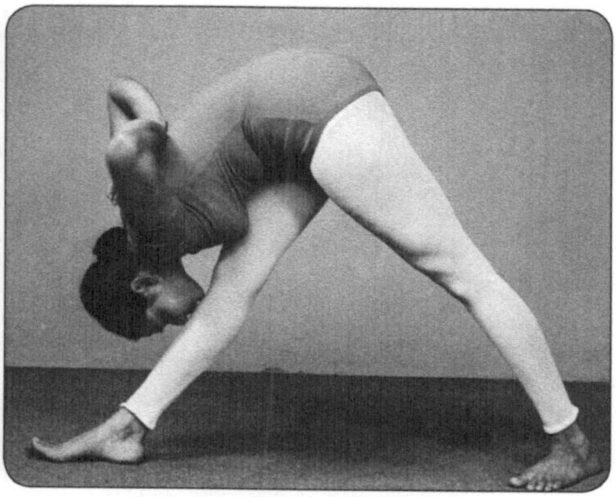

Fig. 15: *Pārśvottānāsana* (Final Stage)

(e) rotate the left side of the abdomen to the right, to bring the navel to the centre of the thigh.

9. Inhale and raise the trunk to position as in Figure 14. Do not take the head back.
10. Turn the right foot inwards and the trunk to the front, as in position 3.
11. Now repeat the posture on the left side by turning the left leg and the trunk sideways to the left.
12. Complete the āsana on the left and come back to *Tāḍāsana* (Figure 1).

Special Instructions

1. Those suffering from rheumatism may find it difficult to do the position shown in Figure 12. They may keep the arms crossed at the back (Figure 13).
2. Pull the abdomen up and broaden the chest as in Figure 14.
3. At first one will not be able to touch the knee. Do not tighten the diaphragm or contract the chest and the waist, but extend towards the head.
4. With every exhalation stretch the spinal column from the navel to the chin and try to reach beyond the knee.
5. Those who cannot perform this āsana with the hands folded behind the back, or those who cannot balance, may rest the palms or the fingers on either side of the right foot and vice versa. It is easy to bend and stretch the trunk now. Gradually learn to fold the hands behind the back.

Effects: This āsana is particularly good for those suffering from arthritis and stiffness in the neck, shoulders, elbows, wrists, and for hunchback. It removes stiffness in the hips. It contracts and tones the abdomen, helps deep breathing, and calms the brain.

11. *PRASĀRITA PĀDOTTĀNĀSANA*

Prasārita means spread apart. Pāda means foot or leg.

In this āsana the legs are spread wide apart and stretched to the maximum.

Technique

1. Stand in *Tāḍāsana* (Figure 1).
2. Place the hands on the hips with the tips of the fingers pointing forward.
3. While inhaling, jump and spread the feet 4 to 4½ feet apart. Tighten the knees and keep the feet pointing forwards.
4. Exhale, bend the trunk and bring it parallel to the floor. Remove the hands from the hips and place them on the floor in line with the feet. Spread the fingers and extend them towards the finger tips tightening the elbows.
5. Raise the head up, keeping the back concave. Stay for 10 to 15 seconds with normal breathing (Figures 16, 17).
6. Exhale, flex the elbows and rest the crown of the head on the floor. Keep the head, palms and feet in one line (Figure 18).

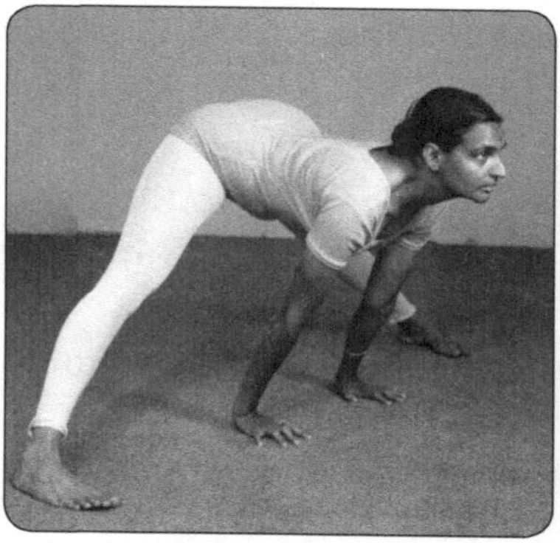

Fig. 16: *Prasārita Pādottānāsana* (Intermediate Stage)

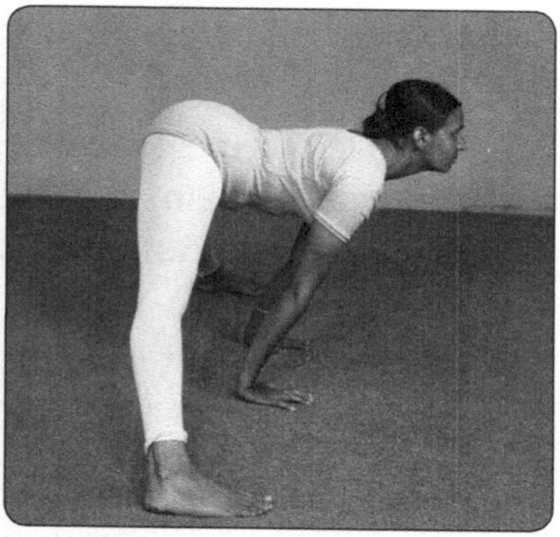

Fig. 17: *Prasārita Pādottānāsana* (Intermediate Stage)

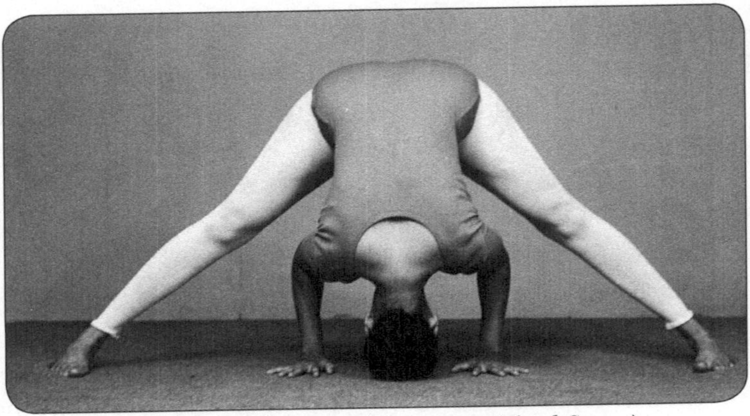

Fig. 18: *Prasārita Pādottānāsana* (Final Stage)

7. Breathing normally, remain in this final position for 20 to 30 seconds, observing the following points:
   (a) do not bend the knees;
   (b) do not throw the weight of the body on the head—it should be on the legs.
8. Exhale, press the hands against the floor, raise the head, and push the thighs backwards. Come to the position as in Figures 16 and 17. Wait for five seconds.
9. Inhale, raise the trunk up, exhale jump to *Tāḍāsana* (Figure 1).

Special Instructions

1. Keep the spine concave, as in Figures 16 and 17 so that the trunk becomes concave from the hips to the neck. Stretch the abdominal cavity and the waist towards the head.
2. Those who cannot keep the head on the floor should keep the palms slightly forward. The head should be kept forward and not in line with the feet.

Effects: This āsana stretches the hamstrings and removes fatigue caused by standing postures.

12. *PĀDĀNGUṢṬHĀSANA*

Pāda means foot. Aṅguṣṭha means big toe. In this posture one catches the big toes with the fingers.

Technique

1. Stand in *Tāḍāsana* (Figure 1).
2. Stand with the feet one foot apart. The outer feet and the outer hips should be in line. Take one or two breaths.
3. Exhale and bend forward. Do not bend the knees.
4. Now, hook the big toes with the thumbs, the index and the middle fingers.
5. Extend the spine from the hips towards the neck and raise the head up (Figure 19). Breathing normally, stay in this position for 5 seconds.
6. Now, while exhaling, bring the head towards the knees (Figure 20).

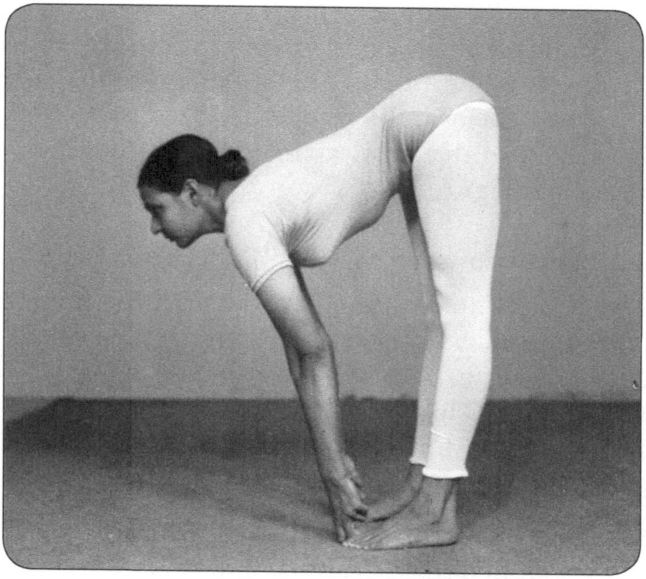

Fig. 19: *Pādānguṣṭhāsana* (Intermediate Stage)

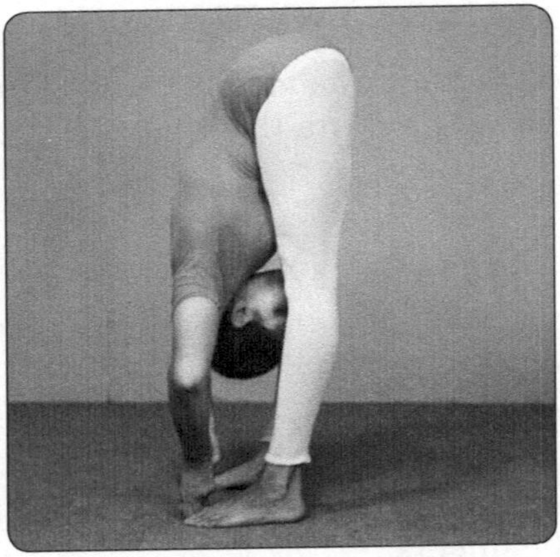

Fig. 20: *Pādanguṣṭhāsana* (Final Stage)

7. This is the final posture. Breathing normally, stay for 15 to 20 seconds, observing the following points:
   (a) pull the spine towards the floor by bending and widening the elbows;
   (b) tuck in the shoulder-blades towards the chest;
   (c) stretch the back and press the abdominal organs towards the thighs; the abdomen and the thighs should be as if fused together.
8. Inhale, raise the head as in Figure 19, and come to *Tāḍāsana* (Figure 1).

Special Instructions

1. Those who cannot catch the toes with the fingers may hold the ankles and later, with practice, catch the toes.
2. Do not try to touch the head to the knee by caving in the chest. This not only causes cramps in the chest and abdomen but it makes the neck stiff and causes headaches.

Effects: This āsana tones the abdominal organs and aids digestion. Slipped discs can be adjusted by doing the posture as in Figure 19.

13. *UTTĀNĀSANA*

'Ut' indicates intensity. Tāna means to stretch. In this āsana the spinal column is intensely stretched.

Technique

1. Stand in *Tāḍāsana* (Figure 1).
2. Tighten the knees, stretch both the legs, and lift both the arms towards the ceiling, palms facing forward. While lifting the arms, stretch the whole body as in *Vṛkṣāsana* (Figure 2). Take 1 or 2 breaths.
3. Extend the spine, exhale and bend the trunk forward.
4. Rest the palms on the floor by the side of the feet. Stretch the trunk forwards by keeping the head up and the spine concave. Take 1 or 2 breaths (Figure 21a).

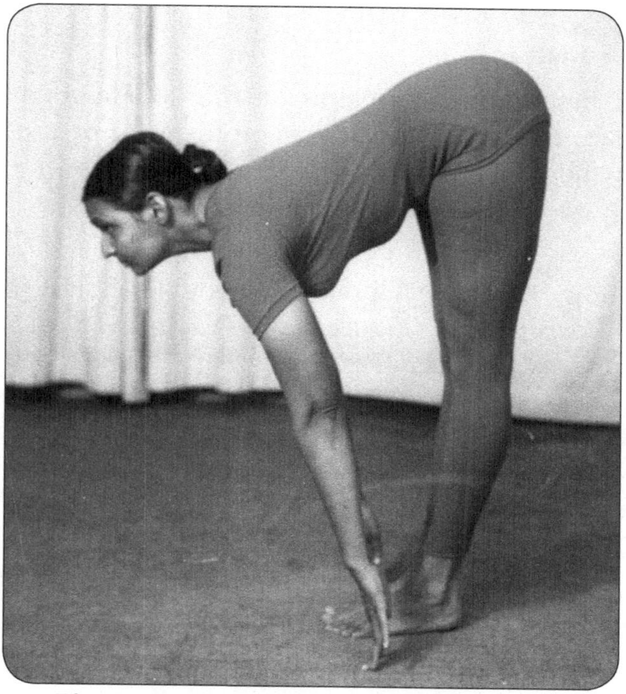

Fig. 21(a): *Uttānāsana* (Intermediate Stage)

5. Exhale and bring the head to the knees (Figure 21).
6. Breathing normally, stay in this final position for 30 to 60 seconds, observing the following points:
   (a) extend the bottom ribs and posterior trunk so that the head touches and rests on the knees;
   (b) pull the abdominal muscles, the anterior trunk, and the diaphragm towards the floor.
7. Inhale, come to the positions as in techniques 4 and 3, and finally come to *Tāḍāsana*.

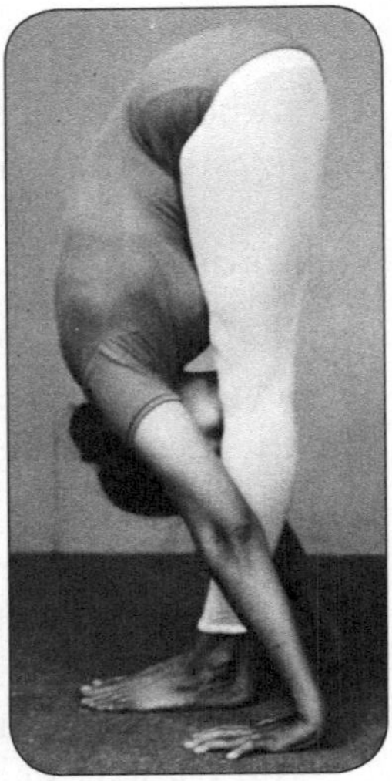

Fig. 21: *Uttānāsana* (Final Stage)

Special Instructions

1. At first resting the palms on the floor is difficult, so place the tips of the fingers on the floor or use bricks by the side of the feet and place the fingers on top.
2. Do not bend the knees to touch the head.
3. Do not constrict the neck and the chest.
4. Those who have slipped disc trouble should practise *Pārśvottānāsana* (Figure 14), *Prasārita Pādottānāsana* (Figures 16, 17), *Pādānguṣṭhāsana* (Figure 19), and *Uttānāsana* (Figure 21a) with the trunk stretched forward so that the spine is concave. There will thus be no pressure on the spine. Do not bend the trunk and touch the knees.
5. Once the body bends correctly in *Uttānāsana* one need not stretch the arms over the head as in position 2. One may go to position 4 straightway.

Effects: This āsana relieves stomach pain, removes depression and calms the brain.

14. *ADHO MUKHA ŚVĀNĀSANA*

Adho means downwards, mukha is face, Śvāna is dog. This āsana resembles a dog stretching himself with his head down.

Technique

1. Stand in *Tāḍāsana* (Figure 1).
2. Exhale and come to *Uttānāsana* (Figure 21). Place the palms on the floor by the side of the feet and in line with them.
3. Bend the knees and take the legs 4 to 4½ feet back, one by one. Keep the hands 1 to 1¼ feet apart and the feet also. Spread the palms and extend the fingers. Keep the feet parallel to each other and extend the toes.
4. Stretch the thighs backwards and pull the knee-caps in; place the heels on the floor. Take one or two breaths.
5. Exhale, stretch the arms and the legs, and push the thighs back. Move the trunk towards the legs.

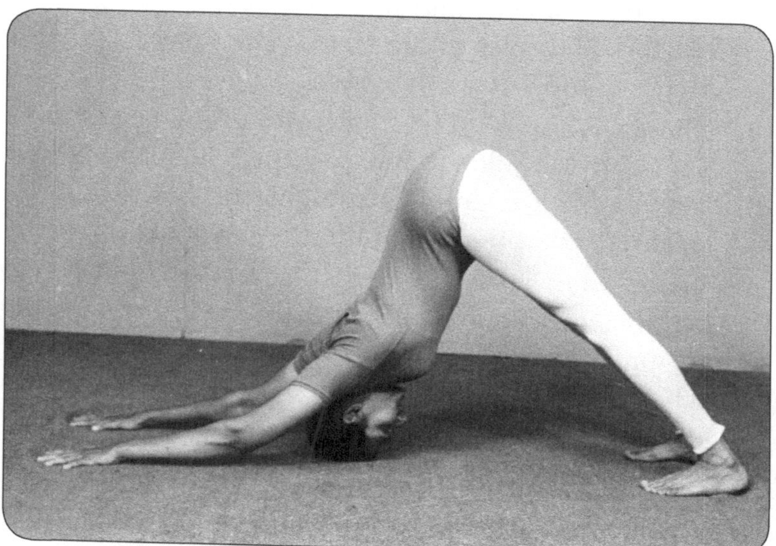

Fig. 22: *Adho Mukha Śvānāsana* (Final Stage)

6. Press the heels into the floor and place the crown of the head on the ground.
7. Remain in this final position for 15 to 20 seconds, breathing normally, observing the following points:
   (a) do not bend the knees;
   (b) tuck the shoulder-blades in and broaden the chest;
   (c) bear the weight on the legs.
8. Inhale, lift the head off the ground, bring the feet nearer the palms, and come to *Tāḍāsana* (Figure 1).

Special Instructions

1. Those who cannot place the palms on the floor in *Uttānāsana* may bend their knees and place the palms on the floor and then walk back.
2. The right arm and the right leg, the left arm and the left leg, must be exactly in line with each other.
3. Those who cannot place their heels on the floor should raise them slightly and place them on a wall, keeping the toes and soles of the feet on the floor so that the arches of the feet are extended.
4. Those who cannot keep the crown of the head on the floor can use pillows and rest their heads on them, keeping the arm and legs straight, the spine stretched inwards and upwards and the chest expanded.
5. Those who suffer from headaches or high blood pressure or who are unable to place the head on the ground should support it as in paragraph 4 above. When the head is thus supported, a calm feeling ensues and blood pressure comes down. Never keep the head hanging loose.

Effects: This posture removes fatigue and brings back lost energy. It is exhilarating.

OVERALL EFFECTS OF ĀSANAS 10 to 14

All these five āsanas increase the supply of blood to the brain. Thus, those who cannot perform *Śīrṣāsana* will get the same benefit of a calm feeling in the brain. In case of breathlessness, extreme fatigue or palpitation, these five āsanas are useful in removing tiredness and restoring high blood pressure and heartbeats to normal. One regains zest. Especially in *Adho Mukha Śvānāsana* (Figure 22), the diaphragm becomes light and soft and the cavity of the chest increases.

The ankle and the knee joints, the spinal column and the hip joints become flexible. The legs become shapely. These āsanas are also beneficial to runners as they gain lightness in the feet. The movements of the ankles and the heels become free. Those who suffer from rheumatism of elbow, shoulder or wrist, or whose movements in these regions are not free, will find *Pārśvottānāsana* (Figures 12, 13) beneficial if the movements of the arms presented in this āsana are followed. The shoulder-joints become free. If one suffers from hunchback, the concave movement of the spine should be performed as shown in Figures 16, 17 and 19 so that the shoulders and the back muscles are stretched and the chest is expanded, thus helping deep breathing and relieving the arthritic condition.

The abdominal organs gain strength; the flow of digestive juices is freed, thus helping the digestive system. They are also extremely helpful for toning the liver and the spleen, relieving stomach-ache and correcting the malfunctioning of the kidneys. For all complaints such as excess of bile, anaemia, indigestion, constipation, heat strokes, obesity these āsanas are of great help.

Circulation is improved by their practice and they correct a displaced uterus, backache, menstrual disorders, hot flushes and strengthen the spinal column.

They tone the nervous system, cure mental disorders, forgetfulness, moods and depressions, and help highly strung individuals and those who get easily tired.

SECTION-II

Āsanas: Forward Bends

The āsanas in this section are to be performed in a sitting position, bending forward. After gaining some proficiency as well as physical strength and endurance by the practice of the āsanas from Section I, practise *Sālamba Sarvāṅgāsana* (Figure 84) and *Halāsana* (Figure 88). Then start to learn the āsanas in this section. The first seven are easy and helpful for gaining elasticity of the body. At first it may be hard to touch the knees with the head. Persistence and perseverance in practice will help achieve the final pose. The remaining āsanas will be easier to perform, once elasticity of the body has been gained.

15. *DAṆḌĀSANA*

Daṇḍa means stick. The āsana resembles a stick or a staff. Like *Tāḍāsana* in Section I, *Daṇḍāsana* is the basic posture for all the āsanas in this Section.

Technique

1. Sit on a blanket.
2. Sit straight with legs extended forwards. Keep the thighs, knees, ankles, and toes together. Extend all the toes towards the ceiling.
3. Keep both the palms on the floor by the side of the hips, with the fingers pointing towards the legs.
4. While inhaling, raise the spine up. Keep the elbows straight, the chest up, the head and the neck erect and look straight forward (Figure 23).
5. This is the final posture. Remain for five seconds, breathing normally, observing the following points:
   (a) pressing the knees and the femur towards the floor, raise the waist;

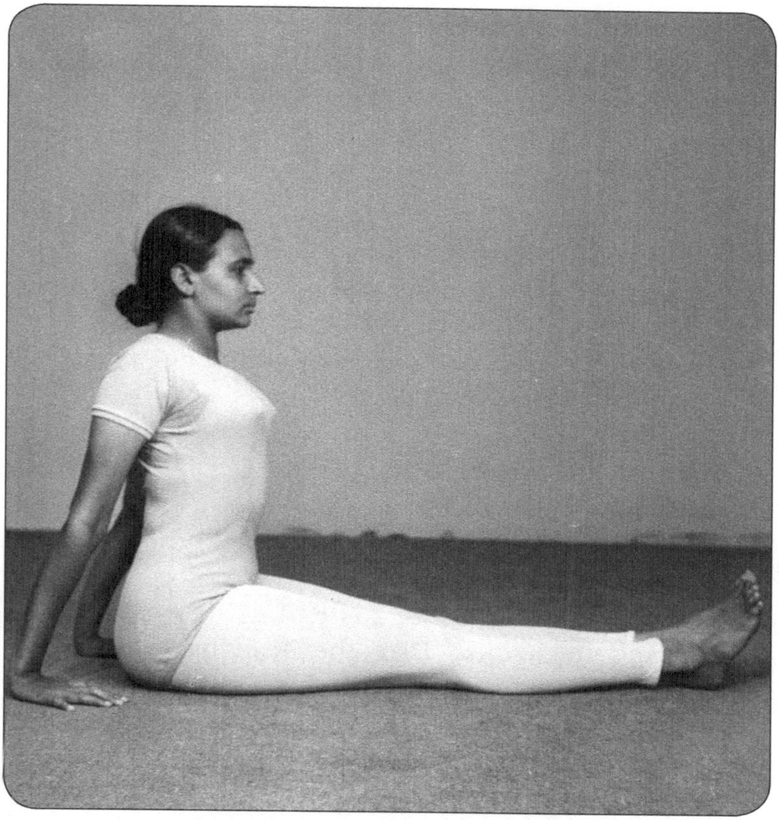

Fig. 23: *Daṇḍāsana* (Final Stage)

(b) keep the buttocks, the back, and the head in one line, perpendicular to the floor;

(c) make the spinal column firm and expand the ribs and the chest;

(d) lift the abdominal organs upwards.

Effects: This āsana stretches the leg muscles, massages the abdominal organs, and strengthens the waist muscles. It tones the kidneys and trains one to sit straight with the spine erect.

16. *JĀNU ŚĪRṢĀSANA*

Jānu means knee, *Śīrṣa* means head. In this āsana there is juxtaposition of the head and the knee, giving the posture its name.

Technique

1. Sit in *Daṇḍāsana* (Figure 23).
2. Bend the right knee and place the right heel near the right groin. Pull the right knee back.
3. Keep the left leg straight. See that the angle between the two legs is an obtuse one.
4. Extend both the arms forward beyond the left foot and catch the right wrist with the left hand. Breathe normally.
5. After holding the palms inhale, extend the spine and lift it up. Press the right knee down and raise the hips up. There should be an angle of 45° between the left leg and the trunk. Take the head back. Breathing normally, stay for 15 seconds (Figures 24, 25).
6. Exhale, bend the trunk forward, and place the forehead on the left knee. Stay in this final stage for

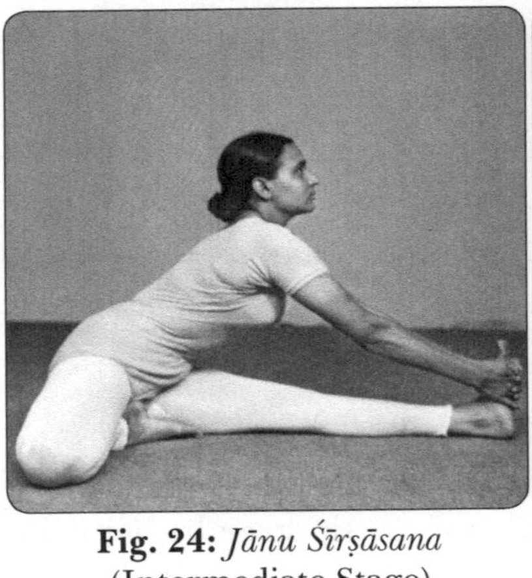

Fig. 24: *Jānu Śīrṣāsana* (Intermediate Stage)

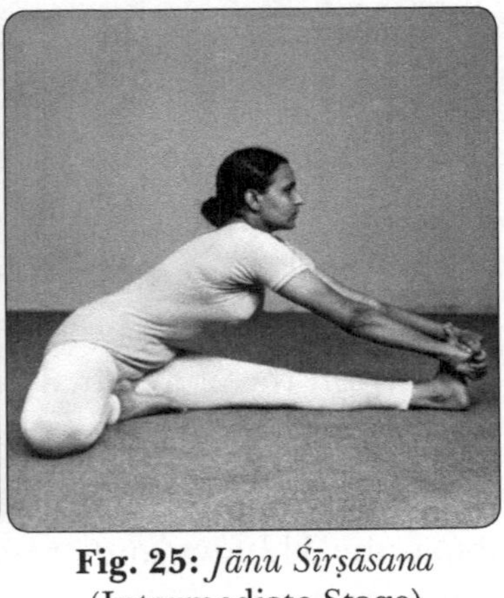

Fig. 25: *Jānu Śīrṣāsana* (Intermediate Stage)

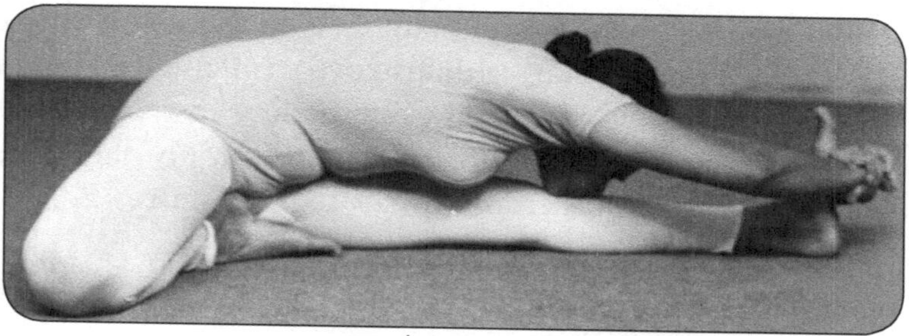

Fig. 26: *Jānu Śīrṣāsana* (Final Stage)

half a minute to one minute while breathing normally (Figure 26). Observe the following points:

(a) keep the elbows out, widening them so as to increase the expansion of the chest and stretch forward;

(b) move the floating ribs forwards and extend them towards the chest;

(c) the sternum and the middle of the abdomen must rest on the left thigh as though the trunk is merged with the leg;

(d) while bending forward, keep the stretched left leg and the right leg firmly on the ground; pull the right knee back as far as possible.

7. Inhale and lift the head and trunk (Figure 25), release the palms and come to *Daṇḍāsana*; then perform the āsana on the other side, following all the techniques but reversing the instructions for right and left. Remain for the same length of time, then return to *Daṇḍāsana* (Figure 23).

Special Instructions

1. Beginners may find it difficult to hold the toes and to place the forehead on the knee. Learn to stretch every part of the body gradually—buttocks, back of the trunk, ribs, spine, armpits, elbows and arms. In the āsanas that follow, the same practice of stretching these various portions of the body should be performed.

2. In the beginning it is difficult to hold the feet with the hands. You may start with instruction (a) as given below and gradually move to the succeeding instructions as the spine becomes more supple and apply the same method to āsanas from No. 17 to 20 (Figures 27, 28, 29, 30):
   (a) Stretch the spine fully so that holding the legs becomes easier.
   (b) First let the hands reach the shin.
   (c) Then hook the big toe of the foot with the forefingers and the middle fingers.
   (d) Now, catch the sole of the foot with the fingers.
   (e) Then clasp the heel with the palm.
   (f) Entwine the fingers of both the hands and encircle the foot (Figure 24).
   (g) Finally catch the wrist of the right hand with the left palm (Figure 25) or vice versa.
3. Keep the abdominal organs lifted up as in Figures 24 and 25.
4. Extend the trunk further and place the forehead, the nose, the lips and the chin gradually on the left knee. Make sure the spinal column is fully extended; this is very important (Figure 26).
5. Those who find it difficult to place the forehead on the knee due to fat around the waist, and suffer from headache and high blood pressure, may use a folded blanket on the knee and rest the forehead on it. Apply the method in the following āsanas (Figures 27, 28, 29, 30).

Effects: This pose tones and activates the liver, the spleen and the kidneys. It is tremendously helpful in the case of persistent low fever when it should be performed for five minutes on each side.

17. *ARDHA BADDHA PADMA PAŚCIMOTTĀNĀSANA*

Ardha means half, Baddha means caught, Padma means lotus. In this posture, one leg is in *Padmāsana* and the other is stretched. The posterior side of the trunk is extended, giving the posture its name.

Technique

1. Sit in *Daṇḍāsana* (Figure 23).
2. Bend the right leg and place the foot over the left thigh so that the outer edge of the foot fits into the pit of the thigh. Bring the right knee as near to the left knee as possible.

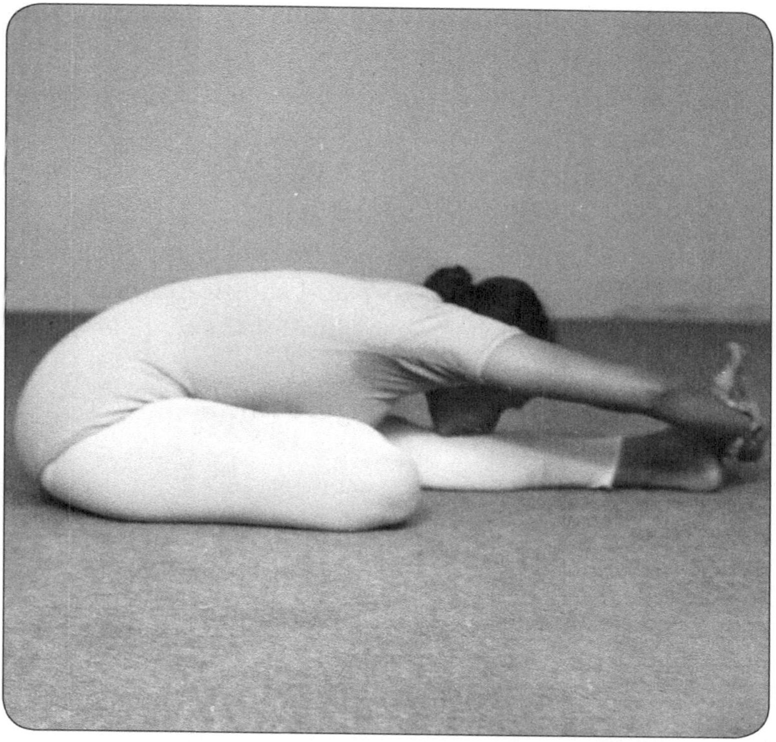

Fig. 27: *Ardha Baddha Padma Paścimottānāsana* (Final Stage)

3. Bring both the arms towards the left foot. Catch the right wrist with the left hand and encircle the foot.
4. Inhale, raise the head, and look up. Extend the spine, expand the chest, and lift up the sternum. Stay for five seconds (Position 1), breathing normally.
5. Exhale, extend the spine forwards, and place the chin on or beyond the left knee.
6. Stay in this final stage for 30 to 60 seconds with normal breathing (Figure 27), observing the following points:
   (a) take the pelvis forward beyond the right foot and ankle;
   (b) rest the stomach and the chest on the thigh, with the chin beyond the knee;
   (c) the trunk should merge more and more into the thighs.
7. Inhale, raise the head up, and come to position 1. Release the hands and the right leg.
8. Now, perform this āsana on the other side, following the techniques from 2 to 7 and substituting the word left for right and vice versa. Stay for the same length of time.
9. Come back to *Daṇḍāsana* (Figure 23).

Special Instruction

In the original pose, the right foot is grasped by the right hand from behind and vice versa. However, here women should hold the extended foot with both the hands so that the back of the trunk can be fully extended. This has a more beneficial effect on the abdominal area.

Effects: This posture is effective for gastric troubles and flatulence.

18. *TRIAṄG MUKHAIKAPĀDA PAŚCIMOTTANĀSANA*

Triaṅg means three parts—foot, knees and buttocks, whereas Mukhaikāpāda means the face and one leg. In this posture all these parts have to play different roles, along with the extension of the trunk, to complete the posture.

Technique

1. Sit in *Daṇḍāsana* (Figure 23).
2. Bend the right leg at the knee. Hold the ankle with the right palm and fold the leg back. Keep the toes of the right foot extending backwards by the side of the right hipjoint. Touch the inner edge of the right calf to the outer edge of the right thigh. The inner edge of the right thigh should touch the inner edge of the left thigh (Position 1). Take one or two breaths.
3. Exhale, bend the trunk forward, and extend the arms beyond the left foot Catch the right wrist with the left hand firmly and encircle the left foot.
4. Inhale, raise the head up, and keep the spine concave. Now, the trunk will be at 45° to the straight leg. Wait in this position for some time. Look straight up (Position 2).
5. Exhale, bend the trunk, and rest the abdomen, the chest, and the chin on the thigh, the knee and the shin.

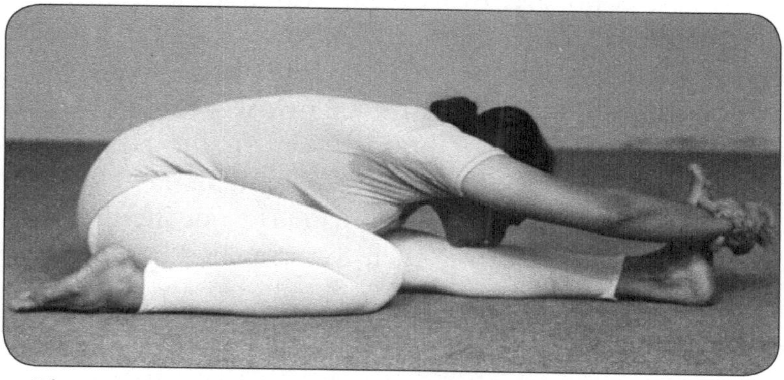

Fig. 28: *Triaṅg Mukhaikapāda Paścimottanāsana* (Final Stage)

6. Remain in this final stage for 30 to 60 seconds, breathing normally (Figure 28). Observe the following points:
   (a) do not tilt the trunk to the left, but shift the weight to the right by bringing the centre of gravity to the middle of the right thigh;
   (b) extend the sides of the trunk forward towards the foot;
   (c) bend the elbows and extend further by pulling the armpits forwards;
   (d) keep the sternum in contact with the thighs.
7. Inhale, raise the trunk up, and come to position 2. Unlock the palms, release the right leg, and keep it straight.
8. Now, bend the left leg at the knee. Repeat the pose on the other side, remaining for the same length of time and following all the techniques but substituting right for left and vice versa. Return to *Daṇḍāsana* (Figure 23).

Special Instructions

1. Do not sit on the right foot for the sake of balancing.
2. In this position, the trunk tends to turn to the left. Those who are overweight will find it difficult to maintain balance. Shift the balance from the left side onto the right side and the weight also onto the right, i.e., the side of the bent knee or use a folded blanket underneath the left buttock, i.e. on the side of the extended leg, so that balance is maintained. The right ankle and foot should be firm. Do not lift the right buttockbone. Keep the left leg stretched and the toes straight.

Effects: This posture cures sprains in the ankles and the knees and is good for flat feet and dropped arches.

19. *MARĪCYĀSANA I*

This āsana is named after the sage Marīcī, son of the Creator Brahma and grandfather of the Sun God Sūrya.

Technique

1. Sit in *Daṇḍāsana* (Figure 23).
2. Bend the left leg with the left knee facing upwards, keep the bottom of the foot on the floor and the inner edge of the foot touching the extended right thigh; the left heel should be close to the back of the left thigh.
3. Keep the left arm on the inner edge of the left knee, stretch the left shoulder forward, and keep the armpit touching the left shin: now twist the arm backwards, encircling the bent knee. Take the right hand back and catch the left wrist. Take one or two breaths.
4. Exhale and extend the trunk upwards (Position 1). Keep the head straight and look ahead. Wait in this position for five seconds, breathing normally.
5. Exhale, extend the trunk further and bend forward so that the stomach and the thigh are in communion with each other. The chin should go beyond the knee. Keep both the shoulders in line with each other (Figure 29).

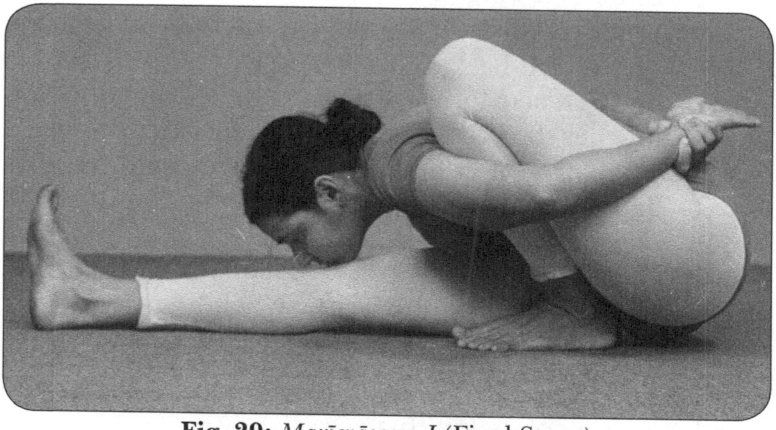

Fig. 29: *Marīcyāsana I* (Final Stage)

6. Remain in this final stage of the āsana for 20 to 30 seconds, if possible for one minute, breathing normally and observing the following points:
   (a) keep the right leg straight; do not allow it to turn outwards;
   (b) grip the wrist firmly to press the trunk against the thigh;
   (c) do not allow the trunk to tilt to the right.
7. Inhale and raise the head to Position 1. Unclasp the hands, stretch the left leg forwards, and come to *Daṇḍāsana* (Figure 23).
8. Now, perform the āsana on the other side, with the right leg bent at the knee and the left leg outstretched, substituting the word right for left and vice versa. Stay for the same length of time, then return to *Daṇḍāsana*.

Special Instructions

1. If one has a large stomach, then the bent leg will tend to drop to the side. See that it is kept upright.
2. In the beginning it is difficult to hold the wrist, so first catch the fingers, then the palm and gradually the wrist.
3. If the thighs and the buttocks are overweight, bear in mind the following instructions:
   (a) While twisting the left arm backwards, the left side of the back and left side of the spine should be stretched forward so that the left hand almost touches the right foot and then encircles the knee.
   (b) The left armpit and the left shin should have no gap between them; in this way the left arm can stretch fully.
   (c) In the beginning hook the fingers, later the palms, and finally clasp the wrist, depending upon your ability and progress.

Effects: In this posture the abdominal organs contract and circulation is increased in that area.

OVERALL EFFECTS OF ĀSANAS 16 to 19

All these āsanas combined have a profound effect on the internal organs of the abdomen. They help digestion and tone and massage the organs of the digestive system such as the stomach, the liver, the spleen, the intestines, the pancreas and the gall-bladder. They are therefore useful in counteracting flatulence, constipation, excessive bile, diabetes and obesity.

They strengthen the urinary system and correct the functioning of the bladder.

After delivery the uterus tends to sag downwards and the internal organs and muscles of the abdomen are in a weakened state. These āsanas strengthen those areas and bring them back to normal. They also help check excessive menstrual discharge.

They strengthen and exercise the entire back, from the lumbar to the thoracic and cervical region, and are good for relieving neck troubles.

They are useful in cases of high blood pressure. They soothe the nerves and exercise a calming effect on the mind.

20. *PAŚCIMOTTĀNĀSANA*

This āsana is also known as *Ugrāsana* and *Brahmacaryāsana*. Paścima means west; applied to the body it means the back. Thus, a posterior extension of the body is indicated in this āsana.

Technique

1. Sit in *Daṇḍāsana* (Figure 23).
2. Exhale, extend the hands, and hold the wrist of either hand beyond the feet.

3. Inhale, stretch the spine upwards making it concave. Raise the back, the waist and the sternum up; lift the head. Stay for five seconds. Take a few breaths.
4. Exhale, bend the elbows slightly and extend the upper arms outwards. Extend the sides of the trunk and bend forward, touching the thighs. The head should rest beyond the knees (Figure 30).

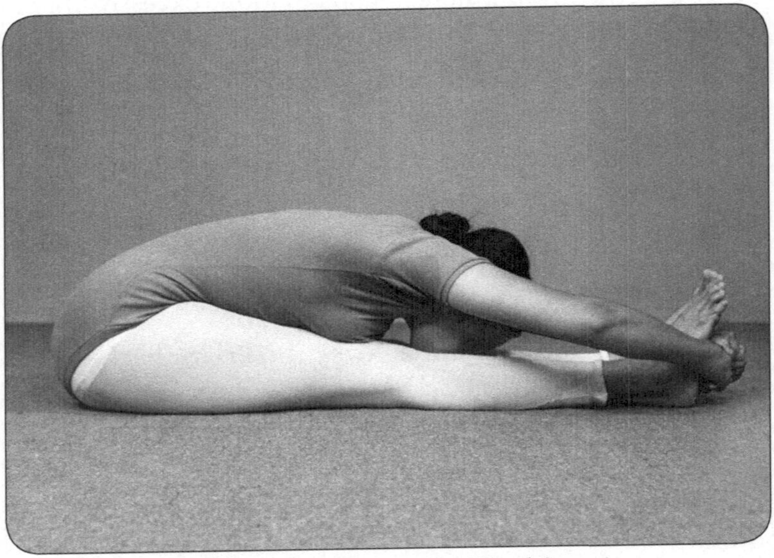

Fig. 30: *Paścimottānāsana* (Final Stage)

5. In this final stage the head and the trunk rest on the legs. Stay in this position for one minute, breathing normally. Gradually increase the time to five minutes, observing the following points:
   (a) widen the elbows so that the chest expands;
   (b) rest the abdomen and the chest on the thighs;
   (c) bend the elbows and lift them upwards; use the handgrip as a lever to extend the trunk;
   (d) do not cave in the chest or draw in the sternum.
6. Inhale, raise the head up (Position I), and come to *Daṇḍāsana* (Figure 23).

Special Instructions

1. In the beginning it is difficult to keep the legs stretched. The knees bend and tension is felt in the hamstring muscles. If the thighs are fat they turn outwards and the feet do not touch each other. Do not be disheartened. Stretch gradually and with practice all these difficulties will be overcome.
2. (a) Beginners should catch the big toes—the right big toe with the right thumb and the index finger, the left big toe with the left thumb and the index finger. (b) Later, gradually learn to encircle the soles of the feet with your fingers. (c) Later still, try to catch the wrist (Figure 30).
3. In the beginning the back may be humped. Raise the trunk from the small of the back and the hump will disappear. Raise the head up or keep a folded blanket on the knees towards the shin-bones and rest the head on it.

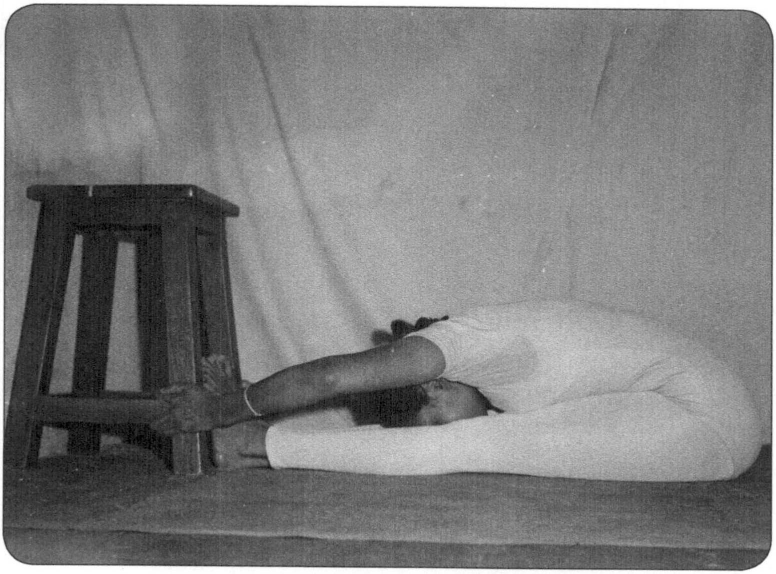

Fig. 31: *Paścimottānāsana* (Final Stage)

4. To stretch the trunk, move a stool or a chair against a wall. Rest your feet on the lower plank of the stool and hold the stool with your hands. This will help stretch the trunk (Figure 31).
5. Do not cave in the chest to touch the knees. Do not rest the elbows on the ground as this hinders the extension of the body.

Effects: This āsana effectively massages the abdominal organs and strengthens them. It is highly beneficial for diseases of the kidneys and for sluggish liver.

Its effects have been described thus:

> *Paścimottānāsana* is the foremost of all āsanas. Its effect is that the life force flows through the very intricate channels called nāḍis, gastric fire is kindled and the stomach becomes free of all diseases.
>
> H.P. I, 29

In this āsana, the pelvic region is stretched and the blood circulation there is stimulated. The ovaries, the uterus and the entire reproductive system are revitalised and their efficiency is enhanced. The posture also helps maintain a balanced attitude to sex.

In the human species, the spinal column is perpendicular to the ground, whereas in animals it is parallel to the ground and the heart is below the spine. Because of the upright position, humans are more prone to strain and to diseases of the heart. In *Paścimottānāsana* (Figure 30) the spine is horizontal and parallel to the ground so that the heart is rested.

The effect of this āsana on the mind is magical: an upset, irritated, and restless mind becomes tranquil, and angry, passionate moods, etc., are calmed down. It sharpens the memory and brings clarity of thought.

21. *PARIVṚTTA JĀNU ŚĪRṢĀSANA*

Parivṛtta means revolved. This āsana is a variation of *Jānu Sīrṣāsana* in which the trunk is twisted around, thereby giving the spine the maximum stretch.

Technique

1. Sit in *Daṇḍāsana* (Figure 23).
2. Bend the right knee and keep the outer edge touching the floor as in *Jānu Śīrṣāsana* (Figure 26). Take one or two breaths.
3. Exhale, twist the spine and the trunk to the right, and bend down sideways so that the left side of the body, especially the left shoulder, rests in front of the left leg and knee.
4. Stretch the left arm and turn it outwards; turn the wrist so that the thumb points towards the floor and the little finger is up. Catch the sole of the left foot, bending the left elbow and resting it in front of the left calf. Keep the elbow further away from the leg.
5. Stretch the right arm over the ear. Hold the outer edge of the left foot with the right palm. Keep the right thumb down and the little finger up.
6. Keep the head between the two arms. Breathe normally.

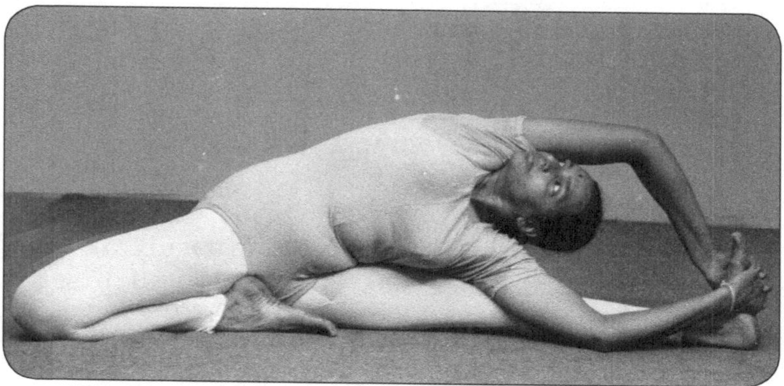

Fig. 32: *Parivṛtta Janu Śīrṣāsana* (Intermediate Stage)

7. Tuck in the left side of the back and the shoulder-blades and twist the waist as much as you can. Turn the right side of the back upwards. Turn the right elbow and the head back and look up at the ceiling. The right side of the trunk will now be twisted to the left (Figure 32).
8. Rotate the trunk further and rest the back of the head on the extended leg (Figure 33).
9. Stay in this final stage of the āsana for 20 to 30 seconds, breathing normally. Increase the time to one minute as you progress, observing the following points:
   (a) tuck in the left shoulder-blade more and more;
   (b) turn the right side of the trunk upwards and backwards;
   (c) do not bend the left knee.
10. Come to *Daṇḍāsana* (Figure 23).
11. Repeat the posture on the other side, following all techniques and reading right for left and vice versa. Stay for the same length of time, then return to *Daṇḍāsana*.

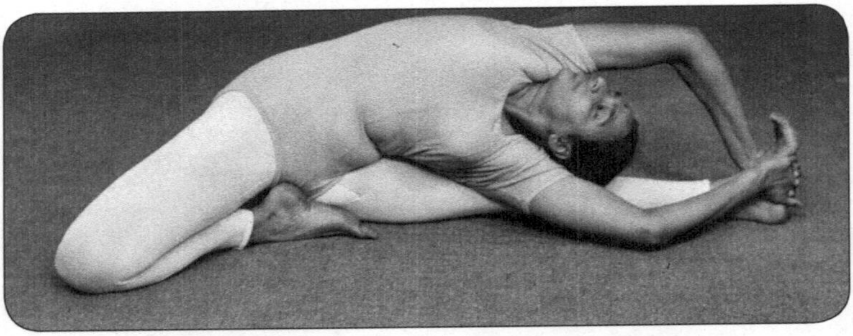

Fig. 33: *Parivṛtta Jānu Śīrṣāsana* (Final Stage)

Special Instruction

Beginners will find the position given in Figure 32 easier than that in Figure 33. They must learn to progress gradually.

Effects: Blood is well circulated in the whole of the back. This āsana is a boon to women because it relieves backaches.

22. *PARIVṚTTA PAŚCIMOTTĀNĀSANA*

This āsana is a variation of *Paścimottānāsana*. Here the trunk is twisted laterally in a forward extension.

Technique

1. Sit in *Daṇḍāsana* (Figure 23).
2. Exhale and twist the right side of the trunk in such a way that it comes over the left thigh and the right hand reaches beyond the left foot. Twist the right forearm and the right wrist so that the thumb points downwards and the little finger up. Hold the outer side of the left foot with the right palm. Take one or two breaths.
3. Exhale again and twist the right side of the trunk a little more so that the left side of the trunk faces the ceiling. Take a breath.
4. Again exhale and extend the left arm over the head, stretching the armpit from the side of the trunk to reach the right foot. Catch the outer side of the right foot with the left hand, thumb pointing downwards.
5. Bend both the elbows, move the head and back in order to twist the left side of the trunk upwards. Twist the spine and rest the right side of the top trunk on the left thigh. Turn the neck and look up.

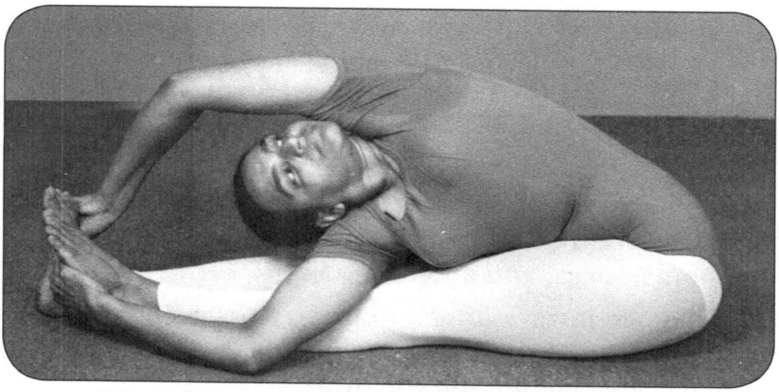

Fig. 34: *Parivṛtta Paścimottānāsana* (Final Stage)

6. Stay in this final position for 15 to 20 seconds with normal breathing. Observe the following points:
   (a) tuck in the shoulder-blades;
   (b) extend the trunk from the navel upwards towards the head;
   (c) the chest should face completely to the left and slightly upwards;
   (d) the right bottom ribs should extend forward towards the feet and away from the right leg.
7. Inhale, raise the head, and come to *Daṇḍāsana* (Fig. 23).
8. Perform this āsana on the other side, by catching the right foot with the left hand and twisting the right side of the trunk upwards and backwards. Stay for the same length of time. Return to *Daṇḍāsana*.

Special Instructions

1. As the diaphragm is compressed in this posture, breathing in and out will be quicker. Beginners may find it difficult to breathe. In that case, they should open that side of the chest which faces the ceiling.
2. In order to twist the spine to the maximum, first bend the left leg and turn the trunk. Then fix the right shoulder-blade beyond the outer edge of the left thigh and knee and hold the left foot with the right hand. Now straighten the left leg and vice versa.

Effects: This āsana tones the kidneys, rejuvenates the spine, relieves backaches, and helps sluggishness of the liver.

OVERALL EFFECTS OF ĀSANAS 21 & 22

In these two postures the waist is twisted and due to this action lower backaches and catches in the waist region are relieved. The spine is strengthened, particularly in the lumbar area, and attains mobility.

They are invigorating and they remove sluggishness, improve digestion, and regulate the functioning of the kidneys, the bladder and the ovaries.

23. *BADDHA KOṆĀSANA*

Baddha means bound or caught; koṇa means angle. In this posture the knees are bent at an acute angle and are taken sideways to the ground. The heels touch each other near the perineum and the feet are caught by the hands.

Technique

1. Sit in *Daṇḍāsana* (Figure 23).
2. Bend both the legs at the knees and bring the feet towards the groins.
3. Bring the soles and the heels together as in Namaste (the Indian way of salutation).
4. Hold both the feet and bring the heels towards the perineum. The outer edges of the feet should touch the ground. Breathe normally.
5. Widen the thighs and touch the floor with the knees.
6. Extend the groins, rest the knees on the floor in line with the thighs.
7. Pull the heels closer towards the perineum, keeping the calf muscles in juxtaposition with the inner sides of the thighs.
8. Hold the feet with the hands, press the knees, the ankles, and the thighs towards the floor, and stretch

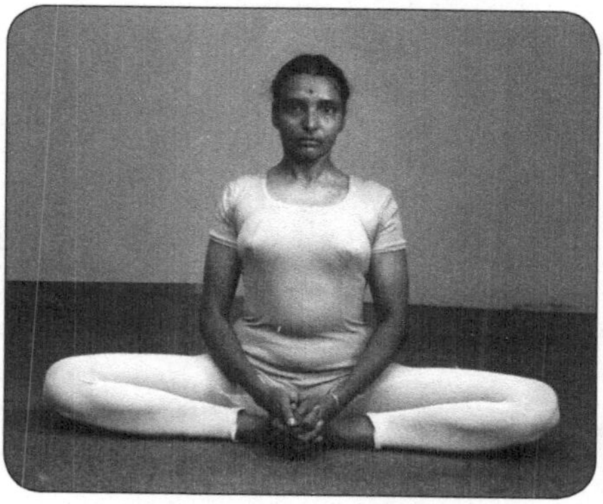

Fig. 35: *Baddha Koṇāsana* (Final Stage)

the trunk upwards. Take care to lift the abdominal region and keep the neck straight (Figure 35).

9. Stay in this final position for 30 to 60 seconds breathing normally. Later increase the time as much as possible. Observe the following points:
   - (a) extend the groins towards the knees;
   - (b) press the sides of the shin bones down;
   - (c) extend the trunk from the navel upwards;
   - (d) the firmer the grip of the hands on the feet, the better the lift of the trunk;
   - (e) keep the shoulders broad and the shoulder-blades tucked in.
10. Press both the elbows against the thighs, exhale and bend the trunk forward. Rest the forehead, the nose and later the chin on the floor, in this order. The chest should rest on the feet (Figures 36, 37).

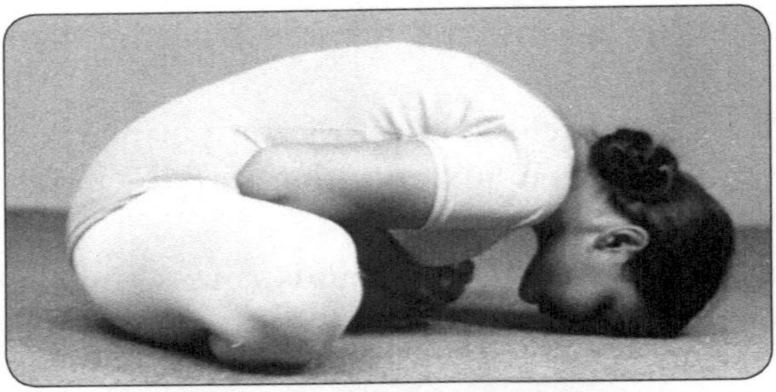

Fig. 36: *Baddha Koṇāsana* (Final Stage)

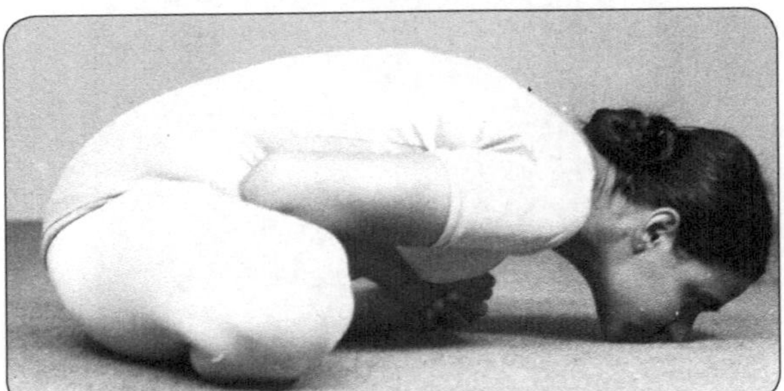

Fig. 37: *Baddha Koṇāsana* (Final Stage)

11. Stay for half a minute to one minute in this final position, breathing normally, observing these points:
    (a) do not tighten the floating ribs;
    (b) do not raise the buttocks from the floor;
    (c) keep the hips, the thighs and the shins firm to extend the trunk forward.
12. Raise the head up and come back to position as in Figure 35. Release the hands and the feet and stretch the legs (Figure 23).

Special Instructions

1. This āsana is very important and one should learn to stay in it as long as possible.
2. In the beginning it is difficult to rest the knees on the ground, due to tension in the groins. The knees should not be forced down, but the groins should be extended towards the knees. With practice, this will become easy.
3. Those who are heavy in the region of the buttocks and abdomen and those suffering from menstrual disorders should place a blanket 3 to 4 inches thick under the buttocks for support so that they can sit up straight with the abdomen lifted up (Figure 183).
4. They may also sit against a wall and use a rope as in Section VIII for lifting the trunk.
5. The positions shown in Figures 36 and 37 should not be attempted unless one first perfects the position in Figure 35.

Effects: This pose is a boon to women as it tones the kidneys, alleviates urinary and uterine disorders, prevents sciatica and hernia. It also strengthens the bladder and the uterus.

24. *SUPTA BADDHA KOṆĀSANA*

Supta means supine, Lying down. This is a variation of *Baddha Koṇāsana* to be performed in a supine position.

Technique

1. Lie flat on the back (Figure 80).
2. Bend the knees and bring the soles of the feet near the buttocks.
3. Spread the thighs and the knees apart, bringing the heels and the soles of the feet together.
4. Now, lower the knees as close to the ground as possible (Figure 38).
5. Stay in this position for 30 to 60 seconds, breathing normally. Gradually increase the duration to any length.
6. Stretch the arms over the head in order to extend the abdomen and the abdominal muscles upwards towards the chest. Turn the palms to face the ceiling (Figure 39).
7. Stay in this final position, breathing normally, for 30 to 60 seconds and later as long as possible. Watch these points in the supine position:
   (a) do not raise the lumbar up;
   (b) keep the pelvic area broad;

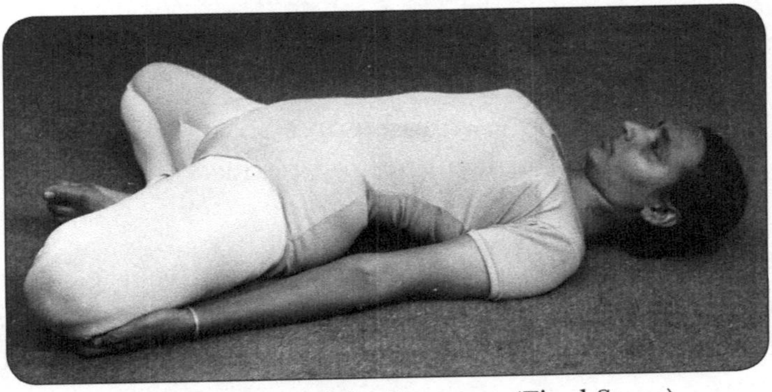

Fig. 38: *Supta Baddha Koṇāsana* (Final Stage)

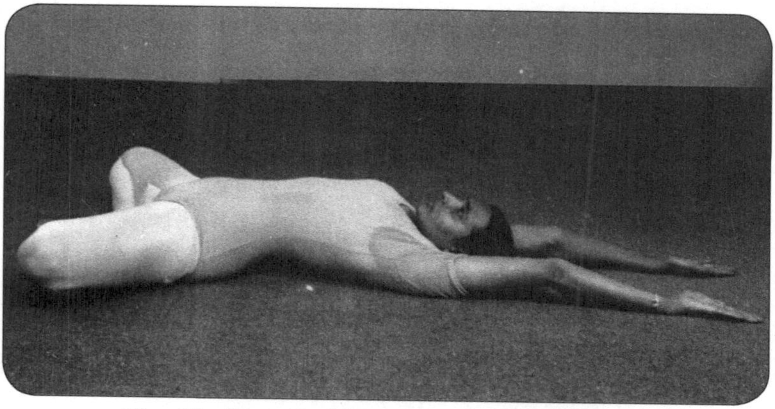

Fig. 39: *Supta Baddha Koṇāsana* (Final Stage)

(c) keep the chest expanded;

(d) allow the knees to go down towards the ground by taking them further sideways.

8. Bring the arms down. Slowly and carefully lift the knees off the ground one by one and stretch the legs.

Special Instructions

1. Sometimes the ankles and the sides of the feet slip and do not stay together. In that case rest the toes against a wall, place the palms underneath the thighs, catch the ankles and pull them towards the thighs.
2. Those who are heavy should place a blanket 3 to 4 inches thick under their back so that the chest opens and the abdomen is at an angle (see *Supta Vīrāsana*, Figure 186).
3. While raising the knees off the ground, allow the groin muscles to relax in order to avoid jerky movements and spasms.

Effects: This āsana gives relief from pains, spasms and burning sensations of the uterine organs during menstruation. It tones the urinary system. It is good for relief from hernia and bleeding piles.

25. *UPAVIṢṬHA KOṆĀSANA*

Upaviṣṭha means seated or sitting. In this āsana the legs are stretched in an obtuse angle while sitting.

Technique

1. Sit in *Daṇḍāsana* (Figure 23).
2. Spread the legs apart and extend them sideways one by one. Increase the distance between the legs as much as you can.
3. Keep the soles of the feet firm, perpendicular to the ground, with the toes pointing upwards.
4. Catch the big toe of each foot with the thumb, the index finger and the middle finger of the corresponding hand, keeping the thumbs on the outer side and the fingers on the inner side of each big toe.
5. Press the legs down raise the waist and the sides of the body up. Stay in this position for some time (Figure 40). Breathe normally.
6. Exhale, extend the trunk, and bend forward, touching the floor with the forehead, the nose, and lastly, if possible, the chin, in this order. Expand the chest and take the sternum nearer to the ground. Rest the chest on the floor and stretch the back of the trunk.

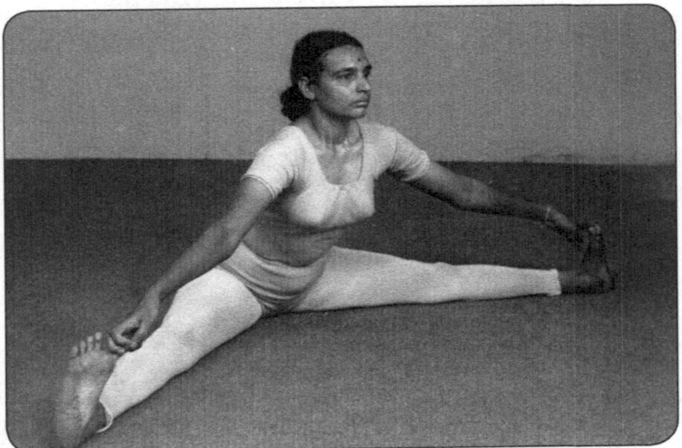

Fig. 40: *Upaviṣṭha Koṇāsana* (Intermediate Stage)

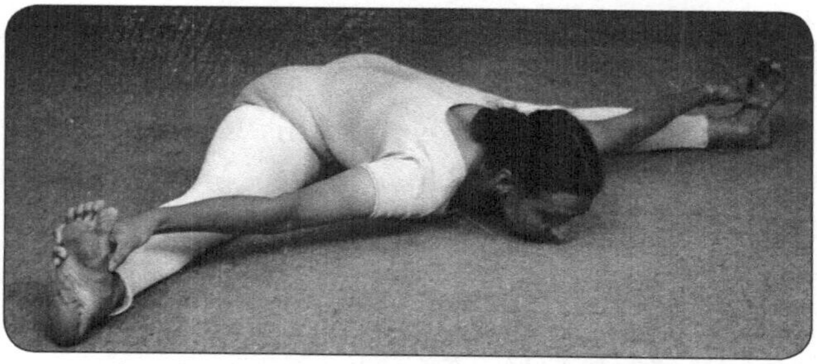

Fig. 41: *Upaviṣṭha Koṇāsana* (Final Stage)

7. Extend the arms and hold the soles of the feet with the hands (Figure 41).
8. This is the final position; remain for 30 to 60 seconds with normal breathing, observing the following points:
   (a) do not lift the thighs off the ground;
   (b) extend the legs further, towards the heels;
   (c) stretch the arms more to broaden the chest;
   (d) extend the trunk forwards, rotating the thighs outwards (towards the outer edges of the legs);
   (e) do not drop the feet to the side.
9. Inhale, raise the head up, release the hands and assume the *Daṇḍāsana* posture (Figure 23).

Special Instructions

1. The entire portion of the back of the legs should touch the ground. The back of the knees have a tendency to bend, so stretch the hamstring muscles.
2. Push the shoulder-blades into the back ribs to open the chest and lift up the front chest so that the gap between the diaphragm and the lower abdomen increases (Figure 40).
3. Do not bend down (Figure 41) until you learn to perfect the position in Figure 40.

Effects: This pose helps the blood to circulate in the pelvic region, regularises the menstrual flow and stimulates the ovaries.

26. *KŪRMĀSANA*

Kūrma means tortoise. This āsana resembles a tortoise and is dedicated to Lord Viṣṇu in his Kūrma incarnation. Legend says that a tortoise balanced the Mandāra mountain on its back. This āsana strengthens the back.

Technique

1. Sit in *Daṇḍāsana* (Figure 23).
2. Spread the legs about 1½ to 2 feet apart.
3. Bend the legs at the knees and raise them a little above the ground.
4. Exhale, bend the trunk forwards, and insert the hands one by one under the knees, then extend the arms sideways. Place the palms on the floor. Now the back of the lower thighs should be resting on the shoulders (Figure 42). Take one or two breaths.
5. Exhale, press the arms under the knees so that they straighten. Rest the chest and the shoulders on the floor. Take a few breaths.

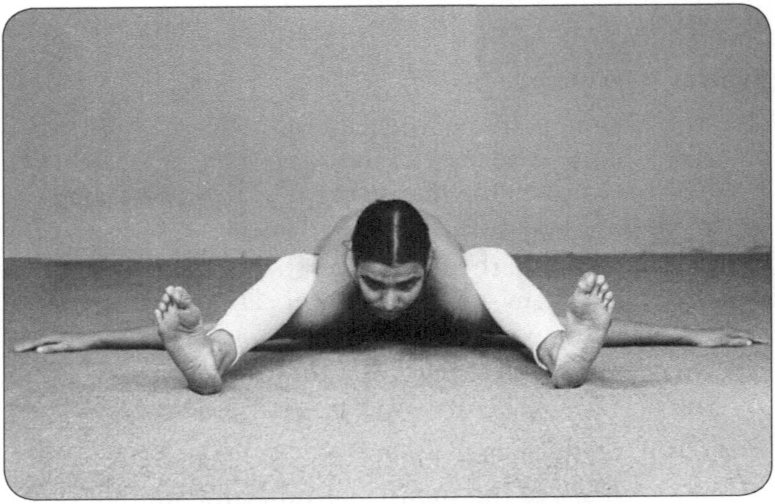

Fig. 42: *Kūrmāsana* (Intermediate Stage)

6. Exhale, extend the trunk forward; the forehead, the nose, and the chin should touch the floor, in that order. Broaden the chest and let it touch the floor (Figure 43).

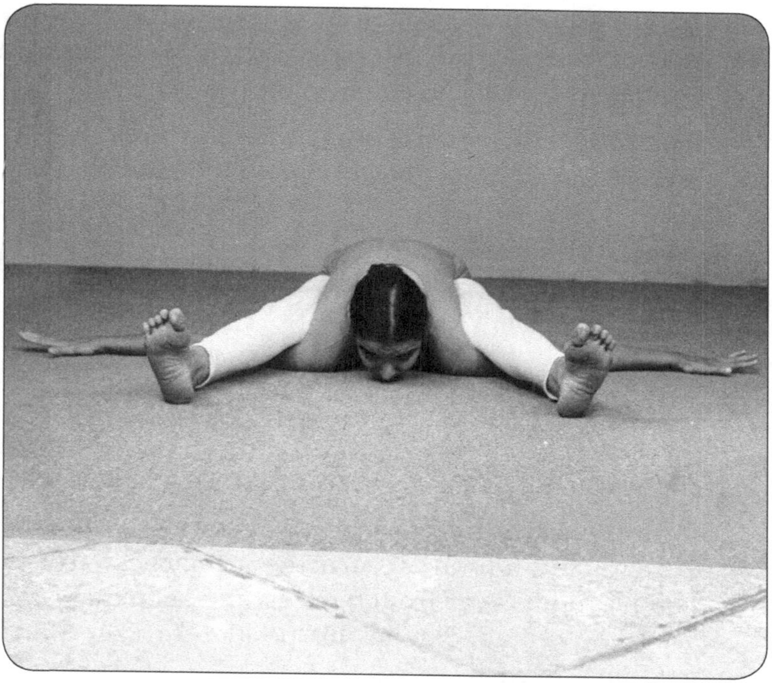

Fig. 43: *Kūrmāsana* (Final Stage)

7. Stay in this final position for 15 to 20 seconds with normal breathing, observing the following points:
   (a) do not allow the distance between the feet to increase;
   (b) press the heels to the ground; do not drop the feet sideways;
   (c) extend the hamstring muscles;
   (d) extend the back of the trunk;
   (e) extend the arms sideways and the legs forwards. Now continue with the next āsana.

27. *SUPTA KŪRMĀSANA*

This āsana resembles a tortoise in a sleeping position with its limbs drawn in. The inner significance of the āsana is the withdrawal of all the senses inside the shield of the back. It is a sacred posture, symbolising the withdrawal of the senses as in pratyāhāra. Lord Kṛṣṇa, while describing the Sthitaprajña (one of stable intellect) to Arjuna, says:

yada saṁharate cāyaṁ kūrmoṅgānīva sarvaśaḥ
indriāṇīndriyārthebhyastasya prajñā pratiṣṭhitā

B.G. II, 58

[He who withdraws his senses from the objects of sense on every side, as a tortoise draws in its limbs, his intelligence is firmly established.]

This āsana helps the mind to be calm and tranquil and aids self-control. It also strengthens the back.

Technique

1. From the position of *Kūrmāsana* (Figure 43) raise the knees slightly upwards, turn the arms backwards so that they point away from the legs, and keep the palms facing the ceiling. Stay in this position for 5 seconds, breathing normally.
2. Bend the elbows, exhale, move the hands towards each other, and entwine the fingers behind the back.
3. Bend the knees and bring the feet nearer the head, lift the left ankle and place it over the right ankle. Now, the hands and the legs seem to be plaited or entwined (Figure 44).
4. Stay in this final position for 5 to 10 seconds, breathing normally and observing the following points:
   (a) tighten the grip on the ankles and hands; do not loosen it;
   (b) watch the firmness and rigidity of the back;

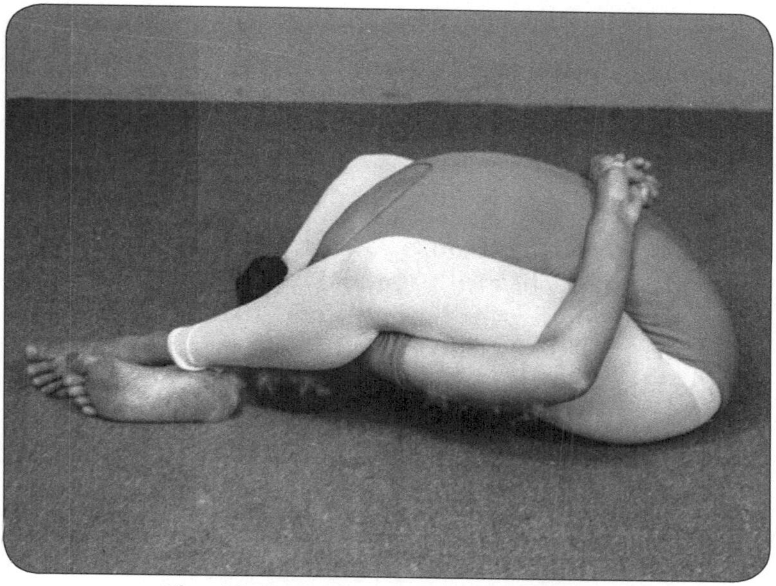

Fig. 44: *Supta Kūrmāsana* (Final Stage)

(c) keeping these grips firm makes the practitioner aware how strong a will-power is needed in order to hold the posture.

5. Release the feet and cross them the other way (right ankle on left). Stay in this position for 5 to 10 seconds, breathing evenly. (By changing the position of the feet, the waist and thighs are exercised equally.)
6. Release the hands and the feet and sit with straight legs as in *Daṇḍāsana* (Figure 23).

Special Instruction

In the beginning, if it is not possible to entwine the fingers behind the back, place the palms on the buttocks.

Effects: These two postures tone the spine, activate the abdominal organs, and keep one energetic. They check the menstrual flow and relieve one from abdominal pains. They make the mind quiet.

28. *MĀLĀSANA*

Mālā means garland. This posture resembles a garland of hands around the body. In its final stage the head is placed on the floor.

Technique

1. Sit in *Daṇḍāsana* (Figure 23). Raise the knees and squat on the haunches with the feet together and the inner sides of the feet, the thighs, and the calves touching each other. The back of the thighs touch the calves and the hinges of the heels.
2. Stretch the arms forward, in line with the shoulders, with the palms facing the floor (Figure 45).
3. Now, take the arms backwards, entwine the shins, and hold the back of the ankles and heels with the hands. Exhale and stretch the spine forward (Figure 46).
4. Stay in this position for 10 to 15 seconds with normal breathing.

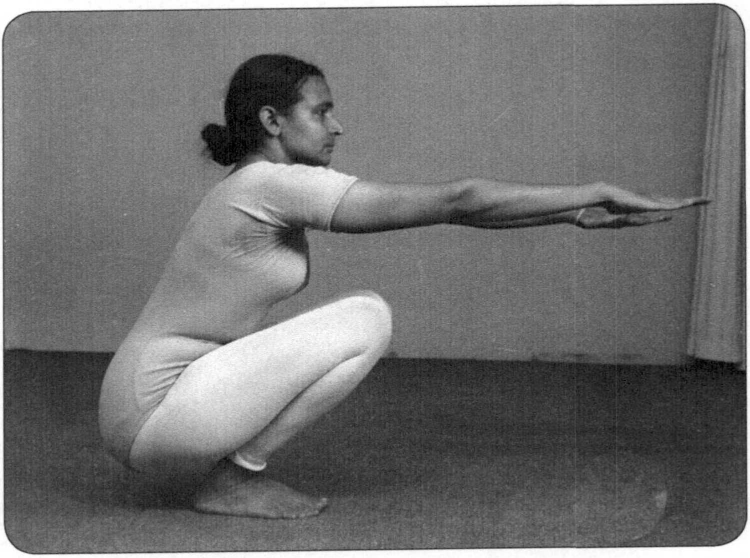

Fig. 45: *Mālāsana* (Intermediate Stage)

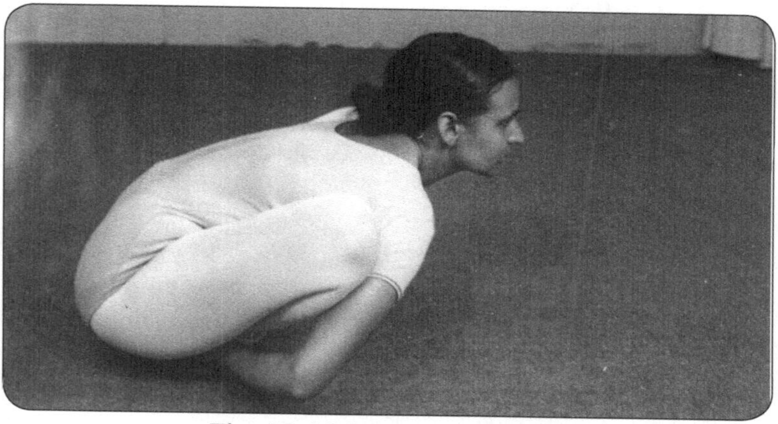

Fig. 46: *Mālāsana* (Easy Stage)

5. Remove the hands from the ankles, bend the trunk forward, take the arms behind the back and clasp your hands. Stretch the spine towards the head so that it is parallel to the floor (Figure 47).
6. Maintain this posture for 10 to 15 seconds, breathing normally. Watch these three points:
   (a) each position is more difficult than the previous one and stretches different parts of the body;

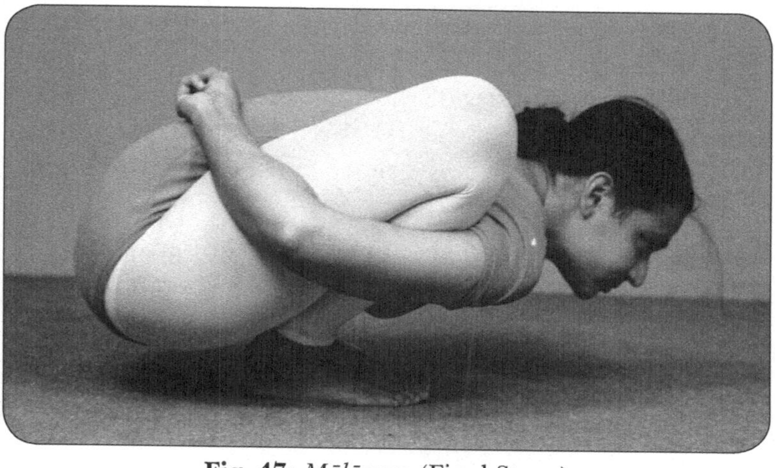

Fig. 47: *Mālāsana* (Final Stage)

(b) watch the range of movement of the ankles;

(c) watch how firmly the palms have to be gripped in order to extend the spine.

7. Release the hands, lift up the trunk, sit on the buttocks, and release the feet.

Special Instructions

1. For those who are overweight, the position shown in Figure 45 is very helpful, as it strengthens the back.
2. Entwine the arms round the legs and rest the head on the knee to relieve backaches.

Effects: This posture is a boon for women as it relieves backache and removes arthritic pains of the knees and the ankles. It is good for providing relief for bleeding piles.

GENERAL EFFECTS OF ĀSANAS 23 to 28

All these āsanas are extremely beneficial for women, especially for those with menstrual problems. With these āsanas the menstrual cycle is regulated and the menstrual disorders are corrected.

These āsanas also tone the abdominal organs, prevent the accumulation of fat in the region of the lower abdomen, and assist in the more efficient functioning of the excretory system.

They strengthen the spine and the muscular system of the lower back and waist. They relieve one from backache and rheumatism.

All these āsanas should be practised regularly and gradually their duration should be increased. They have a soothing and relaxing effect on the brain.

SECTION-III

Āsanas: Sitting and Supine

The āsanas described in this section prepare the body and the mind for prāṇāyāma which leads one further in one's spiritual life. They have a specific role to play in steadying the body and mind to proceed further in the path of Yoga.

Āsanas in the sitting position are necessary for a firm foundation in prāṇāyāma (breath control), dhāraṇā (concentration) and dhyāna (meditation) which lead one towards Samādhi (Self-realisation). They bring firmness of body and steadiness of mind without which self-realisation is impossible. Āsanas in the supine position, bring a soothing sensation to the body and help one recover the lost energy, similar to *Śavāsana* (Figure 212).

These āsanas develop the various actions which are necessary in the practice of prāṇāyāma, dhāraṇā and dhyāna. *Siddhāsana* (Figure 48) and *Padmāsana* (Figure 52) train the body to sit firmly; they extend the spine, bring quietness of the mind, and composure to the body. *Vīrāsana* and cycle (Figures 50, 54, 55), *Parvatāsana* (Figure 59), and *Baddha Padmāsana* (Figure 60) extend and expand the chest so that the thoracic cavity is prepared for breath control; one gains an inner knowledge of how the chest has to function correctly and fully in prāṇāyāma; moreover, one's capacity to sit steadily in an upright position is improved by these postures. Inner control of the spine is gained by the practice of *Yoga Mudrāsana* (Figure 61) which teaches one the anterior extension of the spine as well as giving some control over the movement of the abdominal organs and the diaphragm. In *Supta Vīrāsana* (Figure 58) and *Matsyāsana* (Figure 62) the entire body, from the base of the pelvis to the top of the chest, is extended, bringing control over the pelvic and the thoracic diaphragms which is vital to improve the quality of one's prāṇāyāma practice.

Besides these, each āsana has a particular effect on the body which will be described in the following pages.

29. *SIDDHĀSANA*

Siddha means perfect, accomplished. A Siddha is one who has acquired supernatural powers through penance.

ātmadhyāyī mitāhārī yāvaddvādaśa vatsaram
sadā siddhāsanābhyāsad yogī niṣpattimāpnuyāt

H.P. I, 40

[A Yogi, who contemplates on the Soul, who is moderate in his diet, can attain supernatural powers if he practises *Siddhāsana* for twelve years without break.]

Siddhāsana is one of the important āsanas (the best among 84 lakh āsanas) whose practice purifies the 72,000 nāḍīs in the body. One who has mastered *Siddhāsana* has conquered the Self. It is the most important āsana for breath control, discipline of the senses, concentration, meditation and self-realisation.

Technique

1. Sit in *Daṇḍāsana* (Figure 23).
2. Bend the left leg, hold the left heel, and place it near the perineum. The sole of the left foot should be placed against the right thigh.
3. Bend the right leg and place the right foot on the left ankle; the heel of the right foot should be placed near the pubic bone.
4. Place the right sole and toes between the left thigh and the calf.
5. Lift the lower abdomen so that it does not press on the heel. Keep the heels adjacent to the perineum and the pubic bone.
6. Stretch both the arms. Place the back of the wrists on the knees. Keep the palms open. Breathe evenly.
7. Join the tip of the thumb and the index finger of each hand to form a circle. The other three fingers should be straight and stretched. This is *Jñānamudrā* (Figure 52).

8. The head and the neck should be erect. Close the eyes and look inwards (Figure 48).

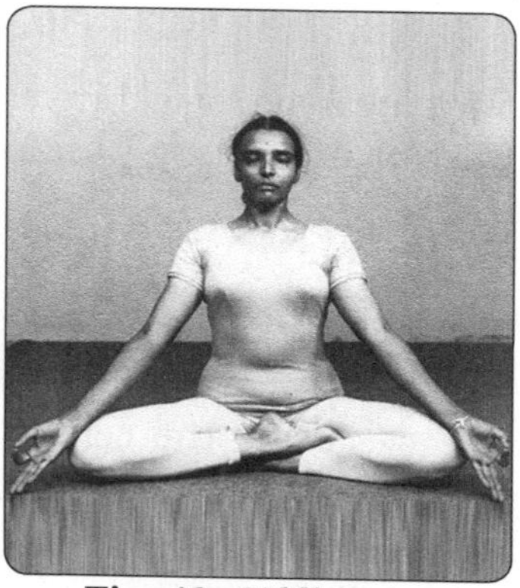

Fig. 48: *Siddhāsana* (Final Stage)

9. Stay in this position for 1 to 5 minutes and later as long as possible and breathe normally, observing the following points:
   (a) straighten the spine; do not bend the lumbar, the lower portion of the back. Keep the sides of the ribs lifted up and both the sides of the trunk parallel to each other;
   (b) keep the shoulder-blades in without tilting the trunk;
   (c) keep both the knees down.
10. Release the right foot and then the left. Now, perform this āsana by bending the right leg first. Stay in the final position as long as possible, for the same length of time, with normal breathing.

Special Instruction

If you find it difficult to straighten the spine, keep a folded blanket under the buttocks. By doing this one relaxes the groins and knees.

Effects: Blood circulates well in the lumbar and the pubic regions. The posture is good for curing stiffness in the knees and the ankles. The erect spine keeps the mind firm, attentive and alert.

30. *VĪRĀSANA*

Vīra means heroic, brave, a hero. This posture resembles a warrior in a sitting position.

Technique

1. Kneel on the floor, keeping the knees together.
2. Take the feet apart and turn them so that the soles are facing the ceiling. Keep the toes and the feet in a straight line, extending backwards.
3. Keep the feet 1 to 1½ feet apart. Lower the buttocks until they rest on the floor, not on the feet. Take one or two breaths.
4. Keep the buttocks touching the floor. The inner side of the calves will now be adjacent to the outer side of the thighs.
5. Turn the palms to face downwards and place them on the knees.
6. Keep the weight of the body on the thighs and raise the waist and the sides of the trunk up.
7. Keep the chest expanded, the neck erect and look straight ahead (Figure 49, side view; Figure 50, front view).
8. Breathe normally and stay in this position for one minute and later as long as possible, observing the following points:
   (a) the body should not lean forwards;
   (b) keep the groins and thighs down.
9. Rest the hands on the floor, lift the buttocks, and come back to a kneeling position. Now, straighten the legs.

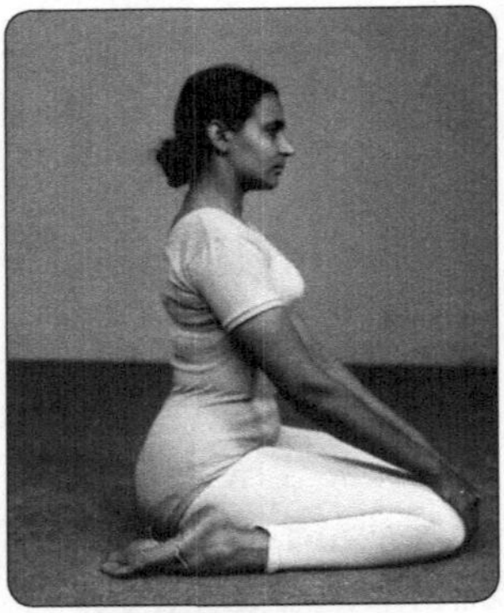

Fig. 49: *Vīrāsana* (Final Stage)

Special Instructions

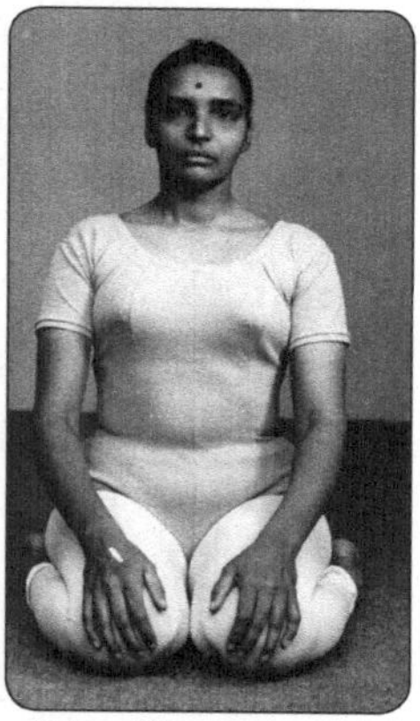

Fig. 50: *Vīrāsana* (Final Stage)

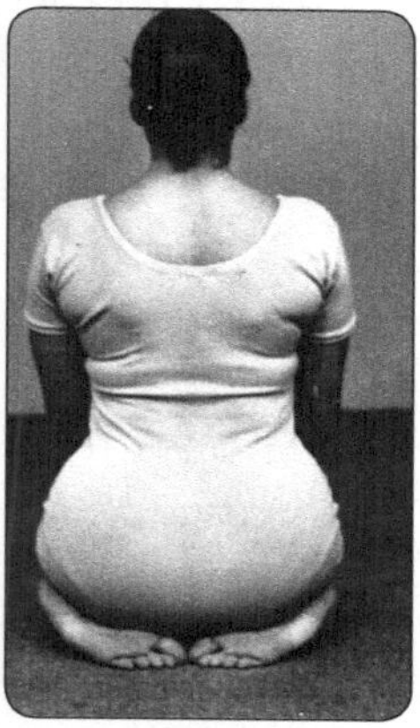

Fig. 51: *Vīrāsana* (Easy Stage)

1. In this āsana there is pressure on the knee and the ankle-joints so that it is sometimes difficult to place the buttocks on the floor. Keep a folded blanket under the buttocks so that the weight of the body is equally distributed in so far as the knees, the feet and the buttocks are concerned. Reduce the height of the blanket gradually (Figure 185).
2. If the legs cannot be bent back, keep them horizontal as in Figure 51. If you find it difficult to bear the weight on the ankles and metatarsals, turn the feet inwards as in Figure 51. This position is suitable for those who have spurs and flat feet.
3. If you find it difficult to keep the body straight, then press the palms firmly on the knees and press the groins down so that the trunk is extended upwards from the base of the pelvis.

Effects: This posture cures rheumatic pains in the knees, relieves gout, helps achieve shapely arches, and is ideal for relieving pain in the feet, the calves, and the heels, for calcaneal spurs and for coldness or exhaustion of the feet. It is good for those who work in water or those who stand for hours on their feet and for inflammation of the blood vessels. This pose can be done with ease even during the menstrual period.

31. *PADMĀSANA*

Padma means lotus. This is the lotus posture, conducive to meditation.

Technique

1. Sit in *Daṇḍāsana* (Figure 23).
2. Bend the right leg using both the hands and place the right foot on the left thigh touching the groin. The toes should remain outside the thigh.
3. Bend the left leg and using both the hands place the left foot on the right thigh, touching the groin. Both the shins will now be crossed. The sides of the heels will touch the pelvis, take one or two breaths.
4. Extend the spine, lift the sides of the trunk upwards, and broaden the chest. Stretch both the arms and place the back of the wrists on the knees. Let the fingers be in *Jñānamudrā* (Figure 52) or keep them crossed, with the palms facing up, on the feet.

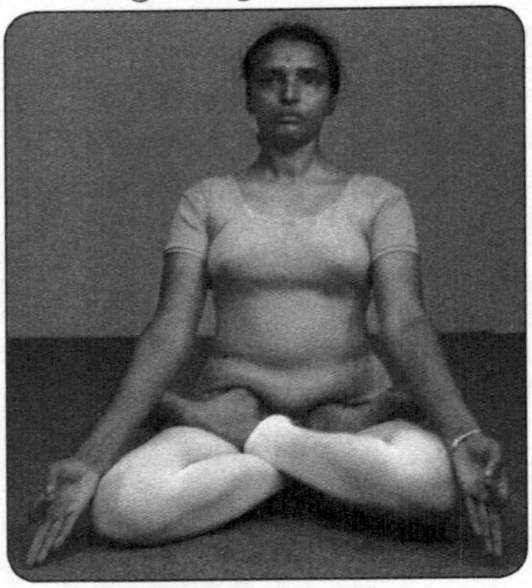

Fig. 52: *Padmāsana* (Final Stage)

5. Breathing normally, remain for 30 to 60 seconds in this final position. Later one can stay as long as possible, observing the following points:
   (a) press the crossed shinbone area firmly so that the spine extends upwards from the base and not from the middle;
   (b) though the top knee (left knee in Figure 25) does not touch the ground, try to lower it as much as you can, but do not loosen the grip on the shins to take the knee down;

(c) let the knees come closer together to enable the spine to extend more from the small of the back,

(d) keep the centre of gravity on the thighs and the crossed shins, but do not allow the body to lean forwards: it should remain L-shaped.

6. Release the left leg with the help of the hands; then release the right leg. Now, perform the āsana by bending the left leg first and then the right. Stay for the same length of time.
7. Uncross the legs and come to *Daṇḍāsana* (Figure 23).

Special Instructions

1. Those whose thighs, knees and ankle joints are not flexible or who are suffering from rheumatism will find *Padmāsana* impossible to perform. They should follow this procedure:

(a) Bend the left leg as in *Siddhāsana* and place it near the right thigh so that the sole remains under the thigh.

(b) Bend the right leg and place it close to the left foot.

(c) Lift the right foot and place it at the root of the left thigh so that the toes do not project beyond the thigh but touch the groin (Figure 53).

(d) Place both the hands on the knees and press them towards the floor so that all joints become loose.

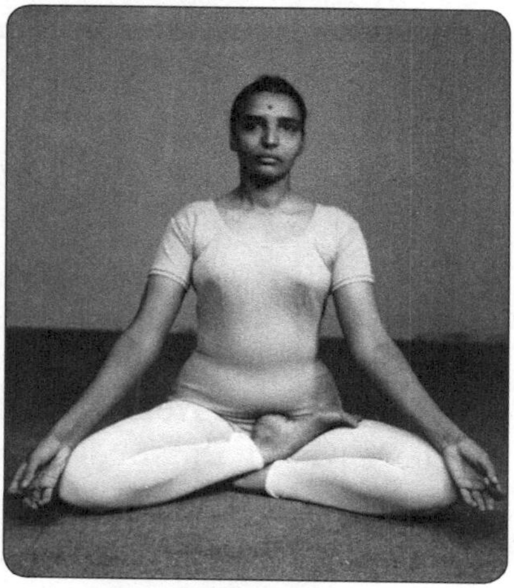

Fig. 53: *Padmāsana* (Easy Stage)

(e) Now, place the right foot as in *Siddhāsana* and the left foot as in *Padmāsana* and press downwards.

2. Often the bending of the knee and the placing of the foot at the root of the opposite thigh is not properly understood. After flexing the knee inwards the calf comes in contact with the back of the thigh. Because of this thickness and hardness, the foot does not reach the groin. In that case one has to keep the hamstrings soft and turn the calf muscles out so that they face the ceiling and do not rub against the thigh; thus tautness is avoided.

Effects: This posture does not allow one to be sloppy. The erect spine keeps the mind alert and attentive.

OVERALL EFFECTS OF ĀSANAS 29 to 31

This trio of āsanas is extremely helpful in breath control, concentration and meditation. All the three are easy to perform and are helpful in keeping the limbs loose and relaxed. The body is still, the mind is calm, alert, and observant, and therefore fit for concentration and meditation. *Padmāsana* is the best of the three āsanas, as the crossed legs exert a downward pressure, bring firmness, and help the upward extension of the spine. *Padmāsana* and *Siddhāsana* are considered sacred.

From the physical point of view alone, these postures are extremely helpful in rheumatism of the knees and the ankles; they create freedom of movement in these joints and improve circulation in the pelvic region. They relieve pain in the small of the back. One can read or knit in this position.

The āsanas which now follow are variations of *Padmāsana* and *Vīrāsana*.

32. *VĪRĀSANA* CYCLE

These are two variations of *Vīrāsana* and both are very useful.

Technique

1. Sit in *Vīrāsana*. Turn the feet backwards and straighten them to be in line with the shins. Keep the knees together (Figures 49, 50). Take a few breaths.
2. Interlock the fingers, turn the wrists out, and extend the arms forward in line with the shoulders.
3. Now, stretch the arms over the head, keeping the palms turned towards the ceiling (Figure 54).
4. Remain in this position for 20 to 30 seconds with normal breathing, observing the following points:
   (a) straighten the arms from the armpits;
   (b) do not bend the elbows;
   (c) keep the shoulder-blades in and the sternum forward and up;

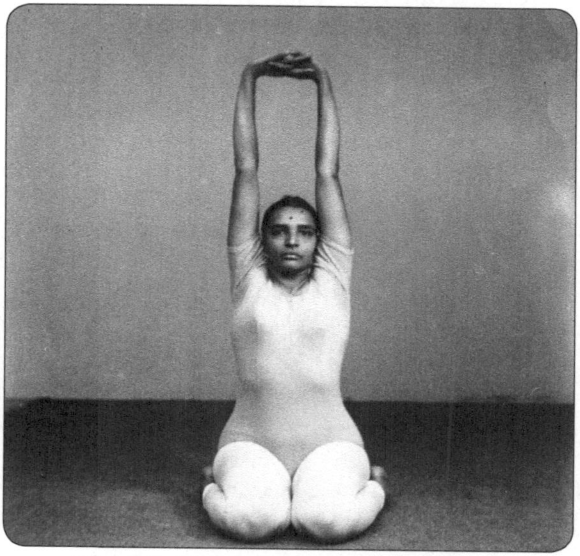

Fig. 54: *Vīrāsana* Cycle (Final Stage)

(d) extend from the floating ribs to the top brim of the chest so that the thoracic cavity extends and expands;

(e) keep the throat relaxed.

5. Exhale and lower the arms.
6. Change the position of the fingers interlocking the other way; repeat the posture and then come back to *Vīrāsana* (Figures 49 and 50).
7. Now, remove the palms from the knees and place them on the soles of the feet with the palms facing down as in Figure 55. Take one or two breaths.
8. Exhale and bend forward towards the thighs. Keep the forehead beyond the knees (Figure 55).
9. Breathe normally in this final position for 30 to 60 seconds and observe the following points:

   (a) do not raise the buttocks and the thighs off the ground;

   (b) do not drop or cave in the chest. The chest should extend from the floating ribs to the top ribs and should remain parallel to the thighs;

   (c) inhale and raise the trunk up, keeping the spine concave;

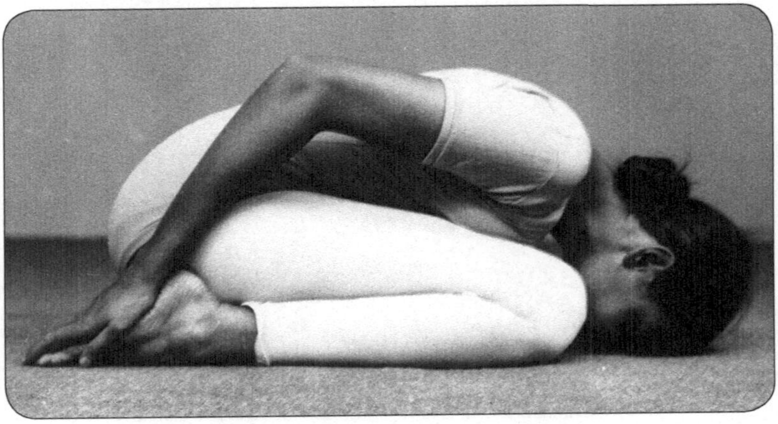

Fig. 55: *Vīrāsana* Cycle (Final Stage)

(d) release the palms, straighten the legs, and come to *Daṇḍāsana* (Figure 23).

Special Instructions

1. According to habit one interlocks the fingers either keeping the left thumb at the free end of the hand, or the right thumb. Observe which thumb comes first when you take the arms up the first time so that you can change the interlock while taking the arms up for the second time.
   - This change in the interlock of the fingers gives one different stretches of the hands and the arms and makes one use unused muscles.
   - Women suffering from arthritic or swollen fingers should perform this version of the āsana and should follow the same technique when performing *Vṛkṣāsana* (Figure 2) and *Parvatāsana* (Figure 59).
   - If interlocking the fingers is difficult, then keep the arms extended over the head with the palms facing forward.
2. If the throat muscles are tensed, bend the head down from the nape of the neck so that it becomes soft. This is especially useful for those with thyroid disorders.
3. Those suffering from backache or unable to bend forward, should keep the knees and the thighs apart; then, stretching the arms up by the side of the head, they should go down, placing the hands on the floor and resting the chest between the thighs. This also brings the breath and blood pressure to normal.
4. The *Vīrāsana* cycle can be performed sitting in the position as in Figure 51, if one has injured the ligaments of the knees.

Effects: This pose relieves backaches and arthritis of the shoulders, the elbows and the fingers.

33. *SUPTA VĪRĀSANA*

This āsana is a variation of *Vīrāsana* and is performed lying on the back.

Technique

1. Sit in *Vīrāsana* (Figures 49 and 50). Hold the ankles with the hands. Take a few breaths.
2. Exhale and lean the trunk backwards so that the back and the waist go down towards the floor. Rest the elbows on the floor, one by one; now the elbows and the forearms are resting on the floor.
3. Lean back further until the crown of the head is on the floor (Figure 56).

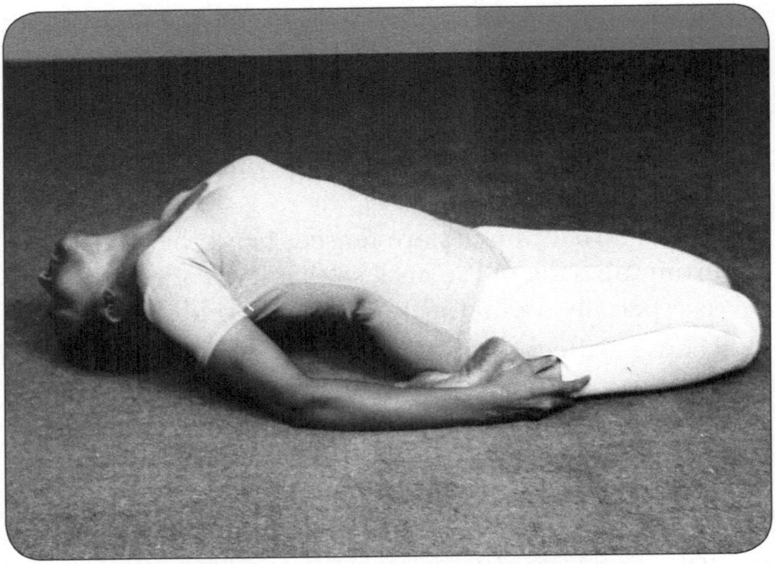

Fig. 56: *Supta Vīrāsana* (Intermediate Stage)

4. Release the back and place the back of the head, the shoulders, and the trunk on the floor. Straighten the arms by the sides of the legs and stay for 15 seconds (Figure 57). Take a breath or two.

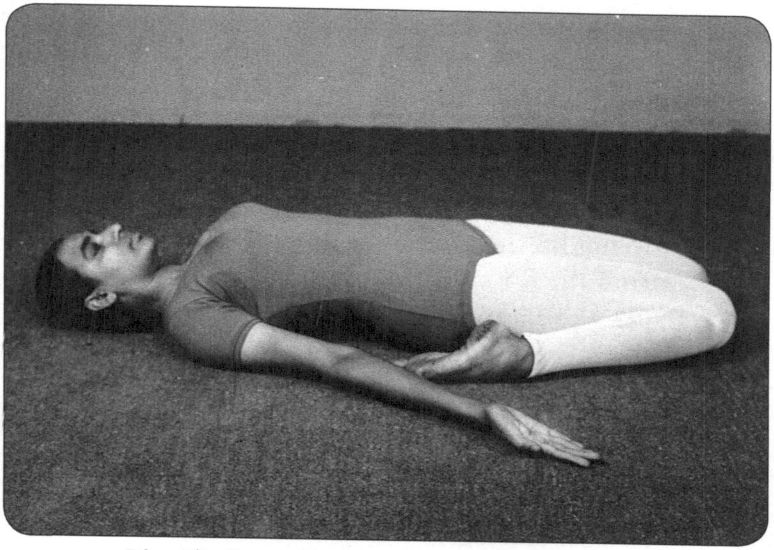

Fig. 57: *Supta Vīrāsana* (Intermediate Stage)

5. Extend the arms over the head with the palms facing the ceiling (Figure 58).

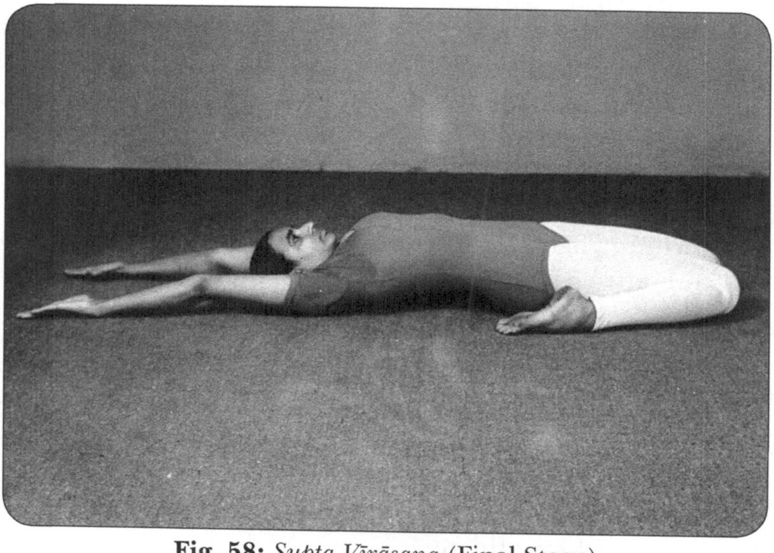

Fig. 58: *Supta Vīrāsana* (Final Stage)

6. Stay in this position for 30 to 60 seconds and later as long as possible, breathing normally, observing the following points:
   (a) stretch the extensors of the arms so that the thighs and the abdomen are massaged and pulled towards the chest;
   (b) do not lift the knees, the buttocks, or the shoulders from the floor:
   (c) take the shoulder-blades in and open the chest;
   (d) the posterior and the anterior trunk should be extended evenly.
7. Bring the hands towards the feet and hold the ankles. Lift the head and the trunk off the ground, supporting yourself on your elbows. Sit in *Vīrāsana* (Figures 49 and 50). Release the legs.

Special Instructions

1. In the initial stages, the knees tend to remain apart. With regular practice it is easy to keep them together.
2. Due to obesity or tension in the thighs and the knees it may be difficult to recline backwards sufficiently. Put a pillow or blanket 4″ to 5″ thick to support the back and the head so that the thighs and the buttocks rest on the floor and the chest is expanded. With this method the tension of the muscles is reduced (Figure 186). Avoid reclining backwards while the feet are in the position as in Figure 51, since one is likely to injure the ankles.

Effects: *Supta Vīrāsana* (Figure 58) stretches the abdomen, the back and the waist. It aids digestion and may be done after heavy meals to obtain lightness in the stomach. It is extremely useful in cases of acidity, rheumatism, stomach-ache, pain in the back, asthma, ulcers, heartburn, disorder of the ovaries and inflammation of the nerves. The āsana is also very good for athletes.

Padmāsana Cycle

34. *PARVATĀSANA*

Parvata means mountain. This āsana is a variation of *Padmāsana*. Here the hands are interlocked and raised above the head.

Technique

1. Sit in *Padmāsana* (Figure 52). Take a few breaths.
2. Interlock the fingers and turn the wrists so that the palms too will be turned out. Keep the arms stretched forward in line with the shoulders.
3. Inhale and raise the arms over the head, perpendicular to the ground and in line with the shoulders (Figure 59).
4. Stretch the arms so that the elbows are straight.

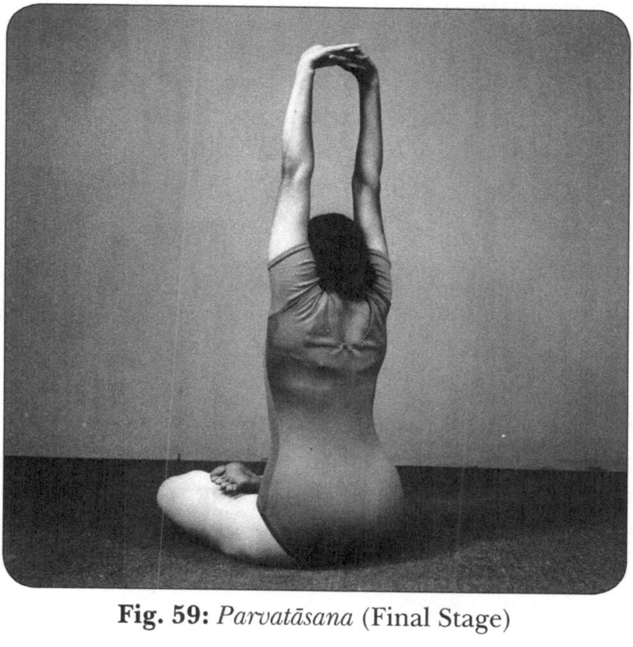

Fig. 59: *Parvatāsana* (Final Stage)

5. Breathing normally, stay in this position for 30 to 60 seconds, observing the following points:
   (a) stretch the sides of the trunk so that the spine is extended;
   (b) tuck the shoulder-blades in;
   (c) expand the chest;
   (d) keep the thighs firm and pressed into the floor to extend the trunk upward.
6. Exhale and bring the arms down, change the interlock, and repeat the posture.
7. Now, perform the āsana, with the legs crossed the other way, following Techniques 2 to 6. However, stay for the same length of time. Bring the arms down and come to *Daṇḍāsana*.

Special Instruction

The arms can be raised over the head in another way. Interlock the fingers and turn the palms up. Rest the back of the hands on the head with the elbows bent outward, then extend the arms towards the ceiling. This method is useful for those with a hunchback. However, it is an advanced method and the first method should be perfected before the advanced one is used. The first method is appropriate when there is neck or back sprain.

Effects: This āsana relieves rheumatic pains and stiffness in the shoulders.

Note: Once this and the following āsanas are mastered, they should be done one after the other without changing the position of the legs in *Padmāsana* (Figure 52). When one cycle of postures has been completed with the legs crossed one way, then all the poses have to be repeated with the legs crossed the other way.

35. *BADDHA PADMĀSANA*

In this āsana the arms are crossed behind the back, the legs are crossed in front, and the toes are caught by the hands—all making a belt round the waist. The posture is a variation of *Padmāsana*.

Technique

1. Sit in *Padmāsana* (Figure 52). Take a few breaths.
2. Exhale and swing the left arm behind the back and bring it near the right hip. Hold the left big toe with the fore-middle fingers. While swinging the left arm, the back will turn slightly to the left. Correct the position by keeping the chest forward. Take one or two breaths.
3. Swing the right arm backwards and hold the right big toe. Bend the trunk slightly forward to make it easier to catch the big toe (Figure 60).

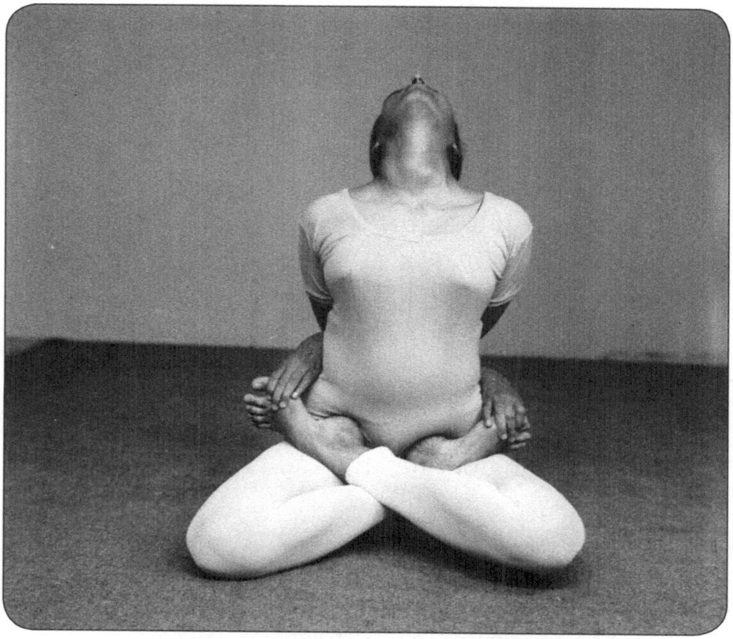

Fig. 60: *Baddha Padmāsana* (Final Stage)

4. Keep the trunk erect and throw the head back.
5. Remain in this final stage for 20 to 30 seconds, breathing normally, observing the following points:
   (a) tuck the shoulder-blades in;
   (b) expand and broaden the chest;
   (c) keep the spine extended;
   (d) raise the sternum while bending the head backwards;
   (e) do not loosen the grip of the fingers on the toes.
6. Inhale, raise the head up, and perform the āsanas on the other side, changing the *Padmāsana* and the arms. Stay for the same length of time, then release the arms and the legs, or proceed to the next āsana.

Special Instructions

1. In the initial stages it will be difficult to catch the toes. Swing the arms back as far as possible and try to hold the garment which you are wearing, or the big toe of the foot which is above, as for example the left big toe in Figure 60 or the right big toe if *Padmāsana* is changed. When the shoulder-joint becomes more flexible it will be possible to hold both the toes at the same time.
2. If *Padmāsana* is performed by crossing the left foot first, then catch the left big toe first and the right toe afterwards; do not catch the right toe first and then the left toe.

Effects: The chest is expanded fully so that one can breathe easily. The thyroids is massaged and the fat around the waist and the hips remains in check.

36. *YOGA MUDRĀSANA*

Mudrā means seal, closing, or control. This āsana is a variation of *Baddha Padmāsana* with a forward bend.

Technique

1. Adopt the position of *Baddha Padmāsana* (Figure 60). Keep the head up, breathing normally.
2. Exhale, extend the trunk forward, and place the forehead on the floor (Figure 61).
3. Stay in this position for 20 to 30 seconds, breathing normally, observing the following points:
   (a) in the initial stage as you bend forward, the big toes tend to slip from the fingers; keep a firm grip on them;
   (b) one can hold the frontal foot instead of the toes (Figure 61).

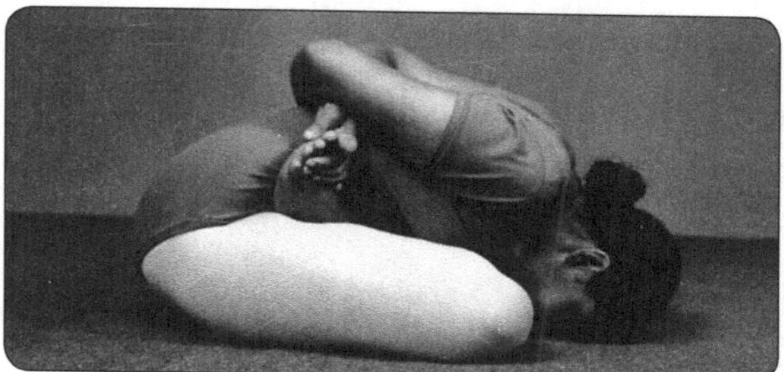

Fig. 61: *Yoga Mudrāsana* (Final Stage)

4. Inhale, lift the head and trunk up, come to *Baddha Padmāsana* (Figure 60), and release the hands and the legs.
5. Repeat the āsana on the other side, changing the *Padmāsana* and the arms. Stay for the same length of time.

Effects: This āsana increases the peristaltic movement, gives good relief from constipation and increases digestive power.

37. *MATSYĀSANA*

This āsana is dedicated to Matsya (fish)—the first incarnation of Lord Viṣṇu.

In this āsana, which is performed lying on the floor, the body forms a slight arch from the waist to the neck and the back of the head rests on the floor. The legs are crossed and held by the hands. But the technique is simplified here to suit the needs of women.

Technique

1. Sit in *Padmāsana* (Figure 52).
2. Exhale, lower the trunk and the waist backwards, place the elbows on the floor, one by one. Incline the trunk still further until the crown of the head reaches the ground.
3. Place the back of the head on the floor and take the trunk down towards the floor. See that the back remains close to the ground and that an arch is not formed. Breathe normally.
4. Extend the arms over the head and straighten them. Keep the palms facing the ceiling. Look up towards the ceiling (Figure 62).
5. Stay in this position for 20 to 30 seconds, breathing normally, observing the following points:
   (a) stretch the arms from the back as well as from the sides of the trunk;

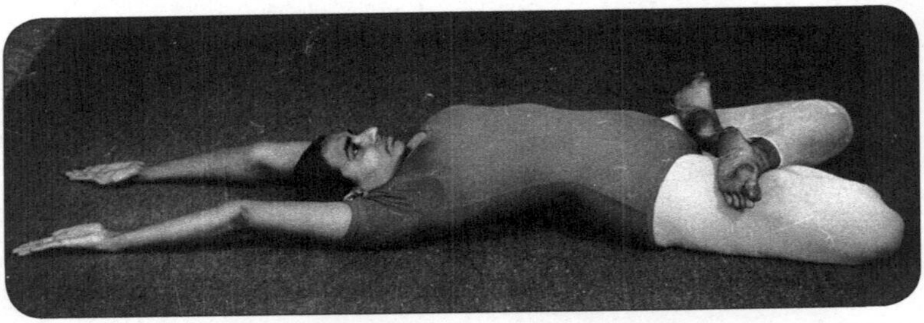

Fig. 62: *Matsyāsana* (Final Stage)

(b) expand the chest;
(c) keep the crossing of the ankles firm.

6. Bring the arms towards the sides of the trunk, press the elbows and the hands into the ground, swing the head and the trunk up and sit in *Padmāsana* (Figure 52). Release the legs. Come to *Daṇḍāsana* (Figure 23), change the position of the legs in *Padmāsana* and repeat the pose on the other side, staying for the same length of time.

Special Instructions

1. As soon as the back touches the floor, sometimes the knees come off. This happens if the buttocks are heavy or if the movement in the sacrum and the coccyx is limited. It may also happen that the shoulders are lifted up if the knees rest on the floor. In that case, place a blanket 4 or 5 inches thick under the waist as mentioned in *Supta Vīrāsana* (Figure 186).
2. Those who find it difficult to swing and raise the trunk up may uncross the legs while lying down.

Effects: This āsana relieves bleeding and inflamed piles; it relaxes the thyroid.

OVERALL EFFECTS OF ĀSANAS 34 to 37

Padmāsana and its variations are effective in curing rheumatism of the shoulders, the elbows, the wrists, and the fingers. They help stretch the spinal column, broaden the chest and cure hunchback. The abdomen, the pelvis and the waist are nicely stretched, causing improved blood circulation. The āsanas are also excellent for relief from stomach-ache, acidity, indigestion, irritation of the liver, the spleen and the gall-bladder, ulcers, backache, menstrual disorders and asthma.

This may be done during menstruation.

SECTION-IV

Āsanas: Inverted

The āsanas in this section are very important, though they are difficult to perform. Many of the diseases of the body and mind are cured by their practice; they help foster an attitude of non-attachment and forbearance. It is essential to master these āsanas and their variations to make our lives materially and spiritually successful. They can be compared to our parents who help us, guide us, and make our lives a success.

38. *SĀLAMBA ŚĪRṢĀSANA*

This is the headstand, which gives balance and equipoise. There are two basic variations—sālamba meaning with support, and niralāmba meaning without support. It is sufficient for women to do *Śīrṣāsana* with support. Read the following instructions carefully before you practise this āsana. Before you start to learn it, however, see that you have mastered all āsanas in Section I and *Sālamba Sarvāṅgāsana* (Figure 84) and *Halāsana* (Figure 88) in this section. It is even easier and safer to maintain balance in *Śīrṣāsana* after gaining proficiency in *Sarvāṅgāsana* and its first five variations. If *Sarvāṅgāsana* is faulty, *Śīrṣāsana* cannot be correct and errors in performing it are difficult to rectify. Bear in mind the following:

1. It is essential to keep the spine straight in this āsana.
2. Once *Śīrṣāsana* has become part of the routine, always practise it before other āsanas, because if other āsanas cause fatigue, then one is liable to get breathless and tremors. It is difficult to maintain balance in such a condition.
3. *Śīrṣāsana* must be followed by *Sarvāṅgāsana*. This is very important. If *Śīrṣāsana* is done alone, without being

followed by *Sarvāṅgāsana*, it will lead to an irritated state of mind and a loss of temper, besides creating emotional imbalance. Therefore, practising *Śīrṣāsana* alone is not good and should be avoided.

4. The duration of both these āsanas should be equal. It is not harmful if *Sālamba Sarvāṅgāsana* is done a little longer, but it should not be the other way round.
5. Technique A should be practised by beginners. One should not jump up and down several times in succession to attempt the āsana; it is a wrong way to practise. The āsana should be attempted only once in one practice session, though it may be done twice a day if one practises morning and evening.
6. Three varieties of technique are given here, which should be followed serially; first, Technique A is to be mastered, then B, and finally C.

Technique A

1. In the initial stages it is helpful to have an assistant. A wall is necessary or, better still, an intersection of two walls or a comer. If *Śīrṣāsana* is performed with the support of a wall balance may be maintained, but the trunk and the legs will not be in line with the head. This maladjustment in alignment is avoided in a corner (Figure 65).
2. Fold a blanket four times and spread it in a corner; let it touch both the walls. Kneel on the floor as in *Vīrāsana* (Figure 49), facing the corner.
3. Interlock the fingers to the pits and keep the thumbs touching each other; this forms a semicircular cup. Place the cupped hands 2 to 3 inches away from the corner. The little fingers and the thumbs should run parallel to each other. If the hands are kept more than

3 inches away from the corner, the following mistakes will occur in the final pose:

(a) the spinal column will bend, losing its extension;
(b) the stomach will protrude;
(c) the weight of the body will fall on the elbows and they will ache;
(d) the eyes will puff and swell;
(e) the face will turn red.

4. Rest the forearms on the blanket so that the elbows remain in line with each other; the wrists should be upright with the ulna touching the blanket and the radius directly above (Figure 63).

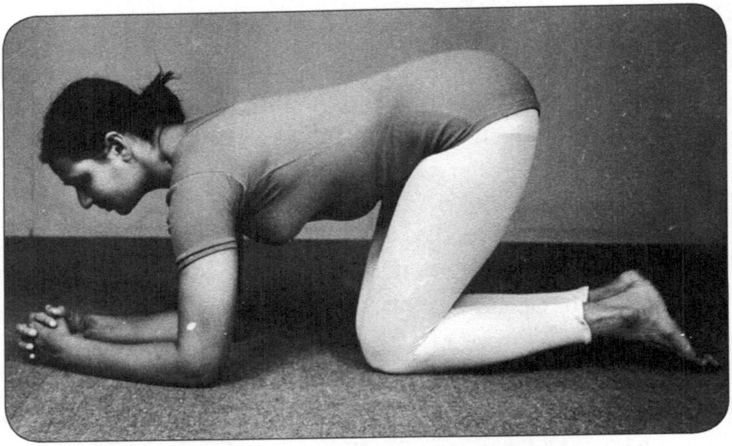

Fig. 63: *Sālamba Śīrṣāsana* (Intermediate Stage)

5. The distance between the elbows should be as wide as the shoulders so that the arms remain straight, slanting neither inwards nor outwards. If the distance between the elbows is too small, this will exert pressure on the side ribs, causing chest pain; if it is too great, the chest will not expand and there will be pressure on the cervical vertebrae.
6. In this position the palms, the forearms, and the space between the elbows and the chest form an equilateral

triangle. Do not move the elbows and the forearms once they are finally adjusted.

7. Raise the buttocks so that the elbow joints and the shoulders are in line with each other and the head is in line with the palms, as in Figure 63. Breathe normally.
8. Exhale and place the crown of the head on the blanket so that the back of the skull remains parallel to the wall and just slightly away from the little fingers so that they do not get pressed underneath the head. Do not keep the head in the cup of the palms—that is wrong. Keep the back of the head adjacent to the cup of the palms. Do not press the head between the wrists. The ears should be parallel to each other (Figure 64). Remain in this position and take a few breaths.
9. Exhale and raise the knees, keeping the toes on the floor. Now straighten the legs and bring the feet in. The trunk should be at right angles to the floor.
10. Keep the legs firm and pull the knee-caps (Figure 64a). Stay in this position for a few seconds and breathe normally.
11. Let an assistant stand to your right or left and support your shins and thighs with her hand. Exhale and move the buttocks towards the corner without bending the

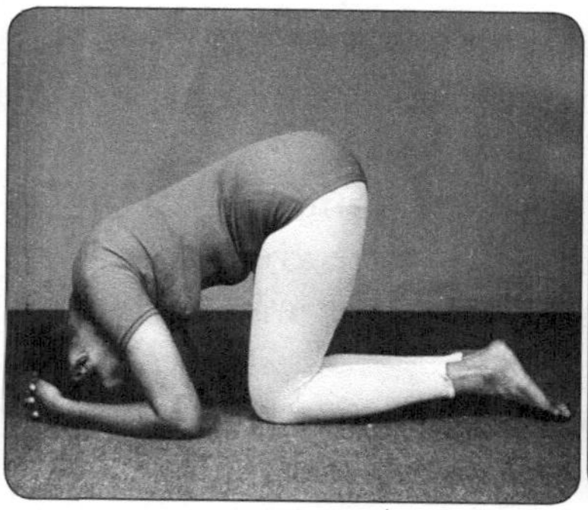

Fig. 64: *Sālamba Śīrṣāsana* (Intermediate Stage)

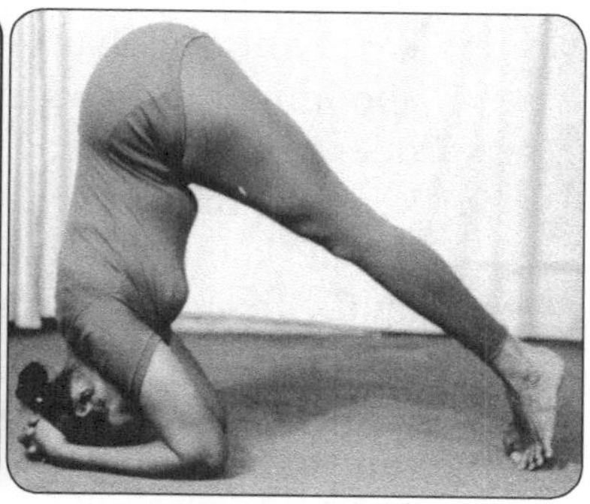

Fig. 64(a): *Sālamba Śīrṣāsana* (Intermediate Stage)

spine. Ask the helper to lift your legs and trunk until the legs rest against the wall in *Śīrṣāsana*. Now, support your trunk against the two walls of the corner. Do not put the weight of your body on the hands of the helper, but on the wall. The outer sides of the heels should touch both the walls (Figure 65).

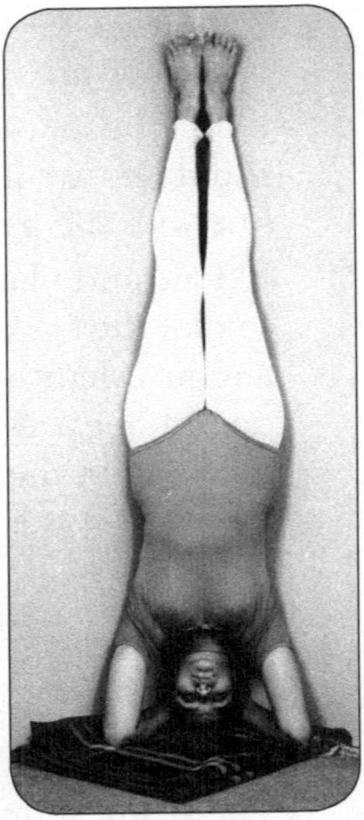

Fig. 65: *Sālamba Śīrṣāsana* (Easy Stage)

12. Now, try to take the buttocks off the wall and learn to bear the weight on the arms, the head and the trunk. Constant support of the wall will lead to a bent spine, so you must learn to leave it. Stay as long as you can, at least one minute, in this final position of *Śīrṣāsana*, breathing normally, and observe the following points:
    (a) lift up the sternum so that the cervical vertebrae are not compressed and the weight of the body is not felt on the head;
    (b) lift the side ribs up and broaden the chest so that the dorsal vertebrae remain concave;
    (c) keep the lumbar vertebrae erect so that the abdominal muscles are stretched and the stomach does not protrude;
    (d) keep the buttocks a little away from the wall so that the neck and the small of the back are balanced;
    (e) let the heels take the support of the wall so that you do not lose balance.
13. As you gain confidence and control, gradually increase the time to five minutes, doing normal breathing.
14. Exhale and rest the buttocks on the wall. Let the assistant hold your shins and thighs, gently lower the

legs and rest them on the floor. Wait for a few moments, raise the head, and then release the hands.

After gaining proficiency in this method of practising *Śīrṣāsana*, gradually increase the duration. If you do not get pain in your head, neck or spine, learn to master Technique B (Pain comes when the chest is not properly lifted up.) However, in case you lack the confidence, concentrate on the position as in Figure 64a. The spinal muscles are strengthened in this position. The weight of the body is shifted from the legs to the trunk and this enables the assistant to help you easily.

Technique B

1. Follow the procedure in Technique A from 1 to 10 (Figures 63, 64, 64a).
2. Bend the knees slightly, exhale, lift both the legs with a jump, and support the back and the buttocks against the wall. In this position the spine may be leaning backwards and has to be extended up. At this moment the legs are bent at the knees.
3. Lift the feet up and rest them against the wall; straighten the legs into *Śīrṣāsana*. In this position the buttocks, the back of the legs, and the heels will be in contact with the wall. The legs should be straightened within a few seconds of jumping into head-balance.
4. This is the final position. Now follow all the instructions given in Technique A 12, breathing normally.
5. Take one foot 3 to 4 inches away from the wall to learn to balance. Keep the leg straight. Tighten the buttocks and bring the other leg in line with the first leg. Learn to keep balance. In the beginning you will be able to balance for 10 to 15 seconds. As soon as you feel that you are losing balance, support the legs on the wall. Then again move the legs away from the wall for a moment and balance. Breathe normally throughout.

6. Come down gradually, following the techniques in reverse order as in Figures 66, 64a, 64. After coming down wait for 5 to 10 seconds before raising the head up.

With the help of this technique, you will learn (a) to jump off the floor and raise both the legs up and (b) to reach the final stage of the āsana without the support of the wall.

After gaining mastery in the above technique, learn Technique C.

Technique C

1. Follow the instructions given in Technique A, 1 to 10, Figures 63, 64, 64a, but without using a wall.
2. Bend the knees slightly; exhale and with a jump raise both the legs up. If the spine leans slightly backwards it has to be brought forward to keep it erect. Lift the knees up so that the thighs are parallel to the floor.
3. Keep the trunk in line with the head (Figure 66). Do not allow the buttocks to drop backwards; keep them in line with the head, otherwise you will topple back. If the buttocks incline forwards, or if they are in line with the elbows or are loose, you will tend to fall forwards. Therefore, when you lift the feet off the ground, the entire action should be upwards—the spine, the buttocks, the thighs, the knees, and the feet all have to be moving upwards so that the weight of the body does not fall on the head and the hands.

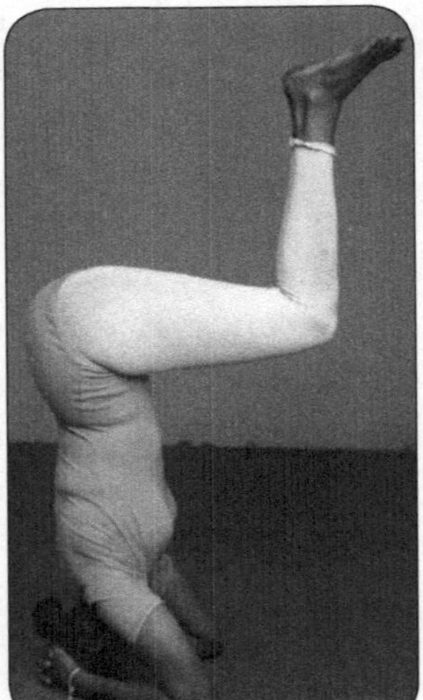

Fig. 66: *Sālamba Śīrṣāsana* (Intermediate Stage)

4. Continue the upward motion, lift the knees up to face the ceiling so that the portion from the navel to the knees remains erect. The lower legs are now bent backwards. Tighten the buttock muscles and tuck the buttocks (Figure 67). The portion from the head to the knees should be in line. Stay in this position for a while, breathing normally.
5. Keeping the body firm from the head to the knees, raise the lower legs up to be in line with the thighs (Figure 68). Extend the shins and the calves completely into *Śīrṣāsana* (Figure 69 side view, Figure 70 front view).
6. The upward movement of *Śīrṣāsana* is thus as follows: The moment the feet are off the floor, keep the movement of the trunk upwards from armpits to buttocks, then from groins to knees, and lastly from knees to feet.
7. Stay in this final position for 5 minutes with normal breathing. Increase this period if possible. *Śīrṣāsana* is

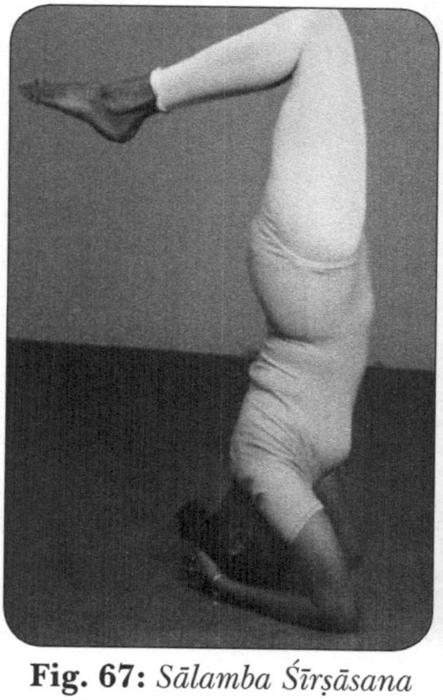

Fig. 67: *Sālamba Śīrṣāsana* (Intermediate Stage)

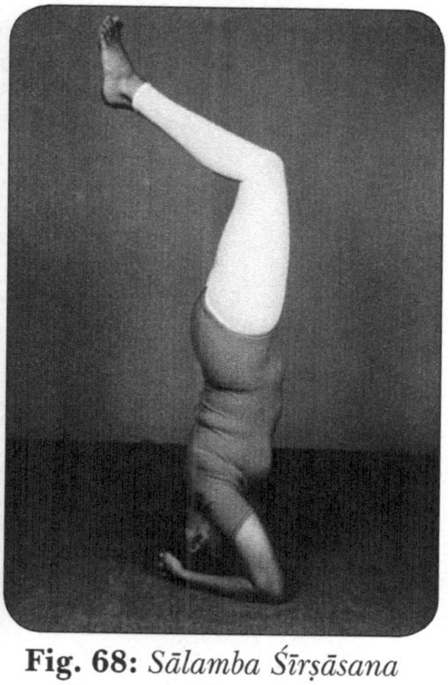

Fig. 68: *Sālamba Śīrṣāsana* (Intermediate Stage)

not just balancing on the head. It should be as natural as standing on the feet. Observe the following points:

(a) press the elbow joints and the forearms down; keep the elbows firm and do not move them; lift the shoulders and the armpits so that the weight does not fall on the ears and neck; keep the shoulders well away from the wrists;

(b) broaden the intercostal muscles and lift them up; keep the armpits well opened and extended upwards;

(c) to lift the sternum and broaden the chest, tuck in the dorsal spine and the shoulder-blades without disturbing the head and the neck;

(d) keep the sides of the trunk lifted up;

(e) keep the middle of the thighs and the knees in line with each other;

(f) press the buttocks together; keep the thighs together and lift the inner sides of the thighs up;

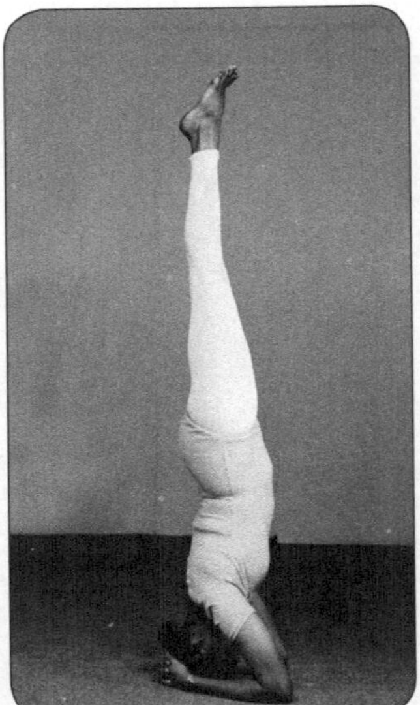

Fig. 69: *Sālamba Śīrṣāsana* (Final Stage)

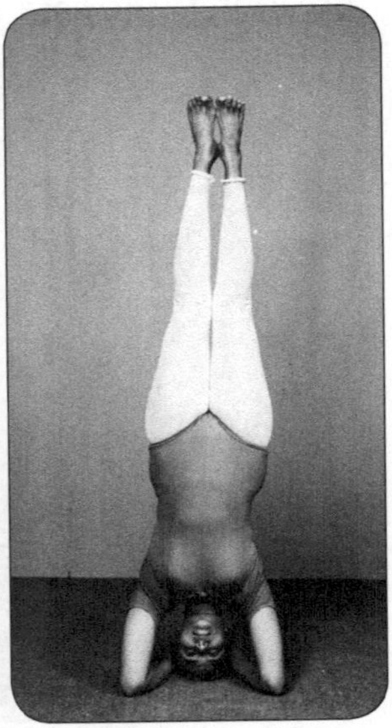

Fig. 70: *Sālamba Śīrṣāsana* (Final Stage)

(g) let the ankles and the toes touch each other; straighten the feet so that they are in line with the legs and not turning in or out and point the toes upwards.

8. Exhale, bend the knees, and come to the position as in Figure 67. Bring the thighs parallel to the floor (Figure 66). Do not jerk the spine, the neck, and the head; rest the toes on the floor (Figure 64a). Bend the knees and kneel on the floor (Figure 64). Wait in this position for 5 to 10 seconds. Lift the head and unlock the fingers.

Advanced Technique

After mastering *Śīrṣāsana* as described above, you may wish to proceed to learn the advanced method. Usually, however, this takes a long time to master. It is given here for those who are interested to intensify their sādhanā. The prerequisites are a strong spine and a strong waist, as the legs are taken up without a jump while being kept straight.

1. Follow the instructions given in Technique A, 1 to 10 (Figure 64a).
2. Exhale, straighten the legs and lift them up. Bring them to a position parallel to the floor. Take a few breaths.
3. Again exhale, lift the legs right up, and come to the final position of *Śīrṣāsana* (Figures 69 side view, 70 front view). Remain for 5 to 10 minutes, breathing normally.
4. Exhale and keeping the legs straight come down without jerking the spine. Release the hands, wait for a few seconds, then raise the head up.

Special Instructions

1. Learn to balance the body using the crown of the head as one pole and the centre of the arches of the feet as

For more details, see description and photograph in *Light on Yoga*.

the other pole. These two should be parallel to each other and perpendicular to the floor.

2. Bear the weight of the body on the head and not on the hands and elbows.
3. While practising *Śīrṣāsana* without the support of a wall, if you think you are losing balance, bend the knees towards the abdomen (Figure 66) and release the hands. Slide down backwards from the neck to the trunk so that you do not fall down with a thud.
4. Those suffering from heaviness or irritation in the uterus, discharge or other menstrual disorders, or hernia should keep the heels apart and the toes touching each other in *Śīrṣāsana*; this will ease the pressure on the uterus and the groins. The knees should also be kept slightly apart (Figure 70a).

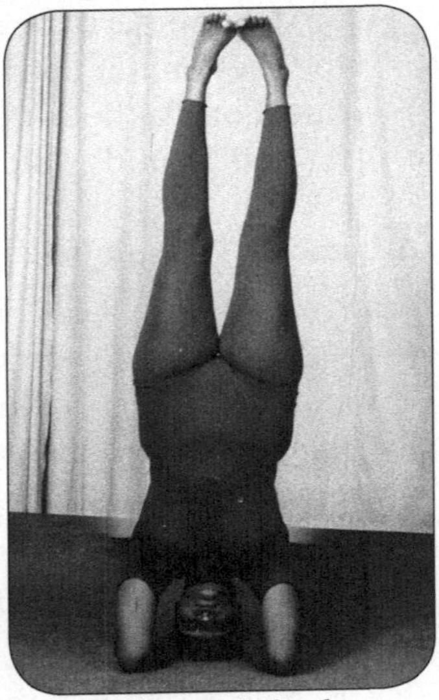

Fig. 70(a): *Sālamba Śīrṣāsana* (Final Stage)

Effects: *Śīrṣāsana* is termed the King of Āsanas. Like the king rules his subjects, the brain rules the numerous systems of the body. It is the controller of the intellect, the will, the memory, the imagination, and the thinking. The origin of the three guṇas is in the brain, the head being the centre of sattvic qualities. It controls the intellect and discrimination. Hence, a brain dominated by sattva can function with clarity.

Śīrṣāsana stimulates the blood supply to the brain and makes it fresh and healthy. It activates the pituitary and pineal glands which affect the health, vitality and development of our body. It is one of the most invigorating of all the āsanas.

The practice of head-balance, if correctly performed, rejuvenates and revitalises the whole body. The upside-down position counteracts the effects of the normal upright position on the internal organs, which have a tendency to drop and to sag and thus to become sluggish. The *Śīrṣāsana* position gently coaxes them to a new life. The body is kept warm with increased blood circulation, the haemoglobin content of the blood is increased, and respiration and digestion are improved.

Many minor ailments such as cold, cough, sore throat, and backache are cured by the practice of *Śīrṣāsana*.

However, its main effects are on the brain, and anyone suffering from tiredness, loss of physical and mental vitality, poor intellect, and weak will-power should practise this āsana religiously and regularly in order to gain mental and intellectual clarity and strength.

In short, *Śīrṣāsana* develops the body and disciplines the mind so that one becomes balanced within.

If you can maintain balance in *Śīrṣāsana* (Technique C, Figures 69, 70) for five minutes without support, you may practise the following variations:

Start with *Pārśva Śīrṣāsana* and *Parivṛttaikapāda Śīrṣāsana* (Figures 71, 72), then do *Eka Pāda Śīrṣāsana* and *Pārśvaika Pāda Śīrṣāsana* (Figures 73, 74). The next two variations, namely, *Upaviṣṭha Koṇāsana* and *Baddha Koṇāsana* in *Śīrṣāsana* (Figures 75, 76), are easy to do and do not require much skill. *Ūrdhva Padmāsana* in *Śīrṣāsana* (Figure 77) is more difficult and should be practised first of all with the support of a wall. Later, when you can do it without support, practise *Piṇḍāsana* (Figures 78, 79). All these variations should be done one after another. The feet need not be brought down every time. Initially, however, you may need to practise and master them one at a time.

39. *PĀRŚVA ŚĪRṢĀSANA*

Pārśva means side or flank. In this variation the trunk and the legs are turned sideways, while retaining the inverted stance.

Technique

1. Be in *Śīrṣāsana* (Figure 70).
2. Exhale and turn the trunk to the right. Do not move the head, the neck and the arms (Figure 71).
3. Stay in this final position for 10 to 15 seconds, breathing normally. Observe the following points:
   (a) the body should revolve on its own axis and should stay perpendicular to the ground when it turns; it should not tilt;
   (b) turn the left side of the trunk more and more to the right so that the right side also continues to revolve backwards;
   (c) from the navel to the feet turn the body to the right;
   (d) lift the left floating rib up and turn it to the right;
   (e) keep the right leg and the right buttock firm;
   (f) lift the shoulders and tuck in the shoulder-blades.
4. Exhale, tighten the muscles of the hips; come to *Śīrṣāsana*, then turn the trunk and the legs to the left and perform the posture on the other side, breathing normally, following the same techniques and staying for the same length of time.
5. Exhale and return to *Śīrṣāsana*.

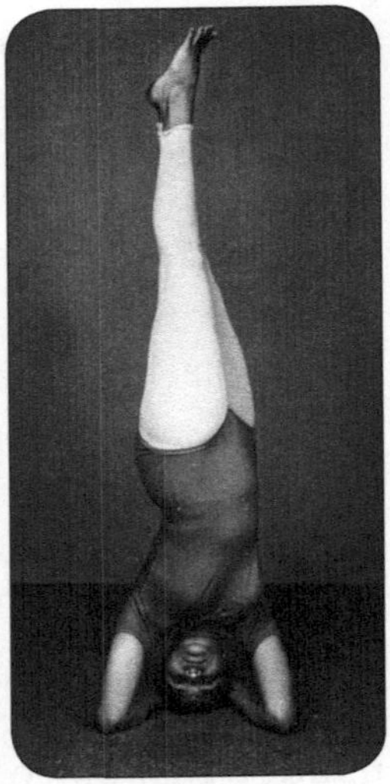

Fig. 71: *Pārśva Śīrṣāsana* (Final Stage)

Effects: This āsana removes backache, pain in the lower back, improves the peristaltic movement of the intestines, and makes the spine strong and elastic.

40. *PARIVṚTTAIKAPĀDA ŚĪRṢĀSANA*

Parivṛtta means revolved, eka is one, pāda is foot. In this variation of *Śīrṣāsana* the legs are spread apart, one backwards and the other forwards, and the trunk is revolved to the side.

Technique

1. Be in *Śīrṣāsana* (Fig. 70).
2. Spread the legs apart, taking the right leg backwards and the left leg forwards; keep the legs straight by tightening the thigh muscles and the knees. Balance for a few moments, with normal breathing.

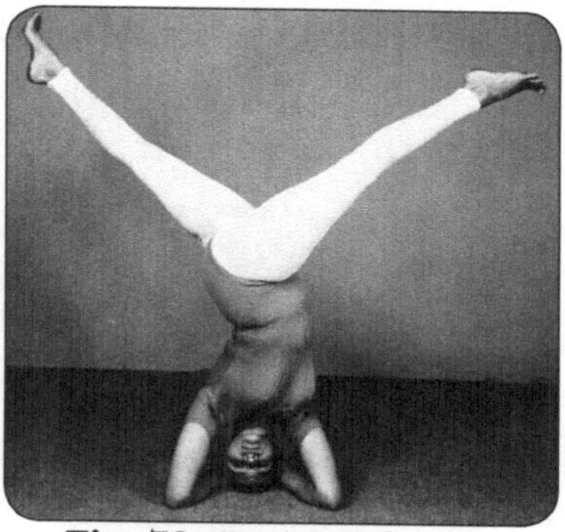

Fig. 72: *Parivṛttaikapāda Śīrṣāsana* (Final Stage)

3. Exhale, turn the trunk to the right so that the left leg is turned to the right and the right leg is turned to the left (Figure 72). The spine is revolved here as in *Pārśva Śīrṣāsana*, but with the legs spread apart.
4. Stay in this final position for 10 to 15 seconds with normal breathing, observing the following points:
   (a) stretch both the legs and make them stiff as rods;
   (b) lift both the sides of the trunk upwards;
   (c) lift the left shoulder and the armpit upwards;
   (d) the trunk should not sag.
5. Exhale, come to the position in Technique 2, then to *Śīrṣāsana* (Figure 70).
6. Now, repeat the āsana on the left side, breathing normally, observing the same points and staying for the same length of time. Return to *Śīrṣāsana*.

Effects: This posture helps digestion and elimination and tones the reproductive and excretory organs.

41. *EKA PĀDA ŚĪRṢĀSANA*

In this variation one has to balance with one leg in *Śīrṣāsana* and one leg down.

Technique

1. Stay in *Śīrṣāsana* (Figure 70).
2. Stretch the left leg from the hip joint up and keep it firm. Keep the trunk lifted up.
3. Exhale and lower the right leg straight down, in front of the face, until the toes reach the floor (Figure 73).

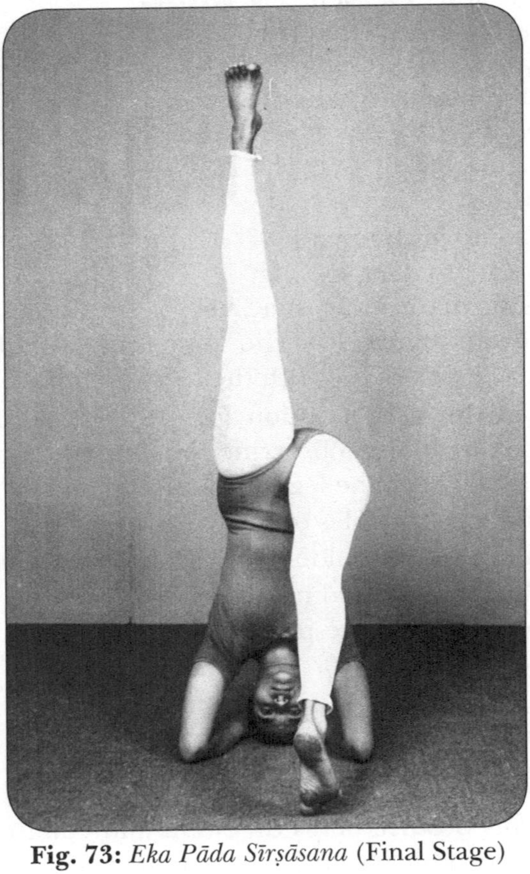

Fig. 73: *Eka Pāda Sīrṣāsana* (Final Stage)

4. Stay in this final position for 10 to 15 seconds, breathing normally and observing the following points:
   (a) tighten both the legs; feel as if the left leg is being pulled up;
   (b) pull the right thigh inwards towards the hip joint, decreasing the distance between the hip and the thigh;
   (c) in this position the following reactions are likely to occur and have to be corrected:
      (i) the spine may become convex, bringing a bend in the trunk;
      (ii) the balance may shift onto the right leg which is on the floor, instead of remaining on the head;
      (iii) the right side of the trunk may move forwards and the left backwards, causing a tilt in the pelvis;
      (iv) the collarbone may not be lifted;
      (v) the neck muscles may contract;
      (vi) the left leg may not remain perpendicular, it may lean forward.
5. Inhale and raise the right leg up, keeping both the thighs taut. Come to *Śīrṣāsana.*
6. Repeat the āsana on the left side by lowering the left leg to the ground. Breathe normally and follow all the techniques, staying for the same length of time. Return to *Śīrṣāsana* (Figure 70).

Special Instruction

If the right leg cannot reach the floor, then keep it halfway down. Do not bend the spine to take the leg down. Repeat the same with the left leg.

Effects: This āsana strengthens the neck and the abdomen, as well as the back. It aids digestion.

42. *PĀRŚVAIKAPĀDA ŚĪRṢĀSANA*

In this variation of *Śīrṣāsana* one leg is lowered to the ground, sideways in line with the shoulder.

Technique

1. Be in *Śīrṣāsana* (Figure 70).
2. Keep the left leg firm. Turn the right leg from the hip-joint to the right so that the femur, the knee, the ankle and the foot turn to the right.
3. Exhale and lower the right leg sideways to the floor, in line with the ear (Figure 74).

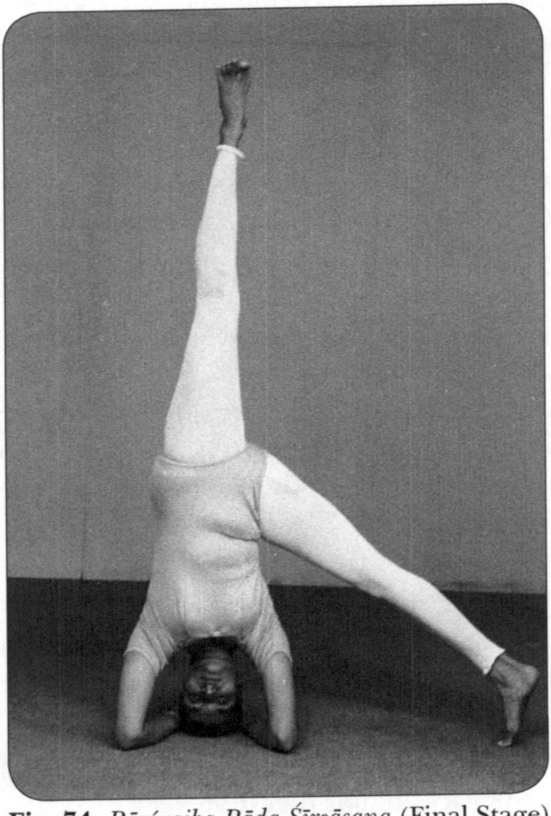

Fig. 74: *Pārśvaika Pāda Śīrṣāsana* (Final Stage)

4. Retain this final position for 10 to 15 seconds with normal breathing and observe the following points:
   (a) do not bend the knees;
   (b) do not contract the back of the right side of the trunk;
   (c) while keeping the right foot in line with the ear, tuck the right buttock in;
   (d) lift the right floating rib;
   (e) do not throw the weight of the body onto the right foot.
5. Exhale and raise the right leg to *Śīrṣāsana* position (Figure 70).
6. Repeat the āsana on the left side by lowering the left leg to the ground, breathing normally, following the same techniques, and staying for the same length of time. Return to *Śīrṣāsana*.

Special Instruction

While lowering the leg to the side, do not allow the body to tilt sideways or forwards. If necessary, keep the leg halfway down and parallel to the floor.

Effects: The effects of this posture are similar to those of the previous one, but more powerful. The neck, the spine and the abdomen become strong. The intestines are strengthened and activated.

43. *UPAVIṢṬHA KOṆĀSANA IN ŚĪRṢĀSANA*

Upaviṣṭha means seated or settled, koṇa means corner or angle. In this āsana the legs are spread apart as in *Upaviṣṭha Koṇāsana* (Figure 40) while performing *Śīrṣāsana*.

Technique

1. Be in *Śīrṣāsana* (Figure 70).
2. Spread the legs apart from the groins (Figure 75).
3. Tighten the thigh muscles inwards, extending the legs towards the feet. Stretch the back of the trunk and the spine normally; and observe the following points:
   (a) do not bend the knees;
   (b) do not cave in the chest;
   (c) do not tuck out the buttocks.
   Keep the toes in line with the knees and stretch them.
4. Stay in this final position for 15 to 20 seconds, breathing normally.

   Now proceed to the next āsana.

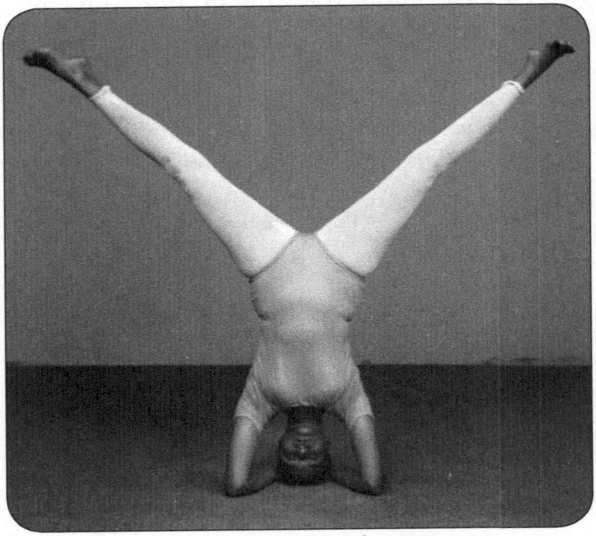

Fig. 75: *Upaviṣṭha Koṇāsana* in *Śīrṣāsana* (Final Stage)

44. *BADDHA KOṆĀSANA* IN *ŚĪRṢĀSANA*

Baddha means caught or restrained. In this āsana the knees are bent outwards and the feet are together. *Baddha Koṇāsana* is performed in *Śīrṣāsana* (Figure 70).

Technique

1. Bend the legs, spreading the knees outwards and bringing the feet together with the soles, the heels and the toes as in Namaste (Figure 76).

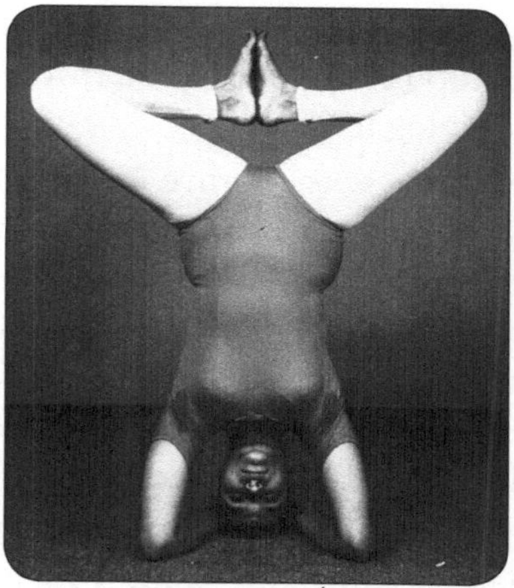

Fig. 76: *Baddha Koṇāsana* in *Śīrṣāsana* (Final Stage)

2. Breathing normally, remain in this final position for 15 to 20 seconds, observing the following points:
   (a) keep the knees wide apart;
   (b) press the soles of the feet firmly against each other;
   (c) keep the hips up and buttocks in.
3. Return to the position as in Figure 75, then to *Śīrṣāsana* (Figure 70).

Effects: These two āsanas are a boon to women. They help regulate the menstrual flow and check leucorrhoea. They are invaluable in urinary disorders and give healthy stretches to the groins and the thighs. They check bleeding piles.

SPECIAL INSTRUCTIONS FOR POSTURES SHOWN IN FIGURES 71, 72, 73, 74, 77, 78

1. These six variations of *Śīrṣāsana* may be done with the support of a wall and resting the heels against the wall, if they cannot be done independently.
2. While attempting *Parivṛttaikapāda Śīrṣāsana* (Figure 72) against the wall, it is not possible to take the legs backwards and forwards as explained in position 2 of the Technique (Figure 72). One has to start with *Pārśva Śīrṣāsana* (Figure 71) and spread the legs apart in that position, taking the frontal leg forwards and the back leg backwards.
3. In *Eka pāda Śīrṣāsana* (Figure 73) and *Pārśvaikapāda Śīrṣāsana* (Figure 74), if it is not possible to rest the toes on the floor or if you are not able to avoid the mistakes that have been listed, you may, in the initial stages, support the lifted leg against the wall, bring the other leg towards the floor as much as possible without losing balance or bending the knee. It is more important to keep the spine erect and firm, rather than to touch the floor with the foot while bending the trunk or sagging. The chest, the buttocks, and the legs should not be allowed to sag. Gradually lower the leg inch by inch. With constant practice and as the body becomes stronger and more elastic you will be able to touch the floor.
4. While attempting all these variations, observe the following points:
   (a) do not change the position of the head;
   (b) do not rub the crown of the head;
   (c) do not tilt or contract the muscles of the neck;
   (d) retain the cervical concavity.

45. *ŪRDHVA PADMĀSANA* IN *ŚĪRṢĀSANA*

Ūrdhva means above, *Padmāsana* is the lotus pose. Here, *Padmāsana* is done in *Śīrṣāsana*.

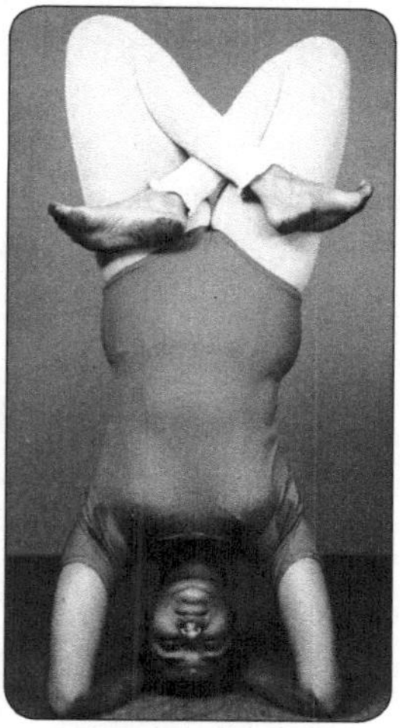

Fig. 77: *Ūrdhva Padmāsana* in *Śīrṣāsana* (Final Stage)

Technique

1. Be in *Śīrṣāsana* (Figure 70).
2. Exhale, bend the right knee and place the right foot over the left thigh. Take one or two breaths.
3. Exhale, bend the left knee, and bring the left shin in front of the right shin. Bring the outer edges of the feet closer to the root of the thighs (Figure 77).
4. Breathing normally, remain in this final position for 5 to 10 seconds, observing the following points:
   (a) keep both the knees facing the ceiling;
   (b) compress the knees and the thighs together;
   (c) tighten the hip muscles;
   (d) keep the chest expanded.
5. Exhale, release the left leg and straighten it and then the right leg.
6. Repeat the posture on the other side, breathing normally, following the above points and staying for the same length af time. Return to *Śīrṣāsana*.

Note: This āsana may be done with the support of a wall if it cannot be done independently.

Effects: In this āsana blood is circulated in the pelvic region and the organs located there are toned. Freedom is created in the abdominal area, thus aiding digestion.

46. *PIṆḌĀSANA* IN *ŚĪRṢĀSANA*

Piṇḍa means embryo. Here *Piṇḍāsana* is done while performing *Śīrṣāsana*. Master *Ūrdhva Padmāsana* (Figure 77) before attempting this posture. Then you can do both in succession.

Technique

1. Stay in *Ūrdhva Padmāsana* (Figure 77).
2. Exhale, maintain the upward stretch of the trunk, and bend the crossed legs downwards. Now the legs are below the groins and the buttock bones are up (Figure 78).
3. Lower the knees towards the arms without tightening the chest muscles (Figure 79).
4. Retain this final pose for 5 to 10 seconds, breathing normally, observing the following points:
   (a) do not cave in the chest;
   (b) do not drop the shoulders;
   (c) do not have a hunch on the back.

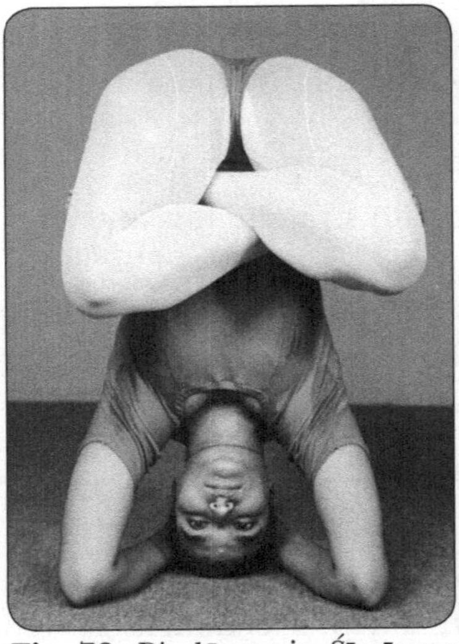

Fig. 78: *Piṇḍāsana* in *Śīrṣāsana* (Easy Stage)

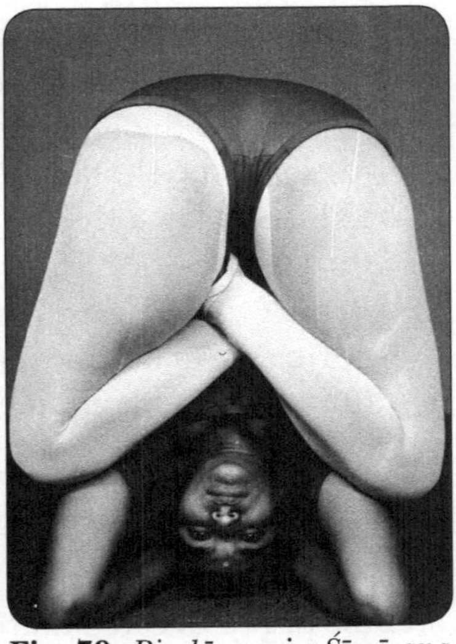

Fig. 79: *Piṇḍāsana* in *Śīrsāṣana* (Final Stage)

5. Inhale and raise the waist moving the knees up and come to *Ūrdhva Padmāsana* (Figure 77).
6. Release the legs one by one and extend them, then change the *Padmāsana* by bending the left knee first and then the right. Repeat the āsana with normal breathing, staying for the same length of time. Come to *Ūrdhva Padmāsana*, then release the legs one by one and stretch them into *Śīrṣāsana*. Then come down.

Effects: This āsana tones the abdominal organs and the pelvic region. It removes stiffness.

OVERALL EFFECTS OF ĀSANAS 38 to 46

The glands situated in the brain control the growth and the health of the body. *Śīrṣāsana* and its variations stimulate the blood supply to the cells of the brain. They help develop a balanced temperament and pure thoughts leading to a contented personality. They are a boon to those who suffer from loss of memory, weakness, uneasiness and brain fatigue due to intellectual pursuits; also to those who suffer from mental disorders such as depression. The lungs develop resistance so that one can get acclimatised to any weather conditions. The haemoglobin in the blood increases.

The spine becomes strong. Diseases of kidneys, bladder, displaced or prolapsed uterus, intestinal disorders, piles, fissures, headaches, complaints of nose and throat are alleviated. The muscular system of the abdomen and the legs is toned.

These āsanas are also a boon for women suffering from emotional instability and general weakness.

47. *SĀLAMBA SARVĀṄGĀSANA*

Sālamba means with support. Sarvāṅga means the entire body. In this āsana the whole body benefits, hence the name. Here two techniques are described; but see also Section VIII '*Yoga Kuruṇṭa*'.

Technique A

1. Spread a blanket, folded fourfold, on the floor. Lie flat on the back with the legs and the feet touching each other. Tighten the knees and stretch the arms alongside the body. Keep the shoulders down and move them away from the head. Keep the palms facing down. The head and the neck should be in line with the spine (Figure 80). Stay in this position for a while, breathing normally.
2. Exhale and bend the knees over the chest. Stay in this position for 5 seconds (Figure 81).

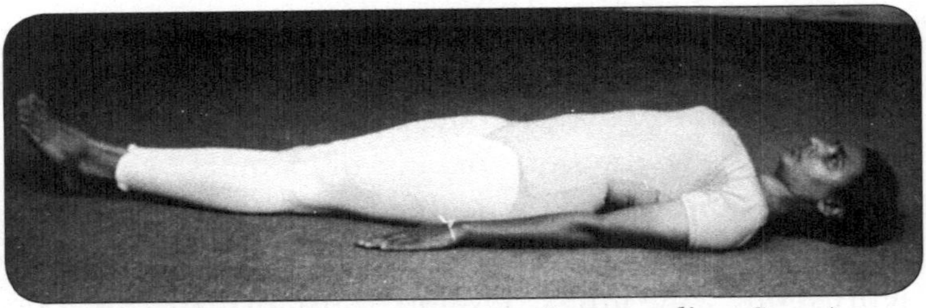

Fig. 80: *Sālamba Sarvāṅgāsana* (Intermediate Stage)

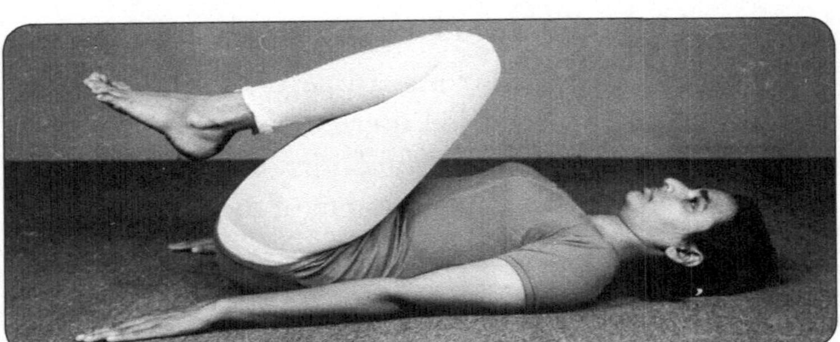

Fig. 81: *Sālamba Sarvāṅgāsana* (Intermediate Stage)

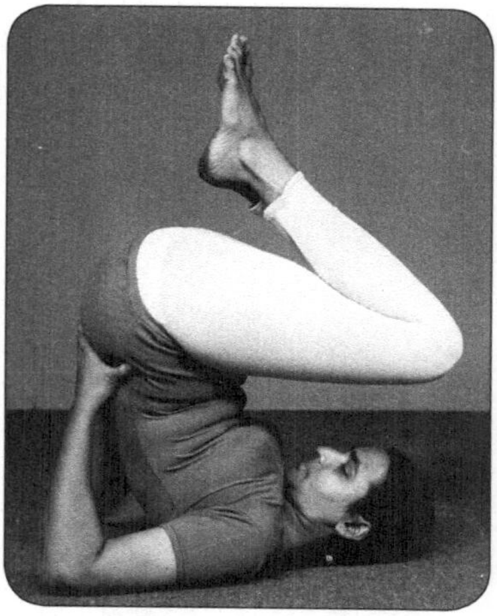

Fig. 82: *Sālamba Sarvāṅgāsana* (Intermediate Stage)

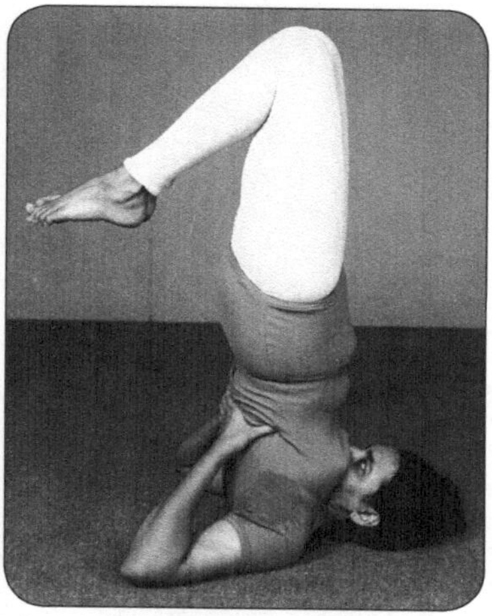

Fig. 83: *Sālamba Sarvāṅgāsana* (Intermediate Stage)

3. Press the hands down and with a slight swing raise the waist and the hips, keeping the knees bent and letting them reach beyond the head. Support the hips with the hands and raise the trunk (Figure 82). Take a breath.
4. Raise the hips and the thighs further and support the back with the hands (Figure 83). The body, from shoulders to knees, is now perpendicular to the ground. The top of the sternum touches the chin. Keep the palms on the back where the kidneys are situated, with the thumbs pointing towards the front of the body and the four fingers pointing towards the spine.
5. Contract the buttocks so that the lumbar region and the coccyx remains tucked in and straighten the legs towards the ceiling (Figure 84).
6. Stay in this final position for 5 minutes with normal breathing. Gradually increase the duration. In the initial stages 2 to 3 minutes are sufficient. Observe the following points:
   (a) press the palms and the fingers into the back to straighten the whole body from armpit to toes;

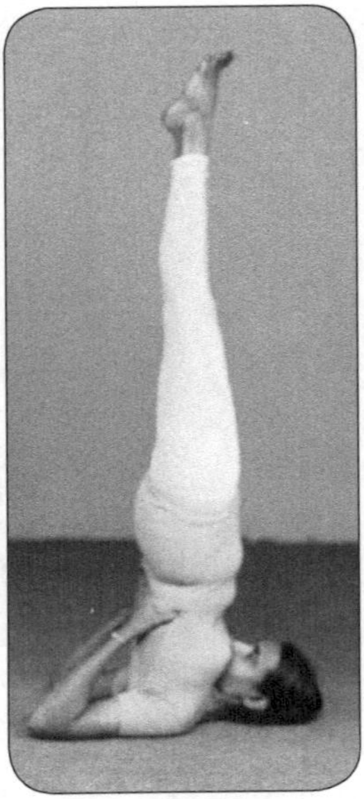

Fig. 84: *Sālamba Sarvāṅgāsana* (Final Stage)

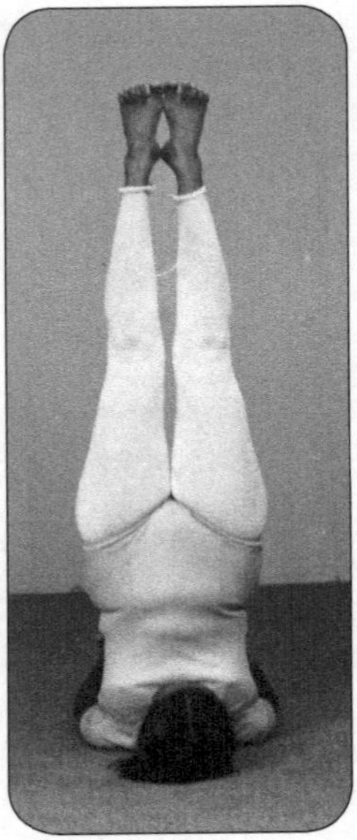

Fig. 85: *Sālamba Sarvāṅgāsana* (Final Stage)

(b) do not allow the elbows to spread outwards, but keep them in as much as possible;

(c) keep the shoulders back and away from the direction of the head; move the upper arms towards each other.

7. Exhale, bend the knees, and gradually slide the buttocks and the back downwards without jerking the spine. After reaching the position as in Figure 82, release the hands from the back, take the buttocks down to the ground and straighten the legs.

Special Instructions

1. Those who cannot do this āsana independently should seek the help of an assistant in the beginning. Come to position as in Figure 81, and ask the assistant to hold the ankles and to push the legs in the direction of the head; at the same time you should raise the hips

and the back and come to the final position of the āsana (Figure 84). Keep the body erect and firm while the helper supports your back and buttocks with the knees.

2. If no assistance is available, a chair or a stool can serve the purpose. Release the hands from the back one by one and grip the chair or the stool while maintaining balance (Figure 86).
3. Or, follow Section VIII '*Yoga Kuruṇṭa*' (Figures 164, 164a).
4. If this is not possible, first learn to perform *Halāsana* (Figures 89, 90; or 88, 91) which is described below. While in *Halāsana*, stretch the legs upwards, one by one, and come to *Sālamba Sarvāṅgāsana*.

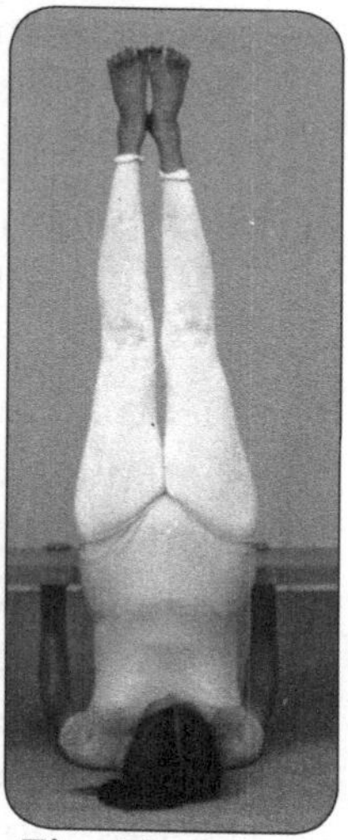

Fig. 86: *Sālamba Sarvāṅgāsana* (Final Stage)

After mastering Technique A, learn Technique B which follows.

Technique B

1. Lie flat on the floor (Figure 80).
2. Straighten the knees and lift both the legs together so that they are at right angles to the trunk. (See *Ūrdhva Prasārita Pādāsana*, Figure 109; in the illustration the arms are extended over the head, but here keep them alongside the body.) Keep the toes pointing upwards. Breathe normally.
3. Exhale and raise the legs higher, in the direction of the head, by lifting the hips and the back from the floor. Support the back with the hands.
4. Keep the trunk at right angles to the floor and extend the legs further up towards the ceiling.

5. Exhale, bring the legs in line with the buttocks. Tuck the back, the waist and the buttocks inwards so that the body is perpendicular to the floor (Figure 84).
6. Breathing normally, stay in this final position for 5 minutes or longer, observing the following points:
   (a) stretch the back of the trunk up;
   (b) broaden the chest;
   (c) tighten and tuck in the buttocks;
   (d) do not bend the knees and do not turn the thighs outwards;
   (e) keep the feet together.
7. Exhale, release the hands and gradually slide down until the back is on the floor and the legs are perpendicular (Figure 109). Lower the legs, keeping them straight.

Special Instructions

1. The elbows should not be more than shoulder-width apart. Widening the distance will result in the collapse of the chest.
2. While lifting the body up, the top of the sternum should touch the chin in *Jālandhara Bandha* (see Ch. XIV, Nos. 29–31), but there should be no choking in the throat; if you cough at this time or on lowering the body, it is a sure sign of pressure on the throat. Do not try to touch the chin to the stemum bone. Rather, the action should be the reverse: lift the chest in such a way that the sternum touches the chin, otherwise the benefits of *Sarvāṅgāsana* are lost.
3. If the chest is not properly lifted, there is difficulty in breathing. Do not turn the neck sideways for easy breathing, but broaden the chest and raise the trunk.
4. Some will experience breathing difficulty due to heavy breasts or improper lift of the chest. They should raise the height of the blanket by folding it again, or by

adding another folded blanket some two or three inches high atop the first one. The fold of the top blanket should come a few inches away from the edge of the lower one to make room for the head to rest on the lower fold so that the shoulders and the lower cervical area (C6, C7) may rest on the upper fold. Now perform *Sarvāṅgāsana*. This additional blanket increases the height by 2 to 3 inches and helps one to breathe freely, relieving pressure on the thyroid glands. This method (Figure 87) makes *Sarvāṅgāsana* easy to perform.

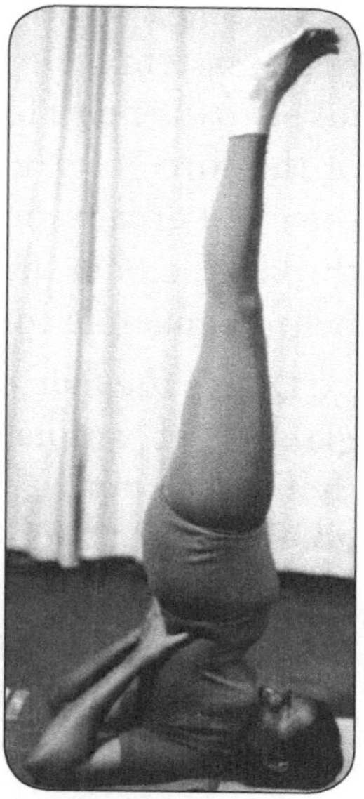

Fig. 87: *Sālamba Sarvāṅgāsana* (Final Stage)

5. Those who have heavy buttocks will find that their legs lean forwards, forming an angle and resulting in heaviness in the chest. They should take the aid of a rope (Figures 164, 164a), a bench (Figure 86), or an assistant.

Effects: *Sarvāṅgāsana* is one of the most beneficial of all the āsanas. If *Śīrṣāsana* is King, *Sarvāṅgāsana* is the Queen of all the āsanas. Where *Śīrṣāsana* develops the manly qualities of will-power, sharpness of the brain and clarity of thought, *Sarvāṅgāsana* develops the feminine qualities of patience and emotional stability. It is considered to be the mother of āsanas. As a mother struggles throughout her life for the happiness of her children, the 'mother of āsanas' strives for peace and health of the body. It is no exaggeration to call this posture 'Trailokya Cintāmani' 'a rare gem among the three worlds'.

Sarvāṅgāsana, as its name implies, has an effect on the entire system. Due to the inverted position, venous blood is taken to the heart for purification without any strain because of the force of gravity. Oxygenated blood is circulated to the chest area, relieving breathlessness, asthma, bronchitis, throat ailments and palpitation. The posture is of great help in anaemic conditions and in cases of low vitality.

Due to the firm chinlock the thyroid and the parathyroid glands get ample supply of blood, thereby increasing their efficiency in maintaining the body and the brain in good balance. Because the head remains firm due to the chinlock, the nerves are soothed, the brain is calmed, and the headaches disappear. Common ailments such as colds and nasal disturbances are cured by the practice of this posture.

Sarvāṅgāsana is very soothing to the nervous system and therefore good to practise when one is tensed, upset, irritated, fatigued, or when suffering from nervous breakdown and insomnia.

It is an excellent aid to digestion and elimination, to free the body of toxins, to rid one of constipation, to cure one of intestinal ulcers, colitis and piles.

It corrects urinary disorders, uterine displacement and menstrual disorders.

It gives peace, strength and vigour to the practitioner and is recommended as the best recuperative treatment after long illness. To avoid prolonged illness and to maintain robust health, practise *Sarvāṅgāsana*.

Note: From the final position of *Sarvāṅgāsana*, practise *Halāsana* direct, as described below. After gaining confidence and poise in *Sarvāṅgāsana* and *Halāsana*, perform the variations of *Halāsana* one after another.

48. *HALĀSANA*

Hala means plough; this posture resembles a plough.

Technique

1. Be in *Sālamba Sarvāṅgāsana* (Figure 84).
2. Lower the legs over the head from their vertical position taking the chest and the hips slightly back to maintain the extension of the body.
3. Exhale, do not bend the knees but extend the legs further, and place the toes on the floor.
4. Remove the hands from the hips and extend the arms beyond the head. Do not bend the elbows. Keep the palms facing the ceiling (Figure 88).

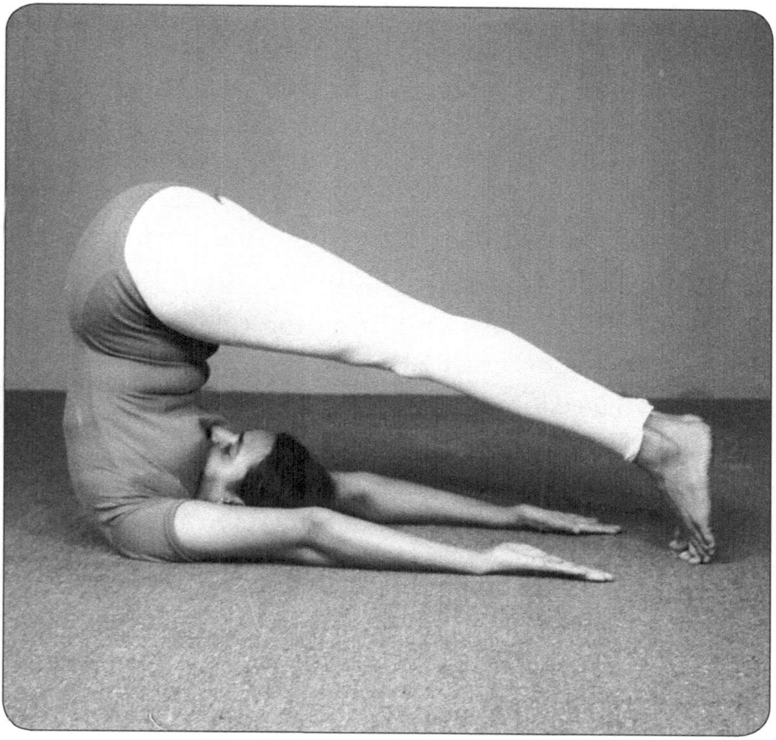

Fig. 88: *Halāsana* (Final Stage)

5. Stay in this final position for 3 to 5 minutes, breathing normally. Gradually increase the duration. Observe the following points:
    (a) extend the trunk towards the ceiling;
    (b) tighten the knees so that there is considerable space between the face and the thighs;
    (c) press the toes firmly to the ground and stretch the hamstrings so that the thighs, the buttocks, and the back of the trunk are raised.
6. Take the buttocks back, bend the legs, and raise the feet upwards; come to position as in Figure 82.
7. Slide down, keeping the palms by the sides (Figure 81). Extend the legs (Figure 80).

Special Instructions

1. Those who are on the heavier side and cannot rest the feet on the floor, or who cannot keep the trunk upright if the feet are down, should follow the technique given below:
    (a) place a stool 1½ to 2 feet high near the head:
    (b) lie flat on the back (Figure 80);
    (c) bend the knees and bring the thighs towards the abdomen (Figure 81); take a few breaths;
    (d) exhale and with a swing raise the buttocks and the back off the floor; keep the hands on the back (Figure 82);
    (e) place the toes on the stool; keep the arms stretched over the head or extended backwards, or hold the edge of the blanket with the hands and press the arms down to raise the trunk (Figure 89);
    (f) stay for 3 to 5 minutes, breathing normally;
    (g) place the hands on the back, bend the knees and take the buttocks back;

(h) lift the feet off the stool and carefully slide down (Figures 82, 81, 80).

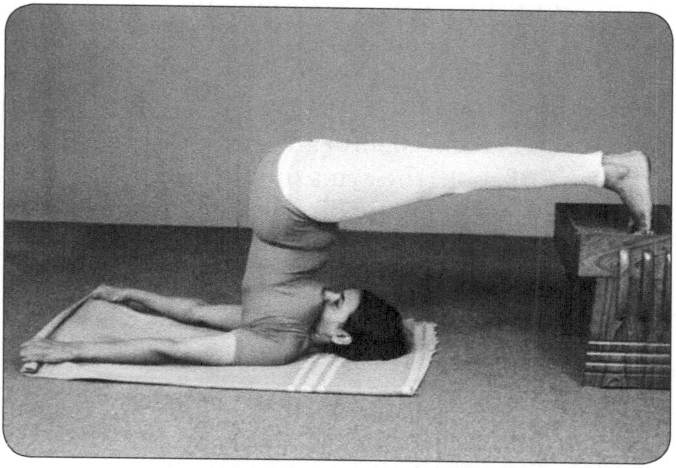

Fig. 89: *Halāsana* (Easy Stage)

2. In conditions where there is much fat around the stomach or the thighs, where there are headaches, migraines, breathing difficulties, high blood pressure, profuse bleeding, or where the nerves have to be rested, *Halāsana* should be practised as shown in Figure 90,

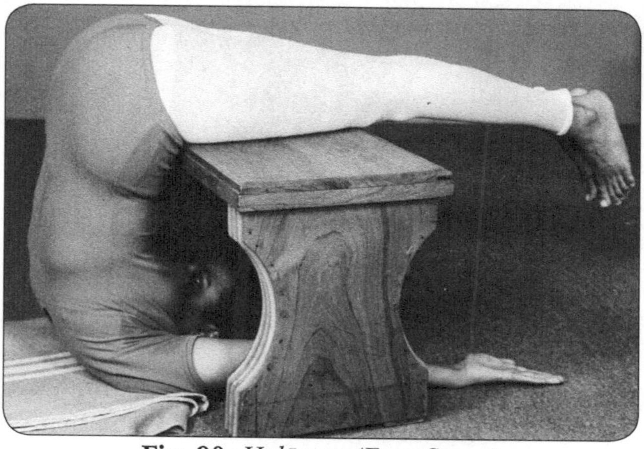

Fig. 90: *Halāsana* (Easy Stage)

with the eyes closed. The thighs should rest completely on the stool. This relieves one from pressure on the diaphragm and from a feeling of tightness in the head. If the breasts are heavy, a blanket on the floor, as described for *Sarvāṅgāsana*, is helpful. The arms should be pointing towards the feet.

3. When you become skillful and can practise *Halāsana* as in Figure 88, both the arms should be extended behind the back, away from the direction of the feet. First hold the side of the blanket and stretch the arms as in Figure 89. In this position the shoulders are stretched and the chest is broadened (Figure 91).
4. For relief from hot flushes, practise *Halāsana* as shown in Figure 90.

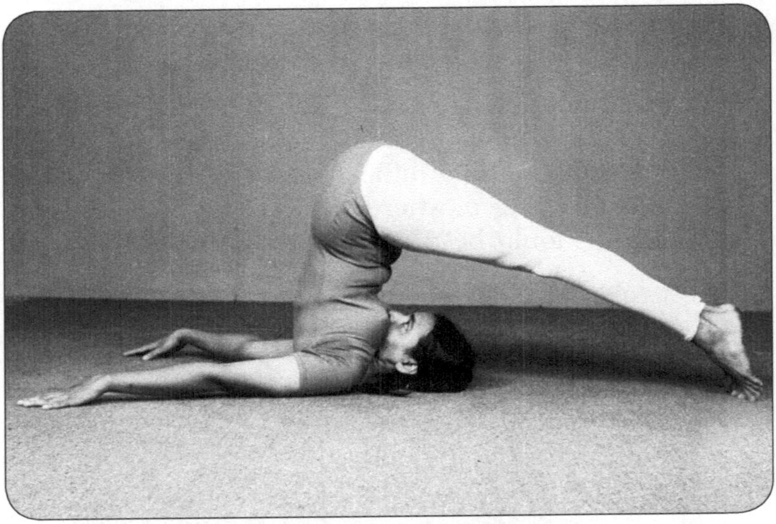

Fig. 91: *Halāsana* (Final Stage)

Effects: *Halāsana* is beneficial in headaches and fatigue; it soothes the brain and the nerves; it relieves hot flushes. It is curative in menstrual and urinary disorders. It is good for those affected by arthritis and stiffness of the shoulders and the arms.

49. *KARṆAPĪḌĀSANA*

Karṇa means ears; pīḍa means pressure; in this posture both the ears are pressed by the bent legs and the outside noise is shut off, which makes one turn inward.

Technique

1. Be in *Halāsana* (Figure 88), place the hands on the back as in *Sarvāṅgāsana*.
2. Exhale, flex the knees and bring the right knee by the side of the right ear, the left knee by the side of the left ear. Rest the knees on the floor (Figure 92).
3. Stretch the toes and bring the feet together.
4. Stay in this final position for 10 to 15 seconds with normal breathing, observing the following points:
   (a) keep the trunk lifted and the spine firm;
   (b) keep the thighs closer to the abdomen so that they remain together.

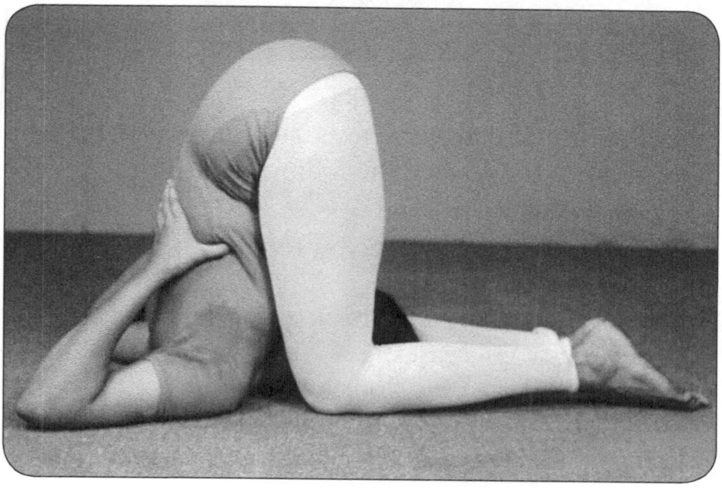

Fig. 92: *Karṇapīḍāsana* (Final Stage)

Effects: This āsana removes backache and relieves flatulence. It rests the heart.

50. *SUPTA KOṆĀSANA*

Supta means lying down, koṇa means angle. In this variation of *Halāsana*, the legs are spread wide apart.

Technique

1. While exhaling, raise the knees from the position of *Karṇapīḍāsana* (Figure 92). Take a few breaths.
2. Exhale and separate the legs, widening them as far from one another as possible, without bending the knees (Figure 93).

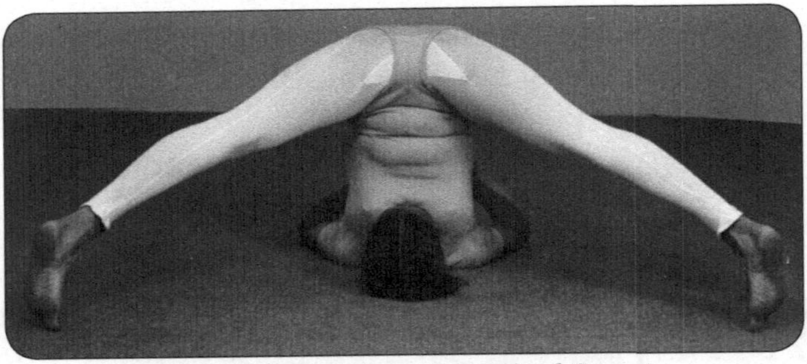

Fig. 93: *Supta Koṇāsana* (Final Stage)

3. Stay in this final position for 10 to 15 seconds, breathing normally and observe the following points:
   (a) keep the chest lifted up;
   (b) raise the back and the buttocks with the help of the hands;
   (c) continue widening the legs further apart as your elasticity increases; the feet should remain perpendicular to the floor and should not drop to the sides.
4. Exhale and bring the legs close together as in *Halāsana*.

Special Instructions

Those who are on the heavier side and cannot rest on the floor or who cannot keep the trunk upright if the feet are down, should follow the technique given for *Halāsana* (Figure (89) under Special Instructions from (a) to (e) on page 239 and do *Karṇapīḍāsana* by bending the knees. However, place the toes on the stool itself. Similarly, do the *Supta Koṇāsana* keeping the toe on the stool or on the bench, so that the legs remain up, level with the buttocks. This method of doing it halfway is of tremendous help for middle-aged women who have problems with the uterus and menstrual cycle.

Effects: This āsana is extremely beneficial to women with kidney and uterus complaints. It checks menstrual flow and white discharge. It removes pain and heaviness in the uterus and corrects the position of the uterus. For maximum benefit, the duration should be extended to 5 minutes.

51. *PĀRŚVA HALĀSANA*

This is a variation of *Halāsana* with the legs taken to one side.

Technique

1. Be in *Halāsana* (Figure 88) with the hands on the back. Take one or two breaths.
2. Exhale and move both the legs to the right as far as possible. Do not move the head and the neck.
3. Extend the right leg and bring it in line with the right shoulder. Bring the left leg close to the right leg (Figure 94). Keep both legs straight with the toes, the heels, and the ankles touching.
4. Stay in this final position for 10 to 15 seconds, breathing normally, and observe the following points:
   (a) lift up the trunk;
   (b) keep both the thighs parallel to each other.
5. Exhale, move the left leg to the centre to *Halāsana* position, then the right leg (Figure 88).

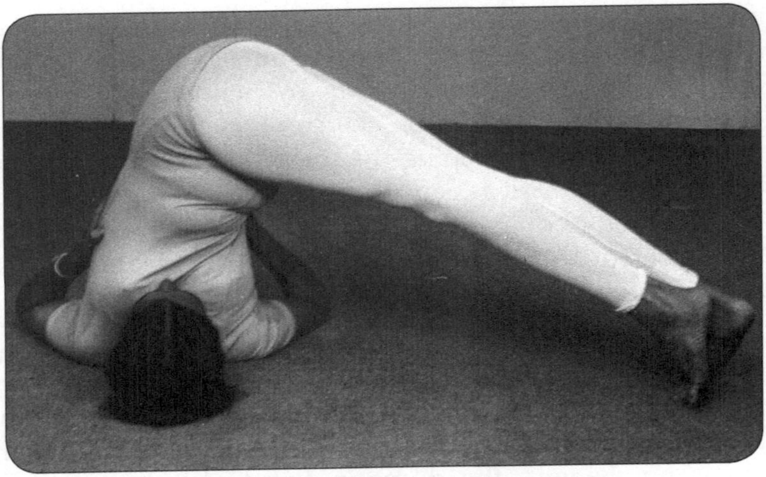

Fig. 94: *Pārśva Halāsana* (Final Stage)

6. Now do the āsana on the left side, moving both legs to the left, breathing normally, following the same techniques and staying for the same length of time. Come back to *Halāsana*.

Special Instructions

1. Move the legs sideways by walking the toes to the side. Do not walk fast, you may lose balance. With each step the trunk should be lifted up, as it has a tendency to drop.
2. This āsana may be done directly from *Supta Koṇāsana* by moving the left leg towards the right leg, returning to *Supta Koṇāsana* and then moving the right leg towards the left leg.

Effects: This āsana is a boon for people suffering from chronic constipation.

Note: After gaining proficiency in *Halāsana* and its variations, practise the variations of *Sarvāṅgāsana* which follow. Each of the variations should first be mastered and then they should be performed in succession.

52. *EKA PĀDA SARVĀṄGĀSANA*

In this variation of *Sarvāṅgāsana* one leg is perpendicular and the other rests on the floor, as in *Halāsana*.

Technique

1. Be in *Sarvāṅgāsana* (Figure 84, side view).
2. Exhale and lower the right leg towards the ground without bending the knee. Place the toes on the floor (Figure 95).
3. Keep both the legs stretched, the left leg upwards and the right leg downwards.
4. Stay in this final position for 10 to 15 seconds with normal breathing, observing the following points:
   (a) stretch the left leg from the groin upwards;
   (b) draw in the left knee and keep it taut;

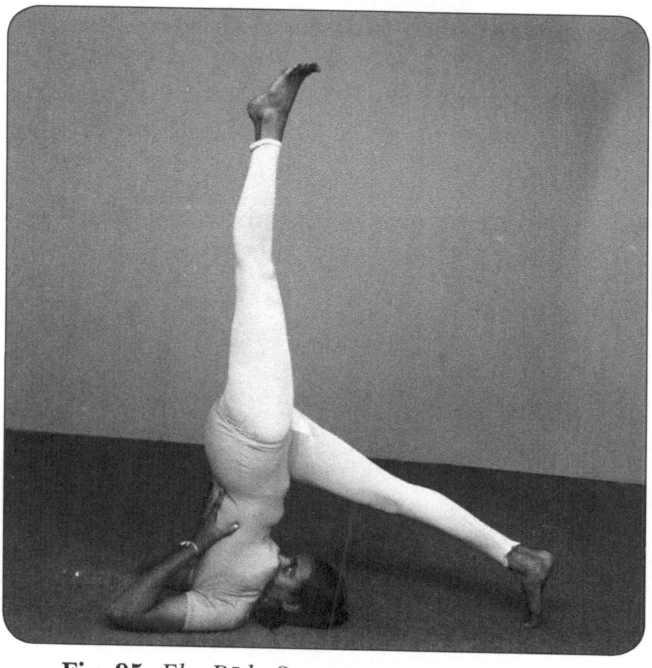

Fig. 95: *Eka Pāda Sarvāṅgāsana* (Final Stage)

(c) the left foot should stay in line with the head and should not tilt forward;

(d) keep the chest expanded and the shoulder-blades tucked in.

5. Exhale, lift the right leg and come to *Sarvāṅgāsana* (Figure 84). Take one or two breaths.
6. Now, do the āsana with the right leg perpendicular and the left leg down, following the same technique and staying for the same length of time.

Special Instructions

1. While practising variations of *Halāsana* and *Sarvāṅg-āsana*, the spine tends to sag. Therefore, straighten it after every variation by adjusting the hands on the back and raising the chest up. Keep the spine firm.
2. If the errors of the final position cannot be overcome, then the leg which goes down should remain parallel to the floor and should not be taken down further. The foot may be supported on a stool (Figure 196). It is important to keep the spine firm without allowing it to become convex.

Effects: This pose relieves pain in the small of the back and tones the back muscles.

53. *PĀRŚVAIKA PĀDA SARVĀṄGĀSANA*

This is a variation of *Sarvāṅgāsana* in which one leg is perpendicular while the other is placed sideways on the floor as in *Pārśva Halāsana*.

Technique

1. Be in *Sarvāṅgāsana* (Figure 85).
2. Exhale, bring the right leg sideways to the right, in line with the right shoulder. Place the toes on the floor (Figure 96).

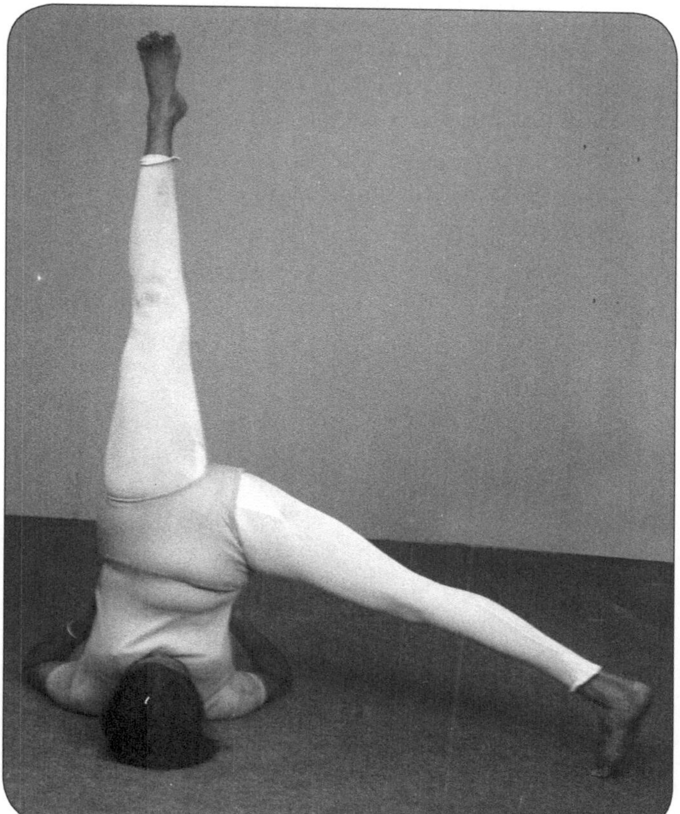

Fig. 96: *Pārśvaika Pāda Sarvāṇgāsana* (Final Stage)

3. Stay in this final position for 10 to 15 seconds, breathing normally and observe the following points:
   (a) keep the left leg upright and stretch it from the groin up; do not allow it to sway to the right;
   (b) do not bend the right knee;
   (c) lift the waist and tighten the buttocks;
   (d) do not allow the right buttock to sag.
4. Exhale, raise the right leg to *Sarvāṅgāsana* and place it near the left leg. Stay in *Sarvāṅgāsana* and take a few breaths.
5. Now do the āsana on the other side, with the right leg upright and the left leg on the floor, staying for the same length of time. Come back to *Sarvāṅgāsana*.

Special Instruction

Those who cannot reach the floor without avoiding the errors as in the previous āsana should keep the downward leg parallel to the floor.

Effects: In this āsana, blood is circulated in the pelvic organs which keeps them toned and healthy. Backaches are relieved.

54. *SETU BANDHA SARVĀṄGĀSANA*

Setu means bridge; bandha means formation or construction. In this variation of *Sarvāṅgāsana* the body is arched backwards as if to form a bridge.

This āsana is difficult; here easy methods of doing it have been described to assist the practitioner. It is essential to learn to bend the spine backwards in order to give it elasticity. By following the easy methods shown here one can gradually learn to achieve the advanced technique. Techniques A and B should be mastered before the Advanced Technique is attempted.

Technique A (1st Method)

1. Lie with the legs bent and the feet touching a wall or stool. The head should be about 4 to 4½ feet away from the wall or the stool.
2. Place the feet at a height of about 1½ to 2 feet on the wall or stool.
3. Press the feet into the wall or stool to raise the buttocks, the back, and the shoulder-blades off the floor. Support the back with the hands (Figure 97).
4. Keep the back of the head and the shoulders firmly on the floor (Figure 97).
5. Straighten the legs, keeping the body arched (Figure 98).

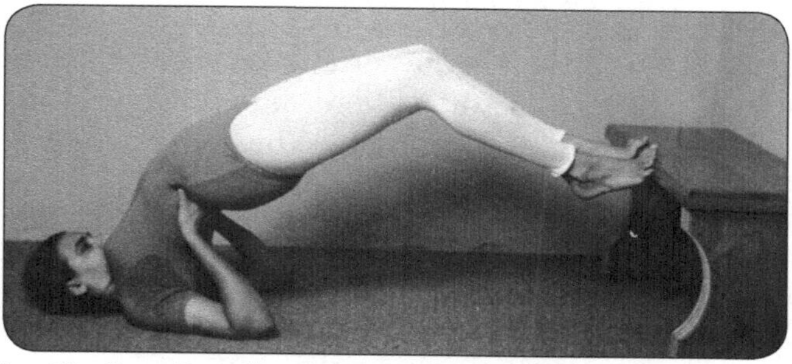

Fig. 97: *Setu Bandha Sarvāṅgāsana* (Intermediate Stage)

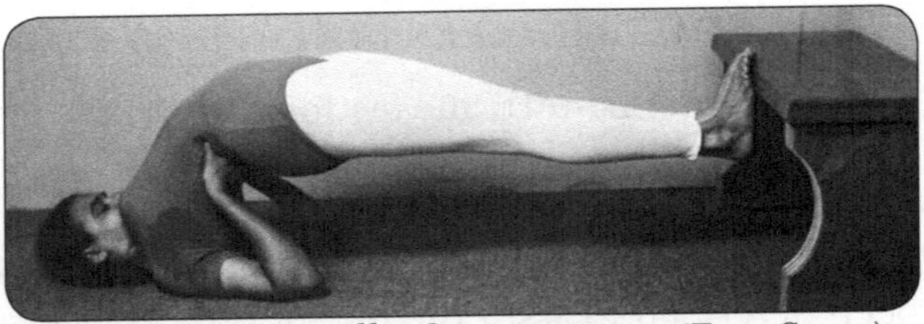

Fig. 98: *Setu Bandha Sarvāṅgāsana* (Easy Stage)

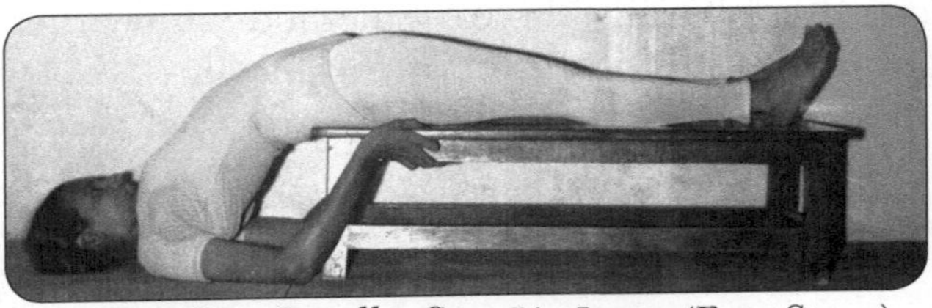

Fig. 99: *Setu Bandha Sarvāṅgāsana* (Easy Stage)

6. Remain in this position for 1 to 3 minutes, breathing normally.
7. Bend the knees as in Figure 97, remove the hands from the back and carefully lower the trunk down.

Technique A (2nd Method)

1. If the limbs are flexible, lie flat on the floor with the head 4 to 4½ feet away from the wall. Bend the knees and place the feet near the buttocks. Exhale and raise the buttocks and back. Support the back with the palms and lift the buttocks, the chest and the thighs still further (Figure 100).
2. Straighten the legs one after another and place the feet on the wall so that you will not slide down. Tighten the buttock muscles and straighten the knees as in Fig. 101.

Effects: This way of doing the posture relieves one from backache and strengthens the back muscles. The organs situated in the pelvic area are rejuvenated. *Setu Bandha Sarvāṅgāsana* is curative in conditions such as inferiority complex, unsteady mental condition in menopause and

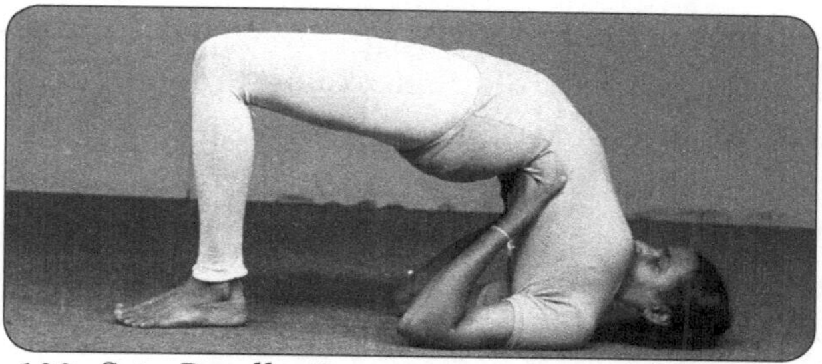

Fig. 100: *Setu Bandha Sarvāṅgāsana* (Intermediate Stage)

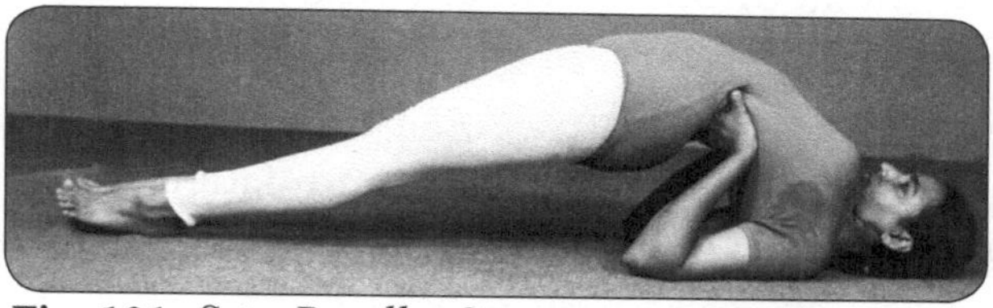

Fig. 101: *Setu Bandha Sarvāṅgāsana* (Final Stage)

high blood pressure. As performed in Figure 101, it is good for relief from hot flushes; however, in this case it should be performed in combination with *Halāsana* (Figure 90).

Technique B

1. Lie lengthwise with the knees bent on a bench 10 inches high, keeping the head and the trunk on the bench. Breathe normally.
2. Exhale and slide down in the direction of the head until the head reaches the ground as in Figure 148.
3. Slide down further until the back of the head and the shoulders touch the floor. Straighten the legs so that the body from the buttocks to the legs remains on the bench (Figure 99).
4. Hold the sides of the bench. Keep the shoulders back and expand the chest, or stretch the arms sideways and relax.
5. Remain in this final position for 3 to 5 minutes, breathing normally. Later one should remain as long as possible. Observe the following points:

(a) keep the face relaxed,
(b) keep the back of the neck and the shoulders down;
(c) keep the sternum bone raised up.

6. Exhale, bend the knees, bring the feet in, and slide down towards the head until the buttocks reach the floor.

Special Instruction

Those who are overweight or who suffer from headaches and intestinal disorders should first master these easy techniques.

Effects: This variation of *Setu Bandha Sarvāṅgāsana* relaxes the nerves, removes headaches and fatigue, and helps asthmatic patients to breathe better.

Technique C (Advanced)

1. Stay in *Sarvāṅgāsana* (Figure 84).
2. Keep the palms firmly on the back. Bend the legs backwards, bringing the heels closer towards the buttocks (Figure 83).
3. Raise the chest and the spine up. Take one or two breaths. Exhale, drop the legs backwards and place the feet on the floor (Figure 100).
4. Keep the feet firmly on the floor. Lift the ribs up so that the chest expands. The moment the feet touch the ground, pressure will be felt on the wrist joints. Lift the buttocks and the thighs upwards a little more to relieve this pressure.
5. Increase the curvature of the spine by lifting it further up. Stretch the legs one at a time. Keep the feet touching each other. Tighten the buttocks and lift the sternum (Figure 101).
6. Place the back of the head, the shoulders, the upper arms, the elbows, and the feet on the floor. Tighten the buttocks.

7. Stay in this final position for 30 to 60 seconds, breathing normally, observing the following points:
   (a) stretch the legs out without dropping the buttocks;
   (b) raise the chest and expand it;
   (c) keep the chin downwards.

   With practice, increase this duration to five minutes or repeat the āsana two to three times.
8. Bend the knees, walk in, and come to position as in Figure 100. Lift the legs off the ground with a jump and come to *Sarvāṅgāsana* (Figure 84).

Special Instruction

In order to facilitate lifting the chest and the buttocks in this āsana, practise the following movements: Lie flat on the floor. Bend the knees, catch the ankles with the fingers and raise the chest, the thighs, and the abdomen (Figure 102). Keep the back of the head and the shoulders on the floor. As the arms are extended in this movement, the chest expands easily. This will enable you to do *Setu Bandha Sarvāṅgāsana* with ease.

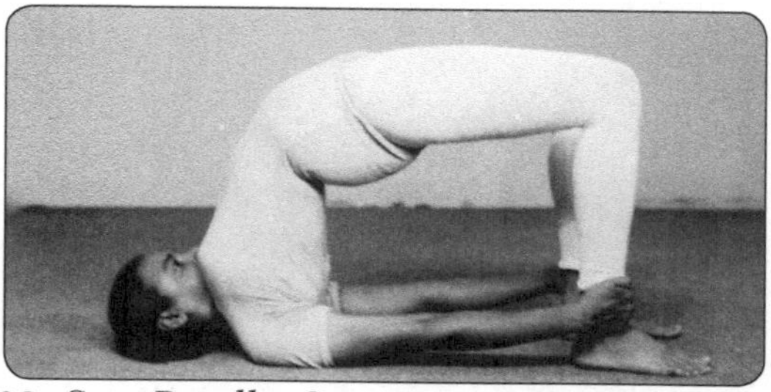

Fig. 102: *Setu Bandha Sarvāṅgāsana* (Intermediate Stage)

Effects: This pose helps the functioning of the kidneys, regulates the menstrual periods, and checks the menstrual flow. It strengthens the back muscles, removes fatigue, rejuvenates the nerves, and improves the circulation around the chest. By the practice of this āsana one develops self-confidence, will-power and steadiness of mind.

55. ŪRDHVA PADMĀSANA IN SARVĀṄGĀSANA

Ūrdhva means upwards; *Padmāsana* is the lotus pose. Here *Padmāsana* is performed in *Sarvāṅgāsana*.

Technique

1. Be in *Sarvāṅgāsana* (Figure 85).
2. Exhale and bend the right knee. Place the right foot at the base of the left thigh. If you are unable to do this, then remove the left hand from the back, use it to place the right foot correctly, then reposition it on the back.
3. Exhale, bend the left knee, and place the left foot at the base of the right thigh, using the right hand if necessary, as above. Then replace the hand on the back.
4. Stay in this position for 5 to 10 seconds, breathing normally and observing the following points:
   (a) tighten the buttocks;
   (b) stretch the thigh muscles upwards;
   (c) bring the knees closer together (Figure 103).

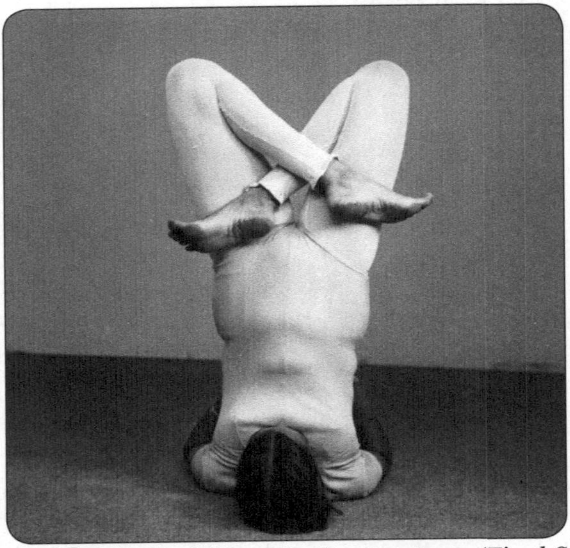

Fig. 103: *Ūrdhva Padmāsana* in *Sarvāṅgāsana* (Final Stage)

5. Release the legs and change the pose by bending the left leg first and then the right leg. Breathe normally and stay for the same length of time.

Special Instructions

1. If the buttocks are heavy, the thighs will remain loose. Therefore, tuck in the coccyx and the lumbar vertebrae and tighten the buttock muscles. The back may be supported against a chair.
2. This āsana must be thoroughly mastered before the next one is attempted. After mastering, however, you should proceed directly to the next āsana without changing the interlock of the legs.

Effects: This āsana broadens the chest muscles, making breathing easy. As it opens the abdominal area, it is good for digestion and tones the abdominal organs.

56. *PIṆḌĀSANA* IN *SARVĀṄGĀSANA*

This āsana resembles an embryo (*Piṇḍa*) and is combined with *Sarvāṅgāsana*.

Technique

1. Be in *Ūrdhva Padmāsana* (Figure 103).
2. Exhale, lower the crossed legs by bending at the groins. Take a few breaths.
3. Now the *Padmāsana* should be lowered further down towards the head.
4. Remove the arms from the back and encircle the crossed legs.
5. Remain in this final position for 5 to 10 seconds. breathing normally, and observe the following points:
   (a) In this position the knees do not touch the floor and the waist has to be lifted up;

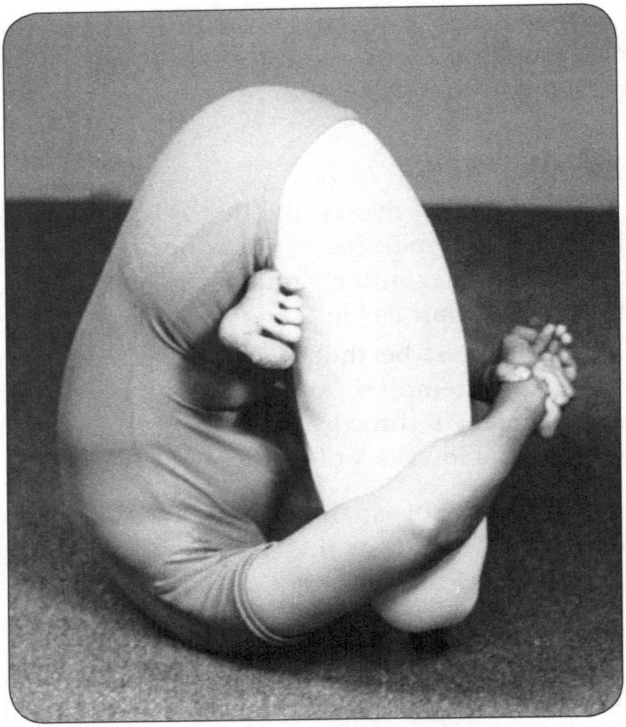

Fig. 104: *Piṇḍāsana* in *Sarvāṅgāsana* (Final Stage)

(b) The front of the trunk, the legs, the chest, and the stomach should merge together, as if forming an embryo.

6. Release the arms and place them on the back.
7. Inhale, return to *Ūrdhva Padmāsana*, release the legs and change the crosslegs. Repeat the āsana breathing normally and stay for the same length of time.

Special Instruction

If you find it difficult to balance when the back is not supported, keep the arms on the back.

Note: This āsana has to be mastered well before the following one is attempted.

57. *PĀRŚVA PIṆḌĀSANA*

In this posture *Piṇḍāsana* is performed on the two sides. It is an advanced pose.

Technique

1. Be in *Piṇḍāsana* with the hands supporting the back;
2. Raise the crossed legs off the forehead by leaning the buttocks slightly back so that the thighs come to the level of the chest. Take one or two breaths.
3. Exhale, turn the trunk to the right and place the right knee by the side of the right arm. Take one or two breaths, balance in this position then continue.
4. Exhale lower the left knee also towards the side of the head so that the crossed legs remain at an angle to the trunk (Figure 105).
5. Remain in the final position, breathing normally, for 5 to 10 seconds, observing the following points:
   (a) keep the back of the body lifted up;
   (b) do not throw the weight of the body onto the bent knees.
6. Exhale, raise the left knee off the ground and then the right knee, revolve the trunk to the left, and do the āsana on the left side breathing normally and staying for 5 to 10 seconds.

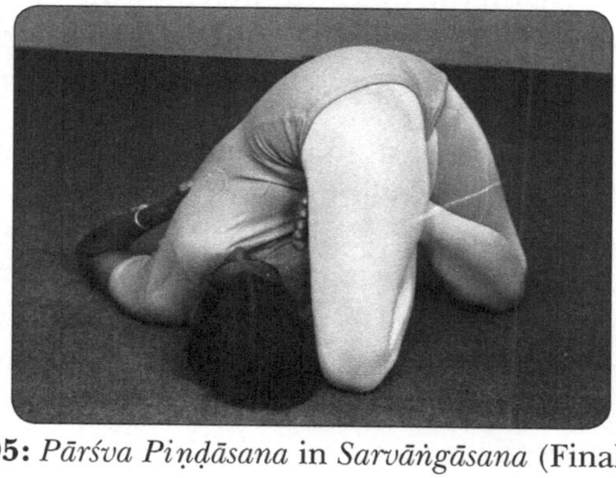

Fig. 105: *Pārśva Piṇḍāsana* in *Sarvāṅgāsana* (Final Stage)

7. Exhale, come to the centre, and then up to *Ūrdhva Padmāsana* (Figure 103). Release the legs and come to *Sarvāṅgāsana* (Figure 85).
8. Change the *Padmāsana* by bending the left knee first and then the other, go to *Piṇḍāsana*, then do *Pārśva Piṇḍāsana* on both sides, breathing normally, following all the techniques and staying for 5 to 10 seconds on each side.
9. Come to *Sarvāṅgāsana* (Figure 85). Follow the movements given in Figures 83 to 80, or slide down carefully and lie flat on the floor.

Special Instruction

In the initial stages, it will not be possible to place the left knee on the floor. If you exert to achieve this, then the left shoulder and the left elbow will shoot off the floor and a somersault to the right will be the result. To avoid this, proceed as follows:

(a) lower the left palm towards the shoulder and press the elbow to the ground;

(b) do not force the left knee if it does not touch the floor; first place the right knee on the floor; raise the left side of the back of the trunk in the direction of the buttock;

(c) if both knees are forcibly placed on the floor, there will be pressure on the diaphragm, resulting in suffocation; therefore the left knee should be kept slightly above the floor to ease the pressure on the floating ribs.

Effects: All these three āsanas tone the abdominal organs and help digestion and elimination.

Note: After thoroughly mastering *Ūrdhva Padmāsana* (Fig. 103), *Piṇḍāsana* (Figure 104), and *Pārśva Piṇḍāsana* (Figure 105), one can perform a cycle of all the three āsanas at a stretch without changing the legs and then repeat all three after changing the legs.

OVERALL EFFECTS OF ĀSANAS 47 to 57

Sarvāṅgāsana and its variations are useful for developing a healthy mind. The nervous system is calmed and one is freed from hypertension, irritability, nervous breakdown and insomnia. They are a boon for combating the stresses and strains of our daily life. They give vitality and self-confidence.

The inverted position of the body in all these āsanas assists the flow of impure blood (venous blood) to the heart and in its purification.

The endocrine glands, especially the thyroid and the parathyroid, are benefited due to the increased blood circulation around them. By the regular practice of these āsanas one is freed from breathing difficulties, asthma, coughs, colds, bronchitis and diseases of the throat.

They relieve abdominal irritations like stomach-aches, diarrhoea, intestinal disorders and ulcers. They relieve abdominal irritation.

In all, the āsanas from this section have a great curative value in diseases of the lungs, disorders of the chest and the throat, biliousness, acidity, diabetes, dysentery, complaints of the liver and the spleen, morbid conditions of the bladder, the uterus and the ovaries. They are valuable for headache, brain disorders, loss of memory and emotional problems.

After a prolonged and chronic illness, *Sarvāṅgāsana* stimulates the life force and helps one to recover vitality. A longer stay in these postures intensifies their beneficial effects.

All these āsanas are a veritable boon to women and should on no account be missed.

SECTION-V

Āsanas: Abdominal and Lumbar

Before starting to practise the āsanas in this section, all the āsanas from Section I should be mastered and also āsanas given in Figures 26, 27, 28, 29 and 30 of Section II and āsanas in Figures 84, 85, 88, 91, 92, 93 and 94 from Section IV.

If the abdominal muscles and the muscles of the lumbar are weak, the āsanas given in this section are too intensive to be attempted immediately. The muscles should first be toned and strengthened by the foregoing practice and then Section V can be commenced.

Women suffering from serious menstrual disorders, displacement of the uterus and leucorrhoea must avoid these āsanas. They reduce fat and for this reason one may be tempted to practise them, but they are harmful for these particular conditions. Therefore, the āsanas recommended for these complaints in Chapter X, Part II, should first be practised until one is completely cured. Then the āsanas from this section can be performed.

If obesity is the result of hormonal imbalance in the glands, the āsanas in the first two sections as well as those from Section IV should be well mastered.

58. *ŪRDHVA PRASĀRITA PĀDĀSANA*

This āsana is done lying on the floor with both the legs extended and stretched upwards.

Technique

1. Lie flat on the back, stretch both the legs, and keep the thighs, the knees, the ankles, and the toes together and the knees tight.

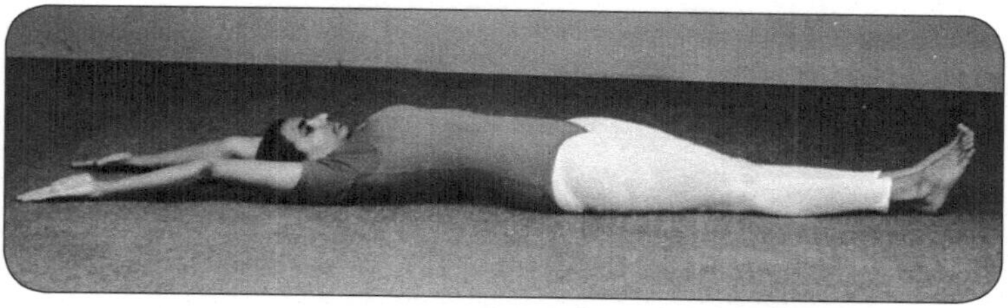

Fig. 106: *Ūrdhva Prasārita Pādāsana* (Intermediate Stage)

2. Stretch both the arms over the head with the palms facing up, and make sure that the back of the body is extending along with the arms (Figure 106). Take one or two breaths.
3. Exhale, raise both the legs to 30° (Figure 107). Stay in this position for 5 to 10 seconds. Breathe normally.
4. Exhale again, raise the legs to 60° (Figure 108). Stay for 5 to 10 seconds, breathing normally.

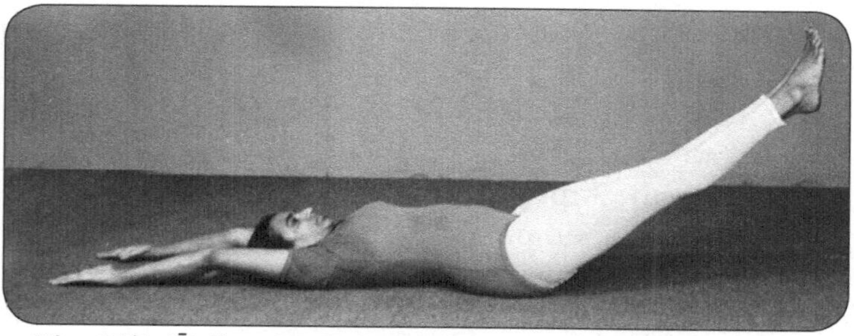

Fig. 107: *Ūrdhva Prasārita Pādāsana* (Intermediate Stage)

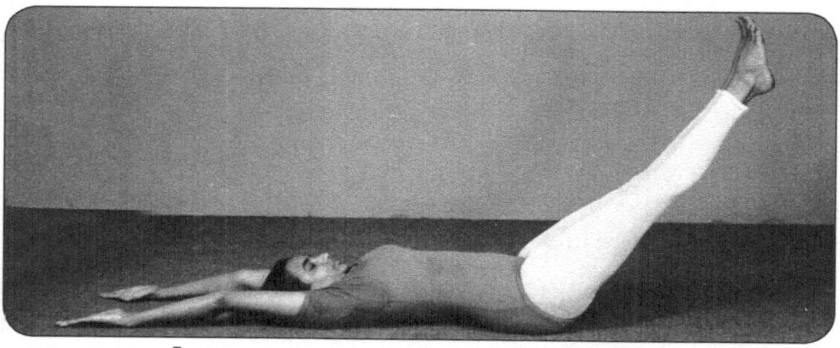

Fig. 108: *Ūrdhva Prasārita Pādāsana* (Intermediate Stage)

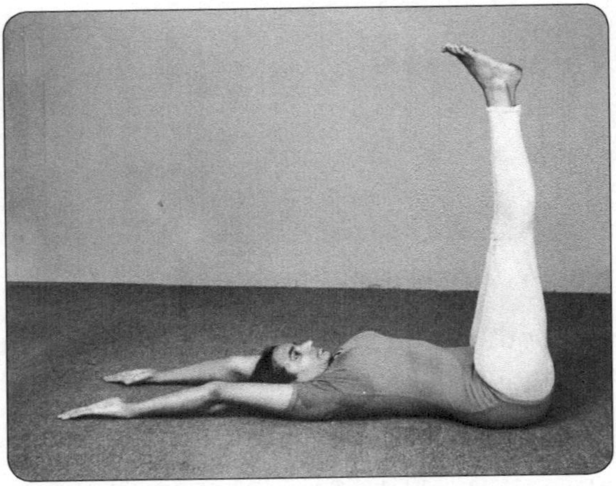

Fig. 109: *Ūrdhva Prasārita Pādāsana* (Final Stage)

5. Exhale and raise the legs to 90° (Figure 109). Remain in this final position for 15 to 30 seconds, observing the following points in all the three steps:
   (a) keep the knees tight, the legs firm and roll them inwards;
   (b) extend the arms more so that the back of the trunk is well stretched;
   (c) keep the hips and the back firmly on the floor so that the abdominal organs are massaged inside;
   (d) breathe normally throughout.
6. Exhale, lower the legs slowly without bending the knees, and come to position as in Figure 106. Then relax.
7. Repeat this āsana three times in the beginning. Once the abdominal muscles are toned one can do it 15 to 20 times.

Special Instructions

1. Those with slipped disc and backache should avoid this method. The muscles in the back are tensed in this āsana and this will cause aggravation of any back complaints. They should do as in Figure 110.

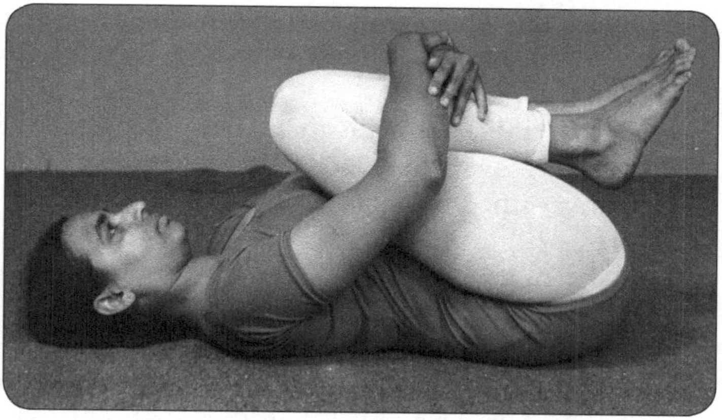

Fig. 110: *Ūrdhva Prasārita Pādāsana* (Intermediate Stage)

2. Beginners and those who are overweight and whose muscles are flabby will be unable to lift their legs without bending the knees. To strengthen the muscles, the following procedure is given:
   (a) Lie flat on the floor and extend the arms over the head as in Figure 106.
   (b) Bend the knees, draw the knees towards the stomach, and keep the heels near the buttocks. Press the knees and the thighs onto the stomach. Stretch the arms further so that the back, the waist and the spine are extended. Now encircle the legs with the arms and press the thighs down onto the stomach (Figure 110). Press the legs in such a manner that the muscles of the back and the hips are pressed into the floor. This relieves backache, weakness in the waist and the legs, and backache during the menstrual period. If you are unable to press the thighs, ask a friend or an assistant to press the shins so that the thighs are pressed down.
   (c) Stretch the arms over the head. Exhale, raise the legs to 90°, keeping the knees straight (Figure 109). Remain in this position for 2 to 5 seconds, breathing normally. Gradually increase the duration.

(d) Bend the knees and bring the thighs onto the stomach. Keep the arms stretched over the head (Figure 106).

(e) If you find it difficult to practise this āsana with the arms over the head, keep them alongside the trunk with the palms facing down; these can be pressed into the floor when raising the legs. It is easier to lower the legs without bending the knees than to raise them up. Hence, to take the legs up one should bend the knees, raise them and then straighten them, but while lowering the legs they may be kept straight. When this method becomes easy, the legs may be taken up without bending the knees.

3. In the beginning, there are tremors in the legs, the thighs, and the abdominal muscles. Do not be alarmed. In the initial stages, the pose should be done once or twice. Later one may repeat it 10 to 15 times.
4. Those who suffer from profuse discharge during menstruation or from leucorrhoea may do the pose while keeping their legs against a wall. The buttock bones, the back of the thighs, the hamstrings, and the heels should rest on the wall, making the body into L-shape. From the head to the hips the body is on the floor, from the buttocks to the heels it is perpendicular, as in Figure 109. When the pose is done in this way, the abdominal organs rest against the spine. The resting of the sacrum on the floor also supports the abdominal organs. As the legs are resting against the wall, there is no cause for tension or pressure. One can remain in this position as long as possible.

Effects: This posture reduces fat around the waist, the buttocks, and the thighs; it strengthens the spine and tones the abdominal organs.

59. *PARIPŪRṆA NĀVĀSANA*

Paripūrṇa means full, complete; nāva means boat. This āsana resembles a boat with oars.

Technique

1. Extend both the legs and sit in *Daṇḍāsana* (Figure 23). Take one or two breaths.
2. Exhale and lean the trunk slightly backwards, simultaneously raising both the legs off the ground.
3. Balance the whole body on the buttocks. Keep the head and the trunk as well as the legs straight. If the back sags, the trunk will drop towards the floor. If the knees are bent, the feet will go down. Hence it is necessary to keep the legs firm and the trunk erect.

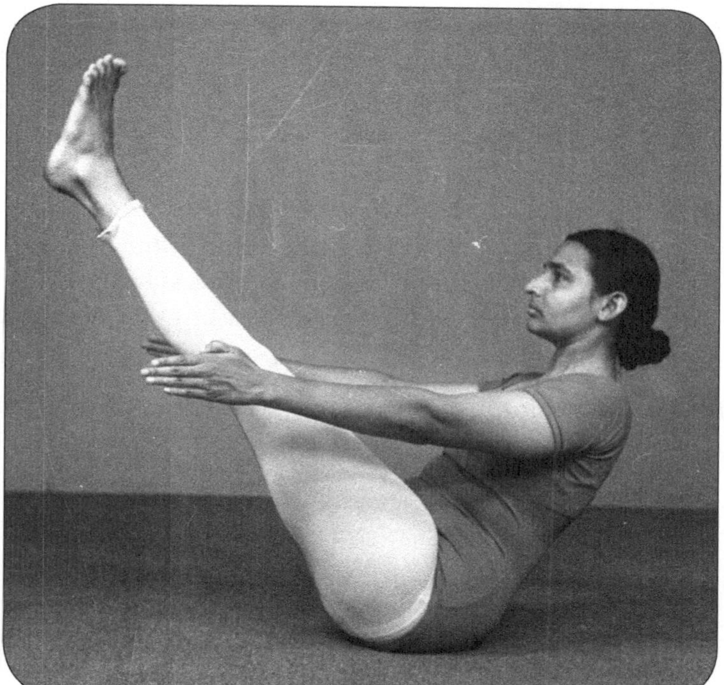

Fig. 111: *Paripūrṇa Nāvāsana* (Final Stage)

4. Raise the hands from the floor; extend them forwards, parallel to the ground. Turn the palms inwards, facing each other. The shoulders and the palms should be in line with each other.
5. Remain in this position for 30 to 60 seconds, with normal breathing, observing the following points:
   (a) keep the legs poker-stiff;
   (b) keep the spine firm, with the head as if floating on it; if the head is bent forward, the neck gets tightened, causing heaviness in the head;
   (c) look straight ahead; do not press the chin against the throat;
   (d) do not cave in the chest nor lower the lumbar for the sake of balance;
   (e) feel as though the body is floating weightlessly like a boat; to do this, keep the spine firm.
6. Exhale, bring the arms and legs down, and assume the *Daṇḍāsana* posture (Figure 23).

Special Instructions

1. Do not touch the legs with the palms.
2. If it is not possible to raise the hands after balancing on the buttocks, attempt all the actions simultaneously, i.e., (a) reclining the trunk, (b) raising the legs, and (c) raising the arms.

Effects: This āsana is good for flatulence and gastric complaints. It reduces the fat and tones the kidneys.

60. *JAṬHARA PARIVARTANĀSANA*

Jaṭhara means stomach, parivartan means turning round, rotating. In this āsana the stomach is given an internal massage.

Technique

1. Lie flat on the back (Figure 80).
2. Stretch both the arms sideways in line with the shoulders, with the palms facing the ceiling. Take one or two breaths.
3. Exhale and lift both the legs together to form a right angle. Do not bend the knees. Wait in this position for some time (Figure 112), breathing normally.

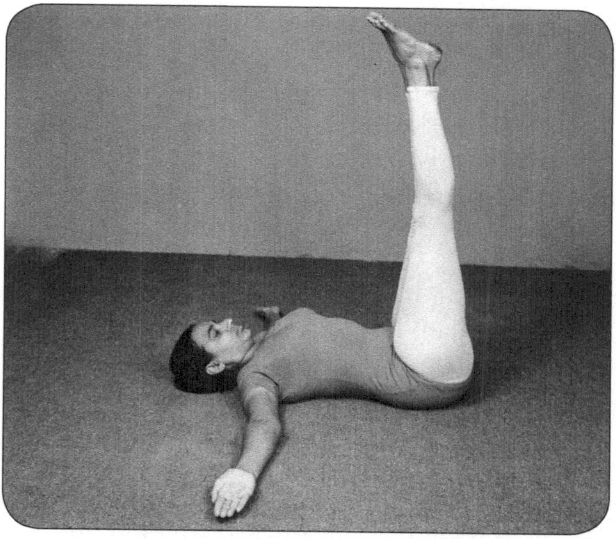

Fig. 112: *Jaṭhara Parivartanāsana* (Intermediate Stage)

4. Exhale, move both the legs slowly sideways towards the right palm, but do not touch the floor with the feet as the abdominal organs lose their grip and do not get the correct contraction. Keep the knees and the thighs touching each other (Figure 113).

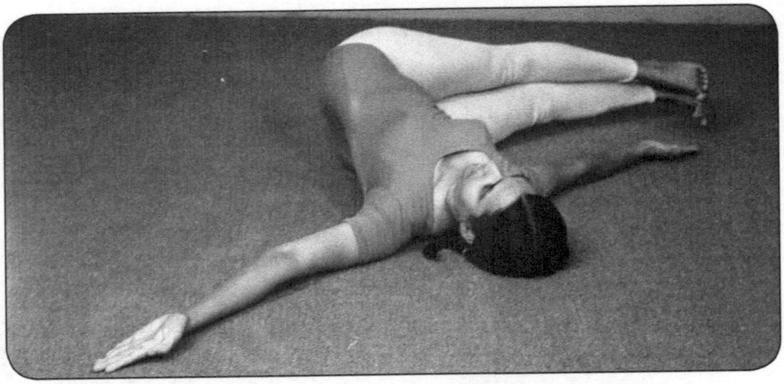

Fig. 113: *Jaṭhara Parivartanāsana* (Final Stage)

5. Keep the left side of the back on the floor as much as possible.
6. Stay in this position for 10 to 15 seconds. Breathe normally, observing the following points:
   (a) as the legs move to the right, revolve the trunk to the left. Stretch both the thighs and pull them· towards the buttocks so that the left side of the back is twisted to the left;
   (b) turn and twist the abdomen and the pelvis to the left so that the abdominal organs are tensed and excercised;
   (c) when going to the right, the right leg tends to lose its grip; keep it firm;
   (d) do not lift the right shoulder from the floor.
7. Inhale and come back to the position shown in Figure 112 by pressing the left buttock and the left side of the trunk to the ground. Stay in this position for a few seconds and then repeat the posture on the left (Figure 114), by moving the legs towards the left and revolving the abdomen to the right.
8. Stay in this position for the same length of time, breathing normally. Bring the legs to the perpendicular position and wait for a few moments. Take one or two breaths.
9. Exhale and lower both the legs slowly to the ground.

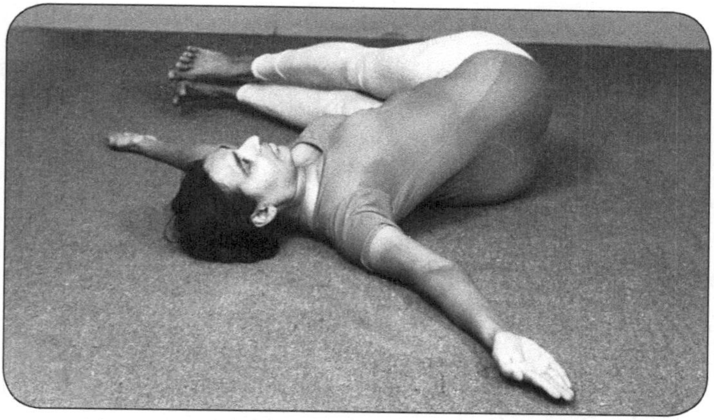

Fig. 114: *Jaṭhara Parivartanāsana* (Final Stage)

Special Instructions

1. Those who cannot raise the legs straight may first bend the knees (Figure 110), then straighten the legs (Figure 109).
2. While the legs are moving to the right side, the left shoulder tends to lift off the floor. Ask an assistant to press it down, or hold a heavy piece of furniture with the left hand. Ask an assistant to press the pelvic bone down if the opposite side comes off the floor. The same has to be done on the other side.
3. All these movements of the legs, whether upwards or sideways, should be done very slowly without any jerking. The slower the movements, the better the action on the abdominal organs. If the posture is done quickly, then only the legs get exercised. In the beginning the āsana should be done only once. Later, with practice, it can be done 2 to 4 times, without lowering the legs down from the perpendicular position. Follow the cycle on the right and left sides.

Effects: The āsana reduces fat, eradicates sluggishness of the liver, the spleen, and the pancreas, cures gastritis and relieves pains and 'catches' in the lower back.

61. *ŪRDHVA MUKHA PAŚCIMOTTĀNĀSANA II*

This is a variation of *Paścimottānāsana*; here the face (mukha) is turned upwards and the posterior stretch is as in *Paścimottānāsana*. As this āsana is difficult, its benefits are intense. See also *Ūrdhva Mukha Paścimottānāsana I* (Figure 173), which is easier.

Technique

1. Lie flat on the back. Extend the arms over the head (Figure 106). Take one or two breaths.
2. Exhale, lift both the legs up to form a right angle to the body. Do not bend the knees (Figure 109). Take one or two breaths.
3. Exhale again, bring the legs over the head and catch the soles of the feet by interlocking the fingers around them. Pull the legs towards the trunk so that the thighs and the abdomen are compressed together. The shins should touch the chin (Figure 115).

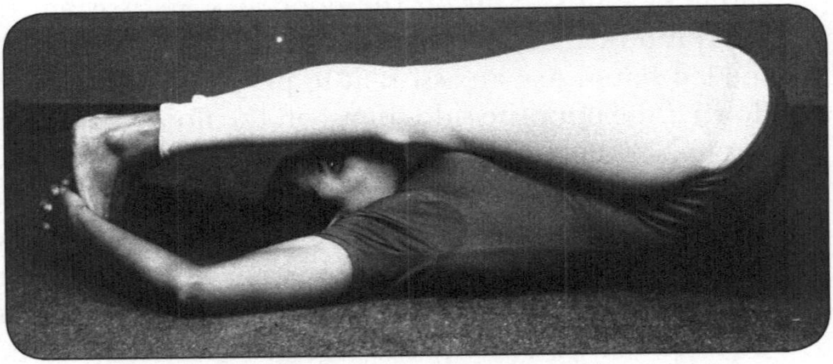

Fig. 115: *Ūrdhva Mukha Paścimottānāsana II* (Final Stage)

4. Remain in this position for 15 to 20 seconds, breathing normally and observing the following points:
   (a) tighten the quadriceps and stretch the hamstring muscles towards the heels;
   (b) do not lift the back and the buttocks up as in *Halāsana* (Figure 88);

(c) extend the elbow-joints by widening them;
(d) stretch the thighs and the buttocks backwards while extending the calves forwards, creating a challenge and response action in the body.

5. Exhale, release the hands and lower the feet.

Special Instruction

1. If the legs do not come closer to the abdomen, then bend the knees, hold the soles of the feet or the big toes firmly with the fingers. Pull the legs towards the abdomen and straighten them by making the knees tight.

Effects: This pose relieves severe backaches and relaxes the back muscles.

62. *SUPTA PĀDĀNGUṢṬHĀSANA*

This is a lying-down posture in which the big toe is caught with the fingers and the legs are extended in three directions.

Technique

Variation A

1. Lie flat on the floor, keep both the legs together and the knees tight (Figure 80). Breathe normally.
2. Inhale, bend the right knee to the chest and catch the big toe with a hook formed by the thumb, the forefinger and the middle finger. Extend the right leg upwards by stretching the hamstring muscle.
3. Stretch the right leg up so that it is perpendicular to the floor (Figure 116). If possible, pull it towards the head. The right hand will now be in line with the right shoulder (Figure 117). Place the left palm on the left thigh.

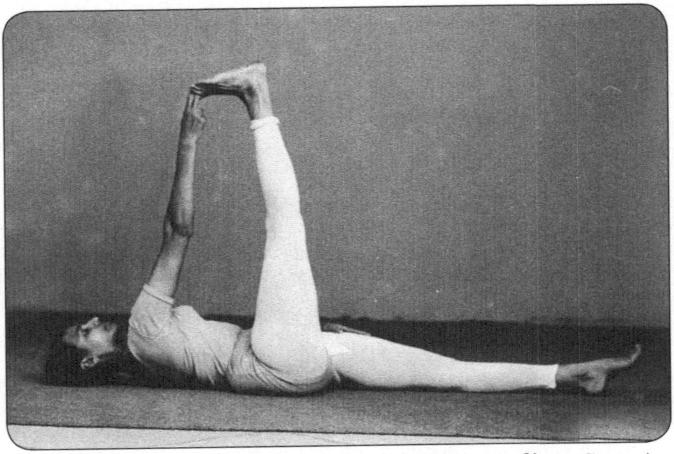

Fig. 116: *Supta Pādānguṣṭhāsana* (Intermediate Stage)

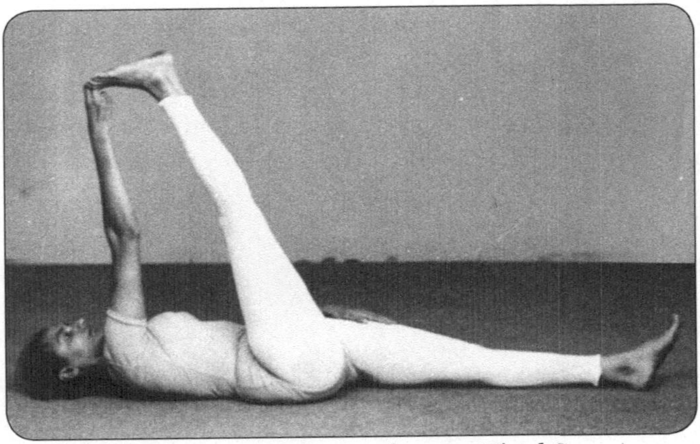

Fig. 117: *Supta Pādānguṣṭhāsana* (Final Stage)

4. Stay in this position for 5 to 10 seconds with normal breathing, observing the following points:
   (a) keep the left leg firmly pressed to the ground without bending the knee. Do not turn the left thigh out;
   (b) do not tilt the trunk to the left;
   (c) press the right buttock down;
   (d) do not loosen the grip of the fingers on the big toe.

Variation B

5. Exhale, take the right leg further over the head and raise the head and the upper trunk from the floor. Touch the leg with the forehead (Figure 118).

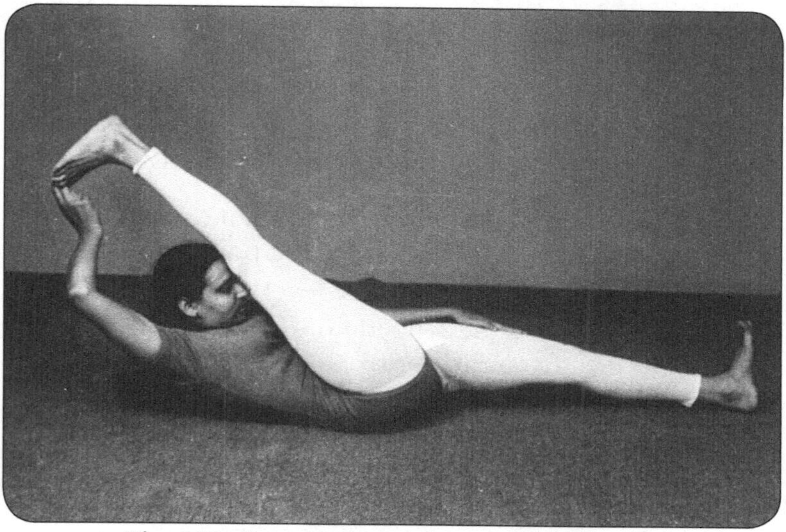

Fig. 118: *Supta Pādānguṣṭhāsana* (Final Stage)

6. Stay in this position for 5 to 10 seconds with normal breathing, observing the following points:
   (a) it is better to take the leg over the head rather than to lift the head and back more;
   (b) do not bend the knees;
   (c) keep the left buttock on the floor so that the trunk does not lean to the right.
7. Inhale, place the head and the back on the floor and come to the position as in Figure 117.

Variation C

8. Exhale, keep the left leg outstretched and pull the right leg sideways to the right until it reaches the floor. Stretch the hamstring muscle (Figure 119).

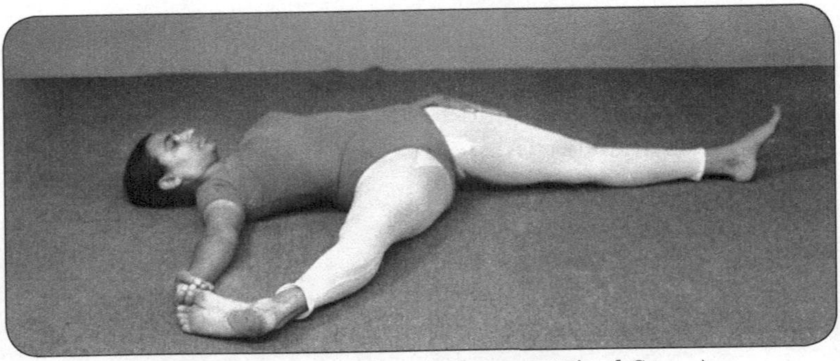

Fig. 119: *Supta Pādānguṣṭhāsana* (Final Stage)

9. Stay in this position for 5 to 10 seconds with normal breathing, observing the following points:
   (a) bring the right foot to the level of the shoulder;
   (b) do not raise the left side of the trunk and the left buttock from the floor.
10. Inhale and come to position as in Figure 117.
11. Release the big toe, lower the right leg and the right arm, and keep the arm by the side.
12. Now, do the āsana on the left side by raising the left leg up and holding the big toe, breathing normally, following all the three movements described above and substituting the word right for left.

Special Instructions

1. Do not loosen the grip of the big toe and the fingers. If it is loose, the knee will bend and the abdominal muscles will be loose.
2. If the outstretched leg on the floor bends at the knee, keep the bottom of the left foot pressed against a wall.
3. In the initial stages it is difficult to pull the raised leg towards the head; therefore, the first variation should be practised more (Figure 116).

Effects: This posture relieves sciatica, stiffness of the hip joints and soothes the nerves around the hips.

63. *UTTHITA HASTA PĀDĀNGUṢṬHĀSANA*

Hasta means hand. This āsana is done by standing on one leg, extending the other leg, catching the big toe with the hands and resting the head on the knees. It is done without any support (see *Light on Yoga*).

Being a difficult posture, it is advisable for women to rest the outstretched leg on a table or a window, as described below. This has more curative value. This āsana is similar to *Supta Pādānguṣṭhāsana*, but is done in a standing position so that there is freedom of movement for the spine. This is more effective in conditions such as slipped disc, backache, weakness in hip muscles, unequal length of the legs.

Technique

Variation A

1. Stand two to three feet away from a table or a window, facing it. Take one or two breaths.
2. Exhale and bend the right knee, raise it and place it on the table or the window sill so that it is parallel to the floor. Stretch the right leg, keeping the foot upright. Extend both the arms and catch a bar of the window for support and lift the trunk (Figure 120).

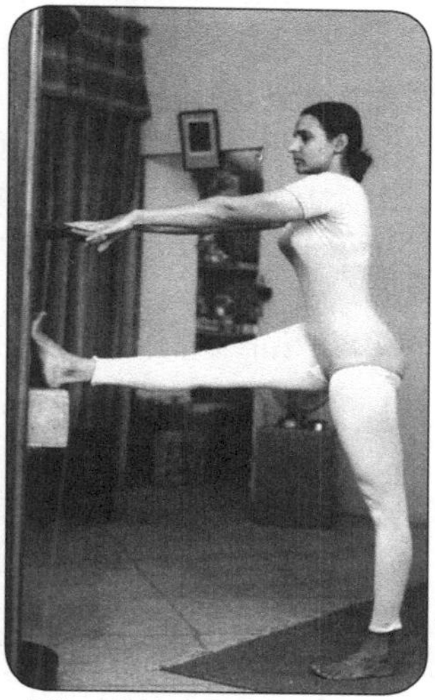

Fig. 120: *Utthita Hasta Pādānguṣṭhāsana* (Intermediate Stage)

3. Keep the head erect and look straight forward.
4. Keep the left leg firmly on the floor and stretch the spine from the coccyx up. Stretch both the hamstring muscles. Stay in this position for 10 to 15 seconds, breathing normally, observing the following points:

   (a) do not lift the shoulders or contract the neck;

(b) do not turn the right buttock out; keep the trunk straight;
(c) do not lean forward;
(d) do not turn the left foot out;
(e) keep both the pelvic bones parallel to each other.

5. With practice, gradually keep the right leg at a higher level. Catch the sole of the right foot with both the hands. Raise the spine and extend the trunk up (Figure 121).

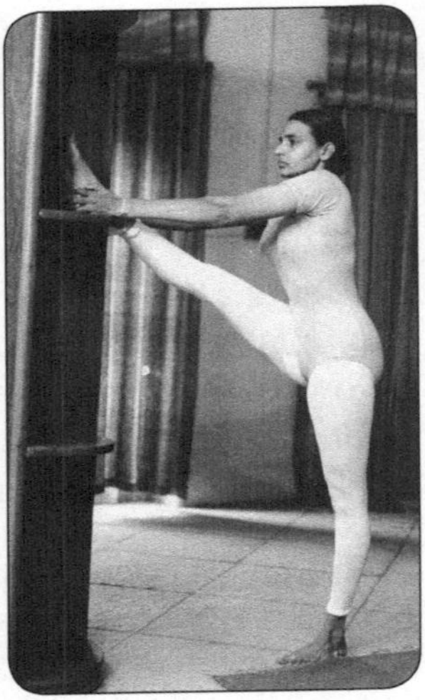

Fig. 121: *Utthita Hasta Pādānguṣṭhāsana* (Final Stage)

6. Inhale and lower the right leg. Now, do the same posture on the other side, standing on the right leg and raising the left leg. Breathe normally.

Variation B

1. Turn the whole body 90° to the left. The feet will now be parallel to the table or the window. Stand 2 to 3 feet away from the table or the window. Take one or two breaths.
2. Exhale, bend the right knee and place the right foot on the table at right angles (Figure 122). Keep the left hand on the hip. Catch a plank or a bar with the right hand, or keep the right hand on the right shin and lift the trunk up.
3. With practice, increase the height and gradually rest the right foot in a raised position at the level of the shoulders. Catch the right big toe or the sole with the fingers of the right hand. Stretch the anterior trunk (Figure 123).

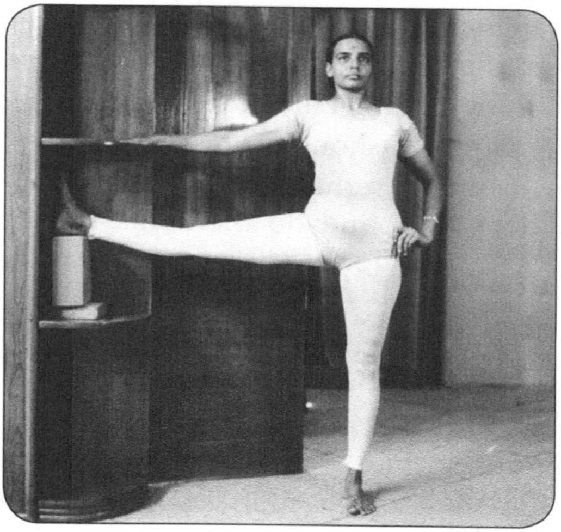

Fig. 122: *Utthita Hasta Pādānguṣṭhāsana* (Intermediate Stage)

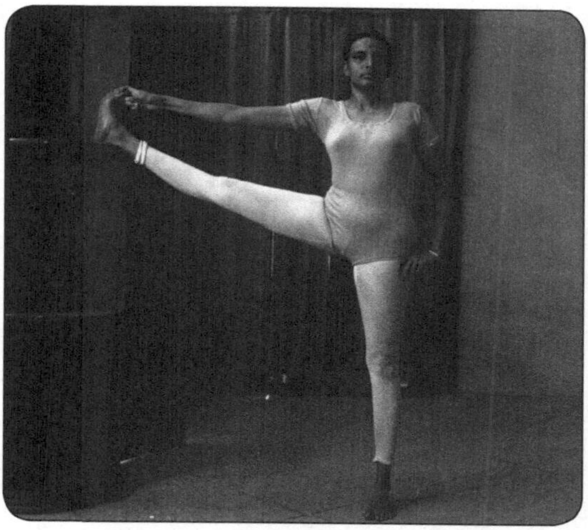

Fig. 123: *Utthita Hasta Pādānguṣṭhāsana* (Final Stage)

4. Stay in this position for 10 to 15 seconds, breathing normally, observing the following points:
   (a) do not lift the right outer buttock upwards. It has a tendency to lift, which can cause backache or cramp in the thighs;

(b) straighten the trunk by keeping the groins firm;
(c) keep the trunk and the buttocks in one line;
(d) lift the abdominal muscles and broaden the chest;
(e) do not lift the shoulders or contract the neck.

5. Exhale, bend the right leg and take it down. Turn the whole body 180° and do the āsana standing on the right leg and taking the left leg up. Breathe normally.

Variation C

1. Come to the position as in Figure 120 or 121.
2. Now, hold the big toe or the heel of the right foot (or the bar or the edge of the table beyond the foot), with the left hand. Keep the right hand on the hip and raise the trunk. Do not bend the knees.
3. Rotate the trunk to the right so that the edge of the left side of the trunk is in line with the right thigh (Figure 124).

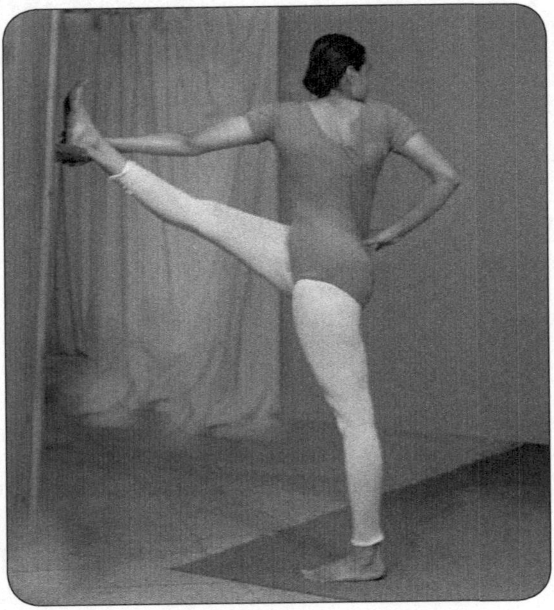

Fig. 124: *Utthita Hasta Pādānguṣṭhāsana* (Final Stage)

4. Keep both the shoulders, as well as the right and the left sides of the body in line with the right leg. Turn the neck to the right and look straight ahead.
5. Stay in this position for 10 to 15 seconds, with normal breathing, observing the following points:
   (a) raise the spine from the coccyx up and rotate it so that the abdomen and the back are well stretched.
   (b) keep an upward lift from the pelvis to the top chest while rotating.
6. Inhale and bring the trunk to the position as in Figure 121. Exhale, lower the right foot and place it next to the left foot.
7. Now, keep the left foot on the table or the window, hold it with the right hand and follow all the movements described above, breathing normally. (The figures depict how to hold the toe, heel, edge of a table, etc.)

Special Instructions

1. In this āsana the hamstring muscles and the muscles of the back of the thighs are pulled intensely, hence the movement of placing the foot on the table or the window should be done gradually. It is better to master the posture by raising the leg to the thigh level as in Figure 120 and not above.
2. Do not be aggressive in the thigh movements while lifting the leg up to a higher level. Any movement done jerkily may cause tearing.
3. It is more important to raise the spine and to keep the trunk firm than to take the leg higher and higher.

Effects: This posture removes backache and relieves lumbago, sciatica, rheumatism and slipped disc.

OVERALL EFFECTS—ĀSANAS 58 to 63

All these āsanas reduce the fat around the waist, the buttocks, the thighs and the lower abdomen. The muscles in the back become firm and the hips and the abdominal organs are strengthened. The arms and the legs gain freedom of movement. They eradicate arthritis and rheumatism of ankle, knee, back, etc. They eradicate the sluggishness of the liver, spleen and pancreas and make them function normally. Those suffering from intestinal disorders, constipation, flatulence, disorders of the kidneys and bladder derive much benefit by the practice of these āsanas.

All these postures bring strength and flexibility to the spine. Women should practice these āsanas after two months of delivery in order to regain strength.

These āsanas especially Figures 119 and 123 are a boon for the women at menopause, which causes stiffness at the pelvic joints, pain in the lower back, burning and itching sensation in the vagina.

SECTION-VI

Āsanas: Twists

The āsanas in this section rotate and twist the spinal column and the trunk laterally. They are extremely beneficial to women and should be practised daily. They tone, massage, and rejuvenate the abdominal organs.

64. *BHĀRADVĀJĀSANA I*

The āsana is named after Bharadvaja the father of Droṇāchārya, who was the Guru of the Kauravas and the Pāṇḍavas.

Technique

1. Sit in *Daṇḍāsana* (Figure 23).
2. Bend both the legs and take the shins backwards to the right so that the feet are adjacent to the right hip.
3. Rest the buttocks on the floor, by the side of the feet and lift the trunk so that the spine is extended upwards. Do not sit on the feet. Take one or two breaths.
4. Exhale and turn the trunk to the left so that the left shoulder moves to the left and the right shoulder comes forward. Turn the chest and the abdomen to the left.
5. Place the right palm under the left thigh with the palm facing the floor.
6. Place the left hand behind the left buttock and turn the spine more. Tuck the right shoulder-blade in and revolve the left shoulder backwards. Take a breath or two.
7. Exhale, move the left arm backwards, from the shoulder, bend the elbow and clasp the right upper arm with the left hand.
8. Turn the head and the neck to the left and look straight ahead (Figure 125).

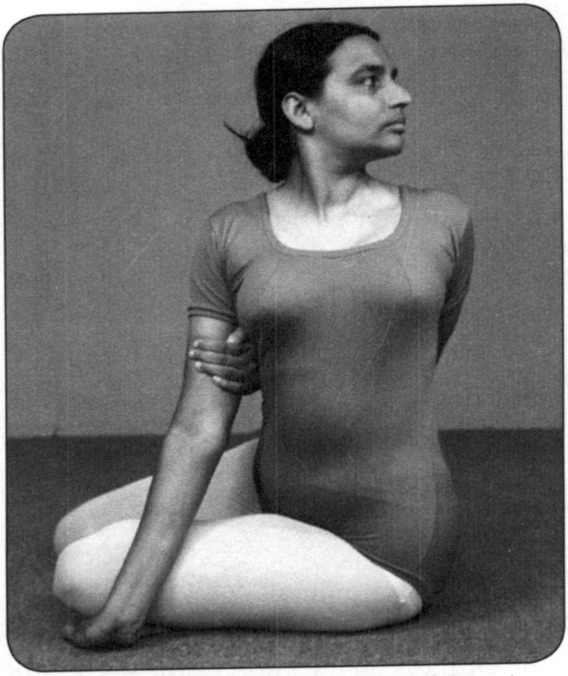

Fig. 125: *Bhāradvājāsana I* (Final Stage)

9. Breathing normally, remain in this final position for 30 to 60 seconds, observing the following points:
   (a) revolve the trunk in such a way that the right side of the body comes almost in line with the left thigh;
   (b) tuck the shoulder-blades in and lift the sternum up;
   (c) keep the spine erect and turn it on its axis;
   (d) do not change the position of the knee while turning, as it tends to move to the left;
   (e) see that the body does not lean backwards. Keep the left hip and the left shoulder in line.
10. Release the hands, bring the trunk forward and straighten the legs (Figure 23).
11. Now, bend the legs and take the shins backwards to the left, adjacent to the left hip. Do the āsana on this side,

following the points of the technique but reversing the instructions for right to left. The duration should be equal on both the sides. Return to *Daṇḍāsana* (Figure 23).

Special Instructions

1. If the left arm does not reach the right upper arm behind the back, swing from the left shoulder and move the left arm more so that it reaches the right arm. However, the swing should be mild and not violent.
2. Often one experiences a cramp in the buttocks; in the right buttock when one is rotating to the left and vice versa. Place a blanket 2 to 2½ inches thick under the buttocks, keeping the feet on the floor. This will help turn the sides of the pelvis more. Instead of holding the arm behind, both the palms may be kept on the floor by the sides of the hips and used as levers to lift the trunk more instead of twisting it (Figure 198).
3. In the beginning this āsana may be practised near a wall so that the hips can twist more easily. *Ardha Matsyendrāsana* (Figure 130) and *Pāśāsana* (Figure 132) are also shown against a wall.
   (a) sit with the left buttock touching the wall;
   (b) place both the feet near the right buttock;
   (c) place the left knee and the thigh adjacent to the wall;
   (d) insert the right hand under the left thigh and place the left palm on the wall in line with the shoulders;
   (e) press the wall with the left palm, raise the trunk and turn it to the left;
   (f) place the right buttock against the wall to do the āsana on the other side.

Effects: This āsana works on the dorsal and the lumbar regions of the spine, removing stiffness and pain. It is a good pose for relief from slipped discs.

65. *BHĀRADVĀJĀSANA II*

This is an intensive variation of the previous pose.

Technique

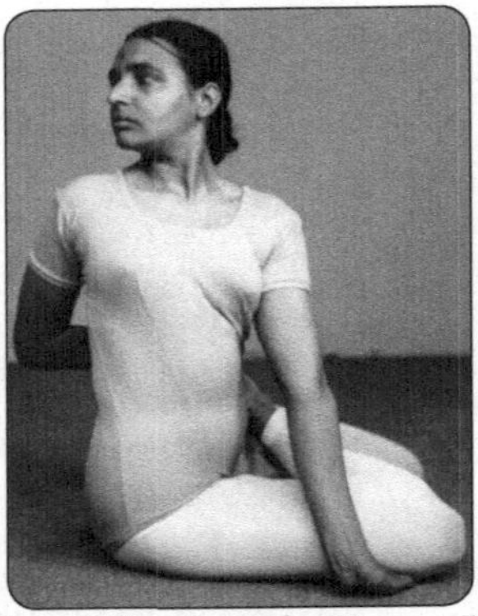

Fig. 126: *Bhāradvājāsana II* (Final Stage)

1. Sit in *Daṇḍāsana* (Figure 23).
2. Bend the left leg at the knee and place it near the left buttock as in *Vīrāsana* (Figure 49).
3. Bend the right leg at the knee and place the right foot at the root of the right thigh as in *Padmāsana* (Figure 52). Do not lift the right knee off the ground. Take one or two breaths.
4. Exhale, rotate the trunk to the right, keeping the spine extending upwards.
5. Place the left palm under the right thigh near the knee. Do not bend the left elbow.
6. Stretch the right arm, take it behind the back and hold the right big toe with the fingers, as in *Baddha Padmāsana* (Figure 61).
7. Turn the neck to the right and look straight ahead (Figure 126).
8. Stay in this final position for 20 to 30 seconds with normal breathing, observing the following points:
   (a) while turning the trunk to the right, keep it perpendicular to the floor;
   (b) broaden the chest and tuck the shoulder-blades in.
9. Exhale, release the right hand and the left arm, straighten the trunk and release first the right leg and then the left leg. Now, do the posture on the other side, reversing the instructions for right to left. The duration should be equal on both the sides.

Effects: In this pose the knees and the shoulders get flexibility and one gains relief from arthritis.

66. *MARĪCYĀSANA III*

This āsana is named after the sage Marici, the grandfather of the Sun God. Here the spine is twisted to the side, whereas in *Marīcyāsana I* it is extended forward. *Marīcyāsana III*, being more effective and intensive for women, is given here; *Marīcyāsana II* is omitted but may, if required, referred to in *Light on Yoga*.

Technique

1. Sit in *Daṇḍāsana* (Figure 23).
2. Bend the left leg at the knee with the shin perpendicular to the ground and pull the foot towards its own thigh. Keep the toes pointing forwards and the sole and the heel on the floor. The left calf and the left thigh should be in close contact. Keep the right leg outstretched. Take one or two breaths.
3. Exhale fully, raise the spine up and rotate the trunk to the left so that the right side of the trunk is close to the left thigh. Rest the left arm 8 to 10 inches away from the buttocks behind the back.
4. Raise the right arm and extend it beyond the left thigh. To do this,
   (a) move the left thigh slightly towards the right leg, or
   (b) push it with the right arm and entwine the arm around the knee. The right side of the trunk and the armpit will now be locked between the left knee and the top of the left thigh.
5. Extend the right arm further towards the right leg so that the right forearm, the armpit, and the right side of the trunk come still closer to the left thigh.
6. Bend the right arm at the elbow, turn it at the wrist, and encircle the left leg, placing the palm on the back. Take a breath or two.
7. Exhale raise the left arm from the floor, extend it backwards from the shoulder. Bend it at the elbow and bring it near the right palm behind the back. Firmly

clasp the fingers, the palm, and the wrist of the right hand with the left hand, in this order. Raise the trunk and turn it to the left. Turn the neck and gaze to the left (Figure 127).

8. Stay in this position for 20 to 30 seconds. At first there is quick breathing because the diaphragm is compressed; within a few moments the breathing becomes normal. Observe the following points:
   (a) stretch the extended leg further;
   (b) tuck in the shoulder-blades;

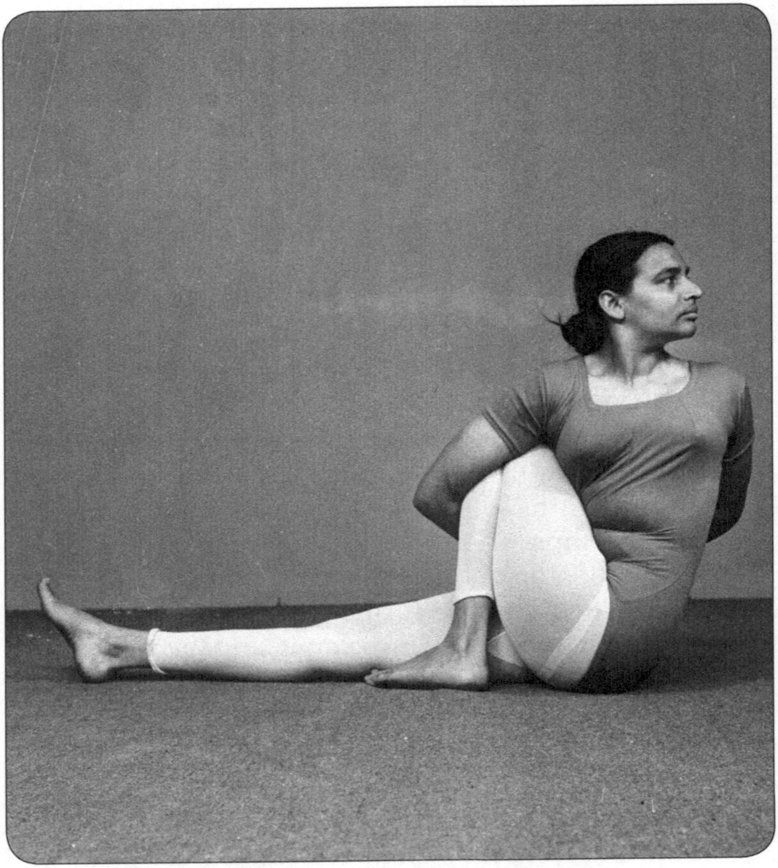

Fig. 127: *Marīcyāsana III* (Final Stage)

(c) there should be no space between the armpit of the intertwining arm and the thigh of the bent leg;

(d) do not loosen the grip of the fingers at the back.

9. Turn the head to the front, release the hands and return to *Daṇḍāsana* (Figure 23).

10. Now, repeat the posture with the left leg stretched and the right leg bent, following all the techniques and reversing the instructions for right to left. Duration should be the same on both sides.

Special Instruction

1. If it is not possible to do this āsana independently, it may be done with the support of a wall, as follows:

   (a) Sit in *Daṇḍāsana* (Figure 23), sideways to the wall so that right leg is extended along the wall;

   (b) bend the right leg at the knee and keep the shin perpendicular; take one or two breaths;

   (c) exhale and turn the trunk to the right so that the left side of the trunk comes closer to the right thigh;

   (d) extend the left shoulder and the left armpit towards the right leg;

   (e) keep the palm of the left hand on the wall and push the right thigh with the right arm;

   (f) raise the right arm and place the palm on the wall;

   (g) press the wall with both the palms, lift the trunk up and turn it;

   (h) now, do the āsana with the left leg along the wall, reversing all the processes.

Effects: This āsana reduces the fat around the abdomen, relieves backaches, lumbago, sprains in the neck and the shoulders and tones the abdominal organs.

67. *ARDHA MATSYENDRĀSANA*

Matsya means fish, Indra is Lord. An interesting anecdote is connected with this āsana. In the Haṭhayoga Pradīpikā, Matsyendra is mentioned as one of the founders of Haṭha Vidyā. Lord Śiva was once expounding Yoga Vidyā to Pārvatī by the side of the river, where a fish was listening intently to the discourse. Lord Śiva sprinkled some water on the fish and it became Matsyendra, Lord of the fishes.

The āsana described here is half *Matsyendrāsana*, For *Paripūrna* or full *Matsyendrāsana* refer to *Light on Yoga*.

Technique

1. Sit in *Daṇḍāsana* (Figure 23).
2. Bend the right leg at the knee and turn it back as in *Vīrāsana* (Figure 49). Lift the buttocks off the floor and place the right foot under them. The foot should be horizontal so that it forms a seat and acts as a cushion for the buttocks to rest on. Place the right outer buttock on the heel and the inner part on the sole.
3. Bend the left leg at the knee and place the shin by the outer side of the right leg so that the left outer ankle is close to the outer side of the right thigh. The left foot and the right knee should point forwards. Keep the hands by the sides of the body as in *Daṇḍāsana*. Maintain balance. Take a few breaths.

   If the buttocks are not properly placed on the right foot, or if the right foot has not formed a good seat, then the body tilts. Or, if the pelvis is heavy, the leg which is perpendicular tilts at an incorrect angle. Take one or two breaths.
4. Exhale and revolve the trunk 90° to the left. Place the left hand 4 to 6 inches behind the left buttock. Turn the spine so that the chest, the stomach, and the pelvis turn to the left, beyond the perpendicular left thigh.

5. Bend the right arm at the elbow and bring it beyond the outer edge of the left thigh so that the right armpit and the right side of the trunk come close to the left knee and the thigh then encircle the left leg with the right arm. Take a breath.
6. Exhale, lift the left hand off the floor, extend it from the shoulder without losing balance, swing the arm back and place the hand on the right hip. Catch the fingers of the right hand with the fingers of the left hand; as the body revolves, gradually clasp further and catch the palm and the wrist (Figure 128).
7. Turn the head towards the left shoulder and look to the left.
8. Stay in this final position for 20 to 30 seconds. In the beginning the respiration rate goes up, but gradually comes to normal. Observe the following points:
   (a) balance in this posture cannot be maintained if the grip of the hands is loose, if the chest is not lifted and broadened while turning both the arms backwards, or if the muscles of the waist and the hips are not stretched upwards;

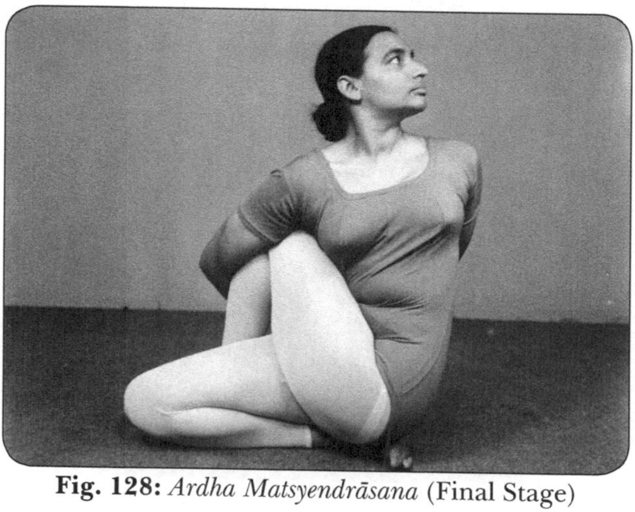

Fig. 128: *Ardha Matsyendrāsana* (Final Stage)

(b) see that the diaphragmatic area does not get caught or compressed against the left thigh, and hinder breathing.

9. Release the hands, bring the trunk forward, straighten the left leg and the right leg in that order.
10. Now, do the āsana on the other side, sitting on the left foot and reversing all the processes from right to left and vice versa. Remain for the same length of time.
11. Come back to *Daṇḍāsana*.

Special Instructions

1. Those who are overweight may find it difficult to sit on the foot: they should place the heel next to the buttock and place a blanket 2 or 3 inches thick under the buttock so that the buttock is up and the heel is on the floor.
2. Those who cannot hold the hands behind the back should place the perpendicular leg near the right knee so that the abdomen is not compressed. Instead of turning the right arm backwards, stretch it and hold the big toe of the left foot as in *Pādānguṣṭhāsana* (Figure 20); with further practice the palm may be placed under the foot. The left arm, however, should be taken backwards round the waist (Figure 129).

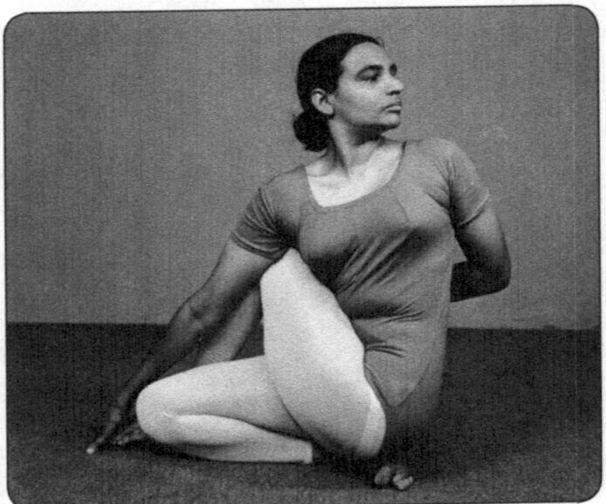

Fig. 129: *Ardha Matsyendrāsana* (Easy Stage)

3. Those who find the above method impossible should practice the āsana near a wall as follows:
   (a) Sit in *Daṇḍāsana* with the right leg along the wall.
   (b) Bend the left leg and sit on the left foot. The right buttock will remain adjacent to the wall.
   (c) Bend the right knee and place the right shin at the outer edge of the left thigh; it will now be away from the wall. Take one or two breaths.
   (d) Exhale, turn the trunk to the right and bring the left side of the trunk towards the right thigh.
   (e) Fix the left upper arm to the outer edge of the right leg bend the elbow and place the palm on the wall. The right arm should not be allowed to slip.
   (f) Raise the right arm and place the palm on the wall.

Press both the palms against the wall, raise the trunk and twist (Figure 130). The abdominal organs and the spine are well massaged by these movements.

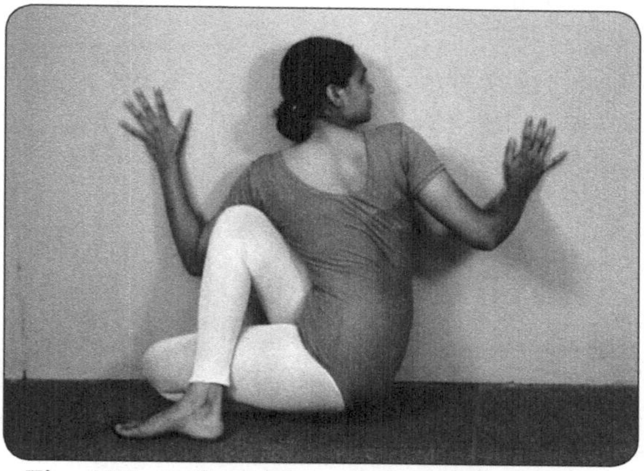

Fig. 130: *Ardha Matsyendrāsana* (Easy Stage)

Those who are able to do the āsana without the support of a wall should also try it against the wall for an intense massage of the abdominal organs and of the spinal column.

Effects: This āsana massages the lower abdominal organs and strengthens the lower part of the back.

68. *PĀŚĀSANA*

Pāśa means noose. In this āsana, the trunk is turned and the arms form a noose around the legs.

Technique

1. Squat with the soles and the heels on the floor as in Figure 45. Take a breath.
2. Place the left hand behind the buttocks, 4 to 6 inches away. Exhale and revolve the trunk 90° to the left, bearing the weight on the left palm and on the feet.
3. Bend the right elbow and bring the arm beyond the left thigh, keeping the armpit as close to the thigh as possible; now, extend the same arm, bend it, then turn it to bring it closer to the right thigh so that the right arm encircles both the legs.
4. Balance on the soles of the feet and raise the ankles; lift the left hand off the ground and take it behind the back. Take a breath. Exhale, revolve the spine more to the left.
5. Entwine both the hands. While twisting the left arm back, do not contract the left shoulder but extend it from the armpit.
6. Turn the neck to the left and look to the left (Figure 131).
7. Stay in this final position for 20 to 30 seconds, with normal breathing.

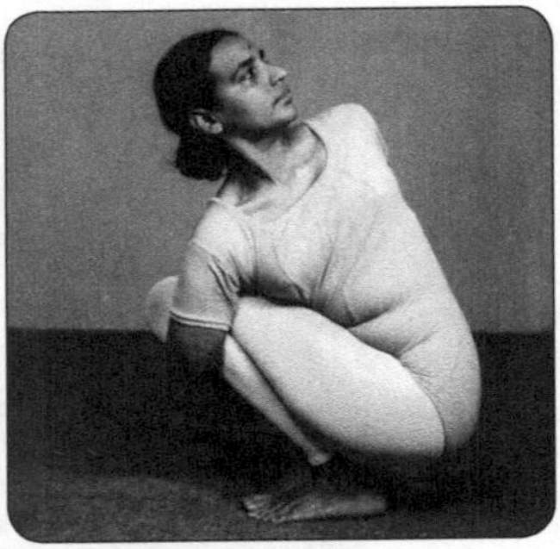

Fig. 131: *Pāśāsana* (Final Stage)

8. Inhale, release the left arm, then the right, and straighten the trunk. Place the hands on the floor.
9. Now, do the āsana on the other side, rotating the trunk to the right, reversing all the processes and staying for the same length of time.
10. Come to *Daṇḍāsana* (Figure 23).

Special Instruction

1. If this āsana cannot be practised independently, do it with the support of a wall (In the Figures, the trunk is twisted to the right in *Ardha Matsyendrāsana*, while in *Pāśāsana* it is twisted to the left.)
   (a) Sit in the position as in Figure 45. The left leg should remain adjacent to the wall and the right leg away from it. The left buttock touches the wall.
   (b) Rotate the trunk to the left so that the right side of the trunk comes closer towards the left thigh.
   (c) Keep the right hand on the outer edge of the left thigh, then place the right palm on the wall, in line with the head.
   (d) Place the left hand on the wall.
   (e) Press both the hands against the wall and revolve the trunk further to the left (Figure 132). Extend and turn the spine so that it becomes flexible.
   (f) Release the hands, sit against the wall with the right leg touching the wall and do the āsana on the other side, reversing all the processes and remaining for the same length of time. Breathe normally.
   (g) Come to *Daṇḍāsana*.

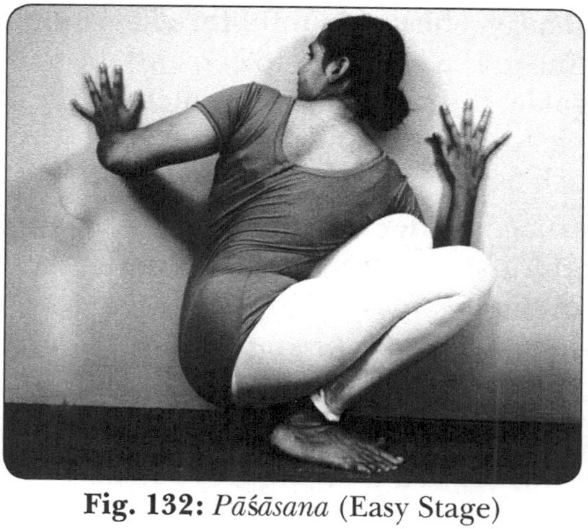

Fig. 132: *Pāśāsana* (Easy Stage)

Effects: The effects of this āsana are, more intense than in the other twisting postures given. It reduces the fat around the abdomen and tones and massages the abdominal organs. The liver, the spleen and the pancreas are revitalised. The āsana removes stiffness in the shoulders

OVERALL EFFECTS OF ĀSANAS 64 to 68

The effects of these āsanas are obvious. They are aimed at obtaining flexibility of the spinal column. In the beginning the spine is stiff, but with practice it becomes flexible.

These āsanas are extremely helpful in relieving rheumatism, backache and pain in the spinal column. They are useful for those with hunchback. For sprain in the back, however, or for slipped disc trouble they should be done against a wall. They increase the mobility of the shoulders and the shoulder-blades and expand the chest. They also give a neat shape to the ankles and the calves. They massage and rejuvenate the abdominal organs.

They are a boon for those who suffer from indigestion, acidity, appendicitis, irritation of the intestines, diabetes and flatulence. They are useful for alleviating disorders of the kidneys, the liver, the spleen and the gall-bladder. They regulate the peristaltic movement of the intestines, strengthen the uterus and the waist, and correct complaints such as the enlarged bladder.

Menstrual disorders, malfunctioning of the endocrine glands and obesity are all remedied greatly by the practice of these āsanas.

They relieve back pain and exhaustion due to overwork or during the menstrual period (Figure 125).

They are beneficial after delivery but should be done with the support of a wall (Figures 130 and 132).

SECTION–VII

Āsanas: Backbends

Our daily tasks often involve forward-bending movements. These stretch the posterior side of the spine. Rarely do we bend the other way. Āsanas in this section stretch the spinal column in a concave movement and are very important, as the anterior spine extends in backbends making the blood circulate more freely. The opening of the chest in these particular postures energises the lungs and breathing becomes deep with the result that oxygenated blood circulates all over the body.

The āsanas from the other sections prepare the spinal column for the movements in this section. The first two āsanas given here are easy to perform and should be practised first along with some preparatory work from Section VIII on Yoga Kuruṇṭa, then the last three āsanas in this section will be easier to do. Some āsanas are described with support and they should be included with this practice.

Do not feel alarmed if you experience dizziness or black-outs in some of these postures, especially when coming up after completing an āsana. Do not close the eyes, keep them wide open and the dizziness or the blackout will disappear.

69. *UṢṬRĀSANA*

Uṣṭra means camel. This āsana is called the camel posture because it imitates the shape of a camel by making the spine concave.

Technique

1. Kneel on the floor with the knees close together and the thighs, the calves and the ankles touching each other. The tops of the feet should rest on the floor with the toes pointing back. This is position 1.
2. Place the palms on the buttocks, push the thighs slightly forward, and bend the trunk back. Push the spine into the body and bend back as far as possible.
3. Throw the head back, broaden the chest and extend both the arms from the shoulders towards the feet. Catch the heels with both the hands and if possible place the palms flat on the soles of the feet (Figure 133).

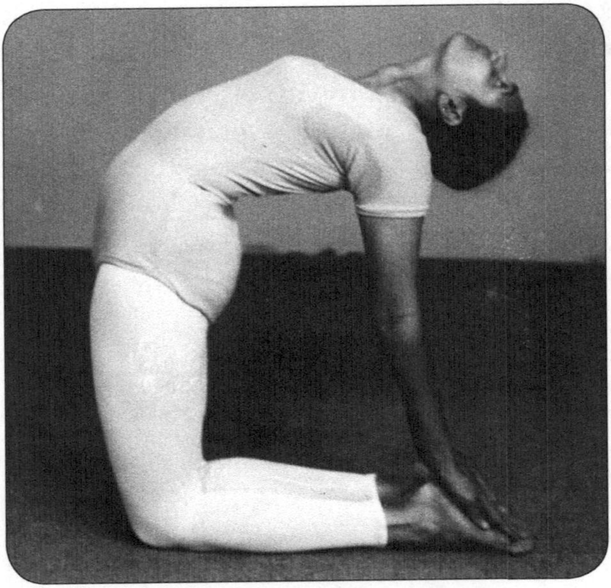

Fig. 133: *Uṣṭrāsana* (Final Stage)

4. Stay in this final position for 10 to 15 seconds with normal breathing, observing the following points:
   (a) stretch the thighs up;
   (b) tuck the buttocks in;
   (c) move the sacrum forward to extend the thighs, the buttocks and the hips;
   (d) broaden the ribs of the chest;
   (e) take the shoulder-blades in and raise the sternum;
   (f) throw the head back from the upper end of the breast-bone;
   (g) press the shins into the floor and the hands into the soles, take the spine into the body, lift it and stretch it so that the entire body forms a good arch.
5. Exhale, lessen the pressure of the hands on the feet; take the thighs and the buttocks slightly forward, raise the trunk and the arms and come to position 1. If both the arms cannot be raised simultaneously, then raise them one after another. The movement for lifting the trunk starts in the thighs and the chest so that the impetus to lift has to come from there.

Special Instructions

1. If it is not possible to catch both the heels simultaneously, catch them one at a time by tilting the shoulders first to one side and then to the other. After both the heels are caught, straighten the shoulders. Learn to take both the arms together as soon as possible.
2. In the beginning, if it is difficult to catch the heels, keep the knees slightly apart so that the movement of the spine is freer and the thighs do not pain. Gradually learn to keep the knees together.

Effects: This posture extends and tones the whole spine. It corrects drooping shoulders and hunchback.

70. *ŪRDHVA MUKHA ŚVĀNĀSANA*

Śvāna means dog. This posture resembles a dog stretching himself with the head up, hence the name.

Technique

1. Lie in a prone position on the floor.
2. Keep the feet 8 to 10 inches apart with the toes pointing back. Keep the knees straight.
3. Place the palms near the floating ribs, extending the fingers towards the head. Keep the chin forward (Figure 134).

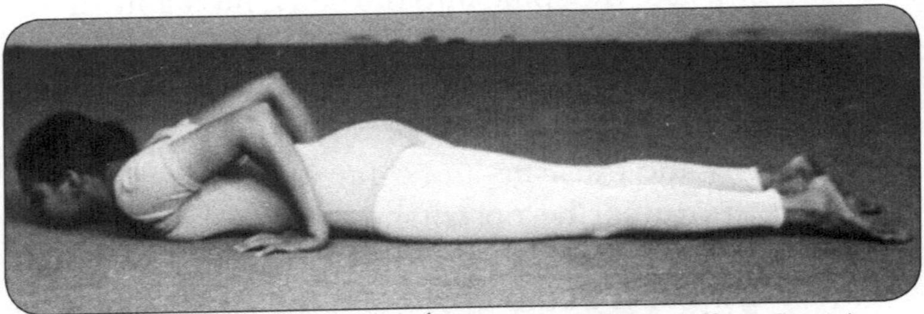

Fig. 134: *Ūrdhva Mukha Śvānāsana* (Intermediate Stage)

4. Inhale, raise the head and the trunk, and let the body weight be borne by the palms.
5. Press the hands into the ground and raise the trunk as much as possible with the thighs off the floor.
6. Throw the head back and look up at the ceiling (Figure 135).
7. Remain in this final position for 15 to 20 seconds, breathing normally and observing the following points:
   (a) compress the buttocks and press the inner thighs towards them;
   (b) expand the chest by raising the sternum up;
   (c) broaden the ribs, especially near the armpits,
   (d) do not compress the ribs with the arms.
   (e) keep the knees and the calves tight.

8. Exhale, bend the elbows, rest the thighs and knees on the floor. Lower the head and the trunk and lie prone on the floor (Figure 134).

Special Instructions

1. Those who are unable to raise the body off the floor should do this āsana as follows:
   - (a) Do *Adho Mukha Śvānāsana* (Figure 22), but do not place the head on the floor.
   - (b) Raise the heels from the floor and keep the front part of the toes down.
   - (c) Move the buttocks down and push the trunk forward onto the arms, towards the head.
   - (d) Do not rest the thighs on the floor.
   - (e) Extend the feet with the toes pointing backwards.
   - (f) Come to the final position as in Figure 135.
2. If this is also impossible, see Section VIII on Yoga Kuruṇṭa, Variation I (Figure 153).

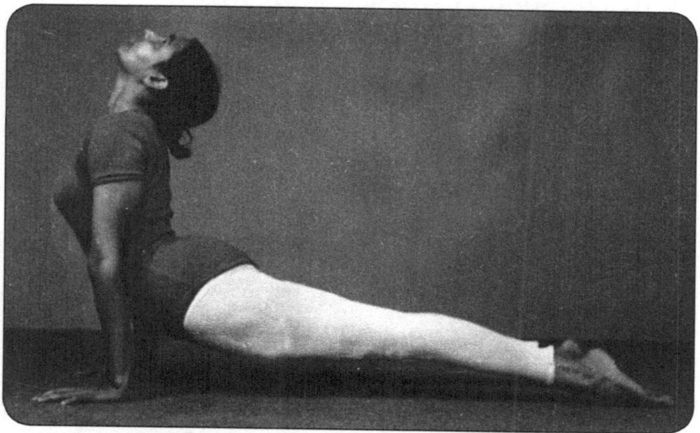

Fig. 135: *Ūrdhva Mukha Śvānāsana* (Final Stage)

Effects: This āsana is helpful for those suffering from slipped or prolapsed discs, lumbago and sciatica. The blood circulates in the pelvic region and keeps it healthy.

71. *DHANURĀSANA*

This āsana resembles a strung bow. The entire body is curved like a bow and is held with the arms as if forming a string to bend the bow.

Technique

1. Lie prone on the floor. Keep both the legs close together, with the toes pointing backwards. Keep the big toes, the heels, the knees and the thighs touching each other.
2. Keep the arms alongside the trunk. Take one or two breaths.
3. Exhale, bend the knees and bring the feet towards the buttocks.
4. Raise the head and the chest slightly off the floor and catch the left ankle with the left hand and the right ankle with the right hand. Hold the ankles tight by encircling them with the palms and the fingers. Remain in this position, taking a few breaths.
5. Now exhale. Raise the shins and the thighs so that the knees do not rest on the floor; at the same time lift the head and the chest off the floor.
6. Hold the ankles tight and straighten the arms. Lift the thighs in the direction of the head.
7. Bend the neck backwards and lift the chin up (Figure 136).
8. Stay in this final position for 15 to 20 seconds, breathing normally and observing the following points:
   (a) the ribs and the thighs should not touch the floor;
   (b) do not be on the pubis;

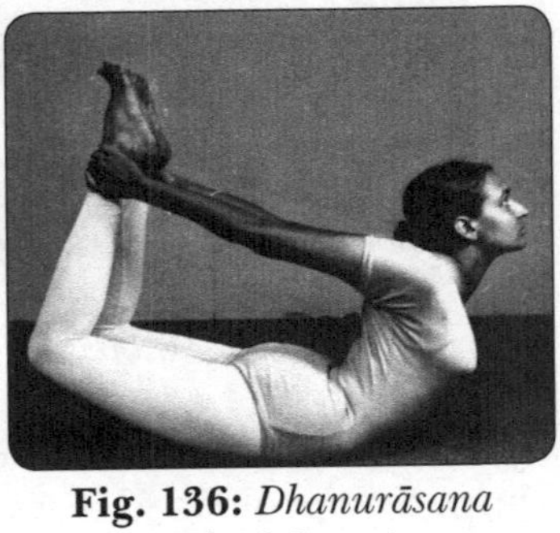

Fig. 136: *Dhanurāsana* (Final Stage)

(c) press the area around the abdomen to the floor and increase the arch which is formed by the arms and the legs.

9. Exhale, bend the knees, lower the chest, release the ankles and straighten the legs. Take the head and the trunk down and lie flat on the floor.

Note: Those who find it difficult to keep the feet together can spread them slightly apart and do this āsana. The important features of this āsana are forming an arch and balancing the torso on the abdomen. The spine has to be curved to the maximum so that the thighs, the waist and the buttocks get exercise.

Effects: This āsana brings elasticity to the spine and tones the abdominal organs.

OVERALL EFFECTS ĀSANAS 69 to 71

The concave movement of the spine in these āsanas is somewhat unusual which is not normally found in our everyday life. They tone and train the spine and the muscles of the back to bend backwards. They rejuvenate the spine and develop physical strength and vitality. They bring freedom of movement and are ideal for those suffering from stooping shoulders, hunchback, slipped disk, stiff spine, rheumatism and backache. They open the chest and improve breathing.

Women are used to bending the spine forwards in doing many of their household chores. These movements tend to make the posterior side of the spine flexible, whereas in these postures it is the anterior or the frontal spine which is worked more.

Elderly people can conveniently do all these poses without inviting any injury to the spine.

Dullness and depression vanish with the practice of these āsanas. They bring courage and will-power and give mental courage to bend backwards.

72. ŪRDHVA DHANURĀSANA

This posture is exactly the reverse of *Dhanurāsana*. An arch of the body is formed with the hands and the feet on the floor.

Technique

1. Lie flat on the back (Figure 80).
2. Bend the legs with the shins perpendicular and take the heels towards the back of the thighs. Hold the ankles with the hands and pull the feet closer to the body.
3. Extend the arms over the head with the palms facing the ceiling.
4. Bend the elbows, turn the wrists, and place the palms on the floor near the shoulders, the fingers facing the feet. Keep the elbows pointing towards the ceiling and the fingers spread out (Figure 137). Take two or three breaths.
5. Exhale, raise the back and the buttocks, lift the chest and place the crown of the head on the floor (Figure 138).
6. Press the palms and the bottom of the feet to the floor and raise the head from the floor. Use the wrists and

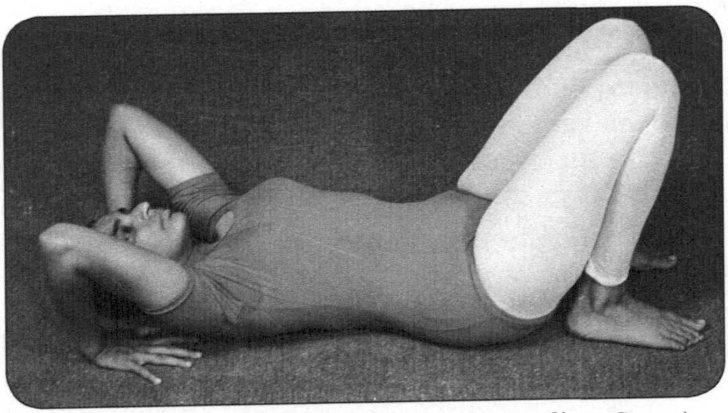

Fig. 137: *Urdhva Dhanurāsana* (Intermediate Stage)

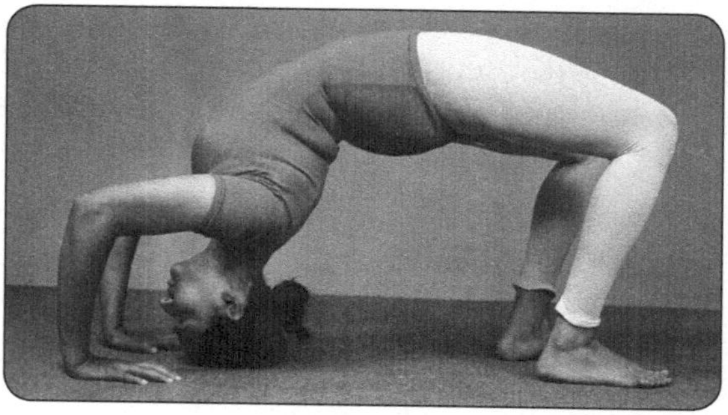

Fig. 138: *Urdhva Dhanurāsana* (Intermediate Stage)

the biceps to lift the head and the quadriceps to lift the legs. Take one or two breaths.

7. Exhale, take the spine and the waist in and straighten the arms to form a fine arch.
8. Turn the head back and look at the floor.
9. Raise the heels off the floor and stand on the mounts of the toes in order to push the spine further in, to contract the buttocks and to stretch the abdominal organs. Now, the whole body will form into a good arch. Without lowering the trunk, stretch the ankles and place the heels on the floor (Figures 139, 140).

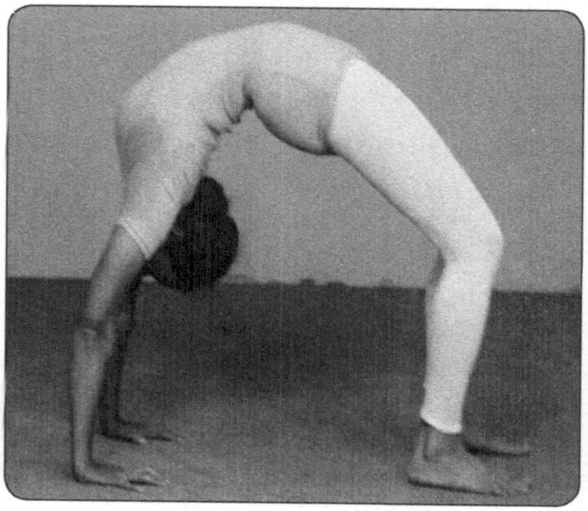

Fig. 139: *Urdhva Dhanurāsana* (Final Stage)

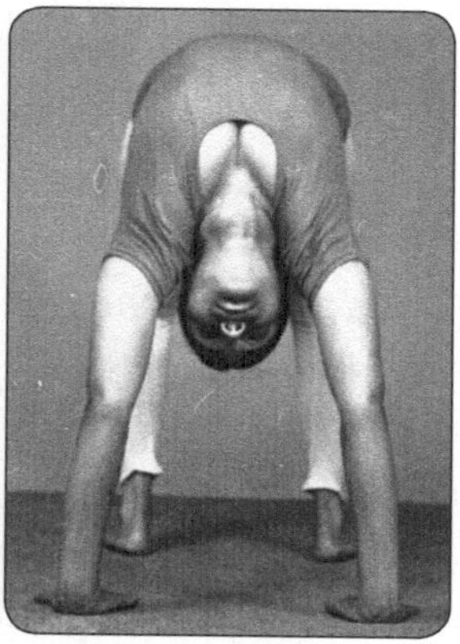

Fig. 140: *Urdhva Dhanurāsana* (Final Stage)

10. Stay in the final position for 5 to 10 seconds. In the beginning, the breathing will be rather fast but with practice it will become normal. Now observe the following points:
    (a) press the palms and the soles into the floor and pull the back of the thighs towards the buttocks;
    (b) contract the buttock muscles;
    (c) push the knees in and lift the thighs up;
    (d) tighten the biceps by pushing the elbows in, so that the arms remain straight and the chest is well lifted;
    (e) push the shoulder-blades in and broaden the chest and the ribs.
11. Exhale, bend the elbows and the knees, and lower the trunk. First rest the crown of the head on the floor (Figure 138), then the back and the buttocks. Take three or four breaths. Repeat this āsana three to five times for greater freedom of movement.

Special Instructions

1. In the beginning it is difficult to raise the head from the floor. In that case follow these movements:
    (a) Place a wooden plank about 5 to 6 inches high on the floor;
    (b) Lie flat on the back, place the palms face down by the edge of the plank; do not have the hands more than shoulder-width apart;
    (c) Place the head on the plank (Figure 141);
    (d) Raise the thighs, the back and the buttocks from the floor (Figure 141a);
    (e) Press the edges of the plank firmly with both the hands and by a lever action raise the chest and the head (Figures 142 and 142a). Form an arch with the body (Figure 143). Figure 142 shows the trunk lifted slightly, while in Figure 143 the trunk

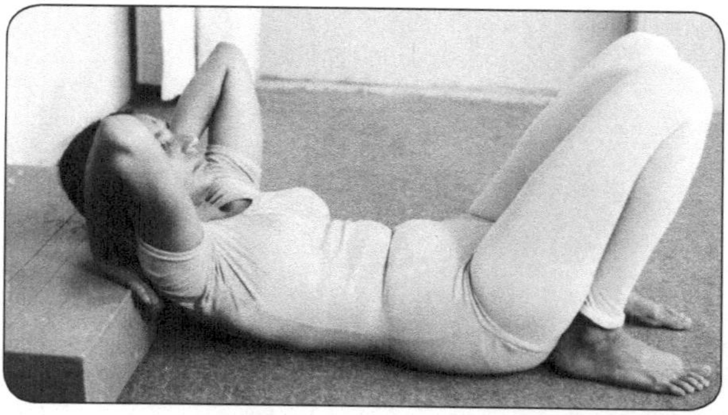

Fig. 141: *Urdhva Dhanurāsana* (Intermediate Stage)

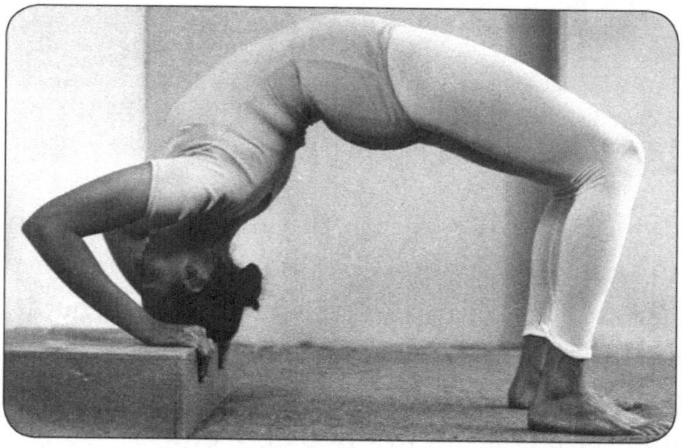

Fig. 141(a): *Urdhva Dhanurāsana* (Intermediate Stage)

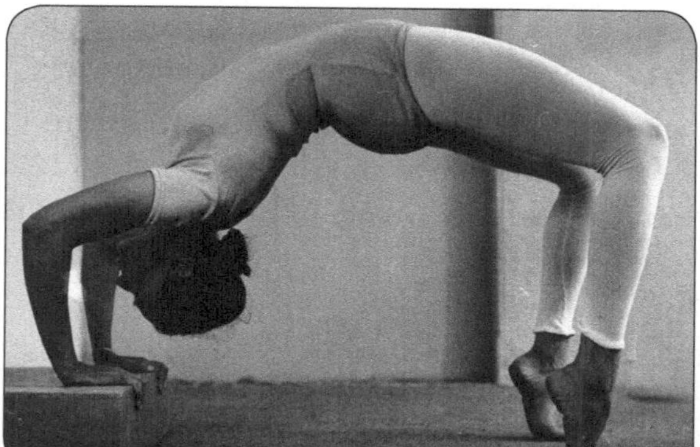

Fig. 142: *Urdhva Dhanurāsana* (Intermediate Stage)

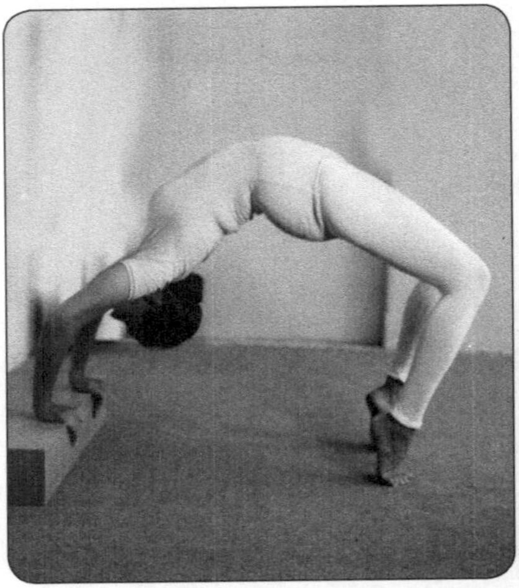

Fig. 142(a): *Urdhva Dhanurāsana* (Intermediate Stage)

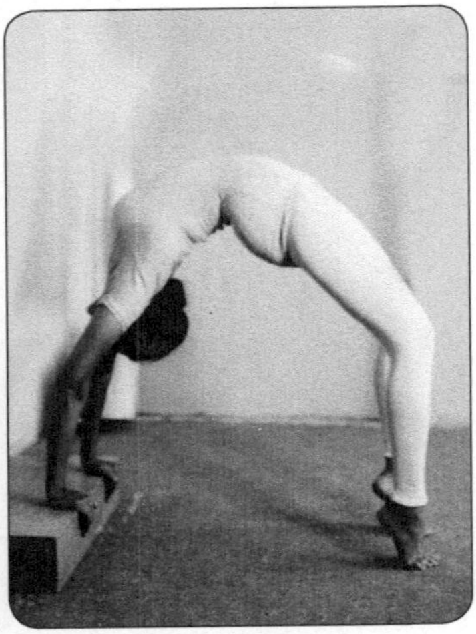

Fig. 143: *Urdhva Dhanurāsana* (Easy Stage)

is shown fully lifted up. After forming a good arch the heels may be kept down, as in Figure 139.

2. In spite of this support, if you find it difficult to raise the trunk up to form an arch, keep blankets or pillows underneath the trunk and follow the same procedure from (a) to (e) as mentioned above. It becomes easier to lift up with the support at the back.

Effects: This āsana tones the spine. It keeps the body supple and alert and gives vitality, energy, and lightness.

The method given under Special Instructions is of great help to strengthen the bladder and the uterus. It keeps the reproductory and the urinary organs healthy. Hernia can be prevented by strengthening the abdominal muscles in this way.

This posture relieves heaviness of the breasts which is felt particularly at the time of menopause. It also reduces the fat around the waist.

If possible, all the methods should be used.

73. *DVI PĀDA VIPARĪTA DAṆḌĀSANA*

In this posture the body is arched on the feet, the hands, and the head—it is a Yogi's salutation.

Technique

1. Lie flat on the floor (Figure 80).
2. Bend the knees and bring the feet close to the buttocks.
3. Bend the elbows, turn the wrists and place the palms on the floor near the shoulders. Keep the fingers outstretched as in Figure 137. Take one or two breaths.
4. Exhale, raise the buttocks and the back from the floor, and rest the crown of the head on the floor (Figure 138).
5. Lift the right arm and place the hand behind the head, keeping the elbow and the forearm resting on the ground. Then lift the left hand and place it similarly behind the head. Interlock the fingers of both hands. The head will be cupped by the hands as in *Śīrṣāsana* (Figure 144).

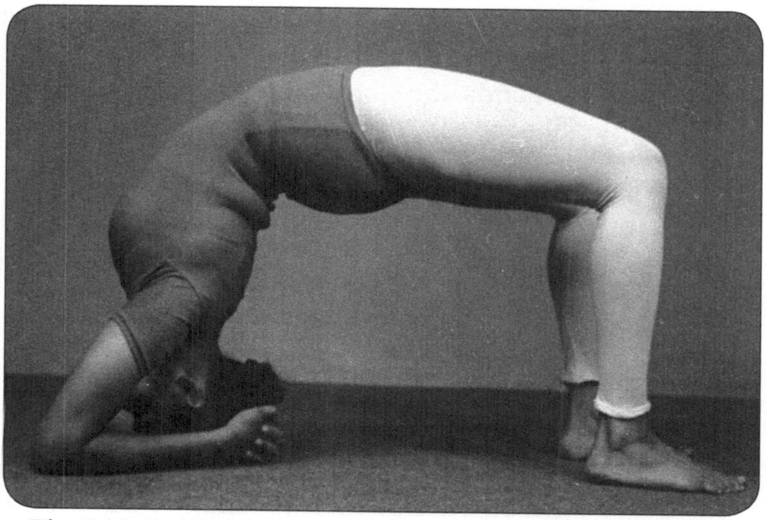

Fig. 144: *Dvi Pāda Viparīta Daṇḍāsana* (Intermediate Stage)

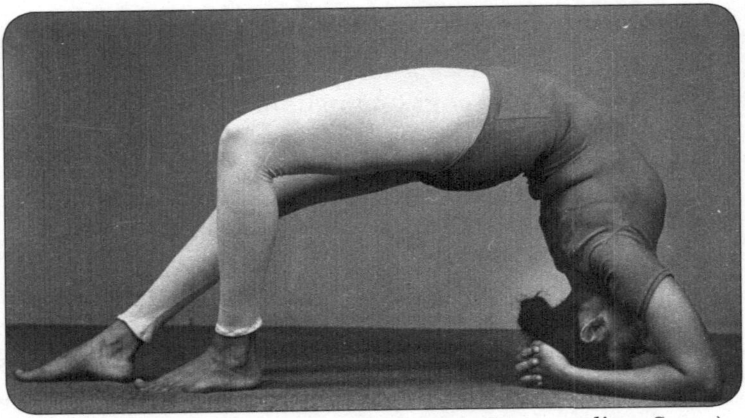

Fig. 145: *Dvi Pāda Viparīta Daṇḍāsana* (Intermediate Stage)

6. Press both the forearms to the ground, raise the buttocks and extend the legs one after the other (Figure 145). In this illustration the right leg is stretched and the left leg is in the process of being stretched.
7. Then stretch the left leg in line to the right (Figure 146). Remain in this final position for 30 to 60 seconds, breathing normally. Gradually this period can be increased to five minutes. In this position observe the following points:
   (a) keep the hands, the elbows and the forearms firmly on the floor;

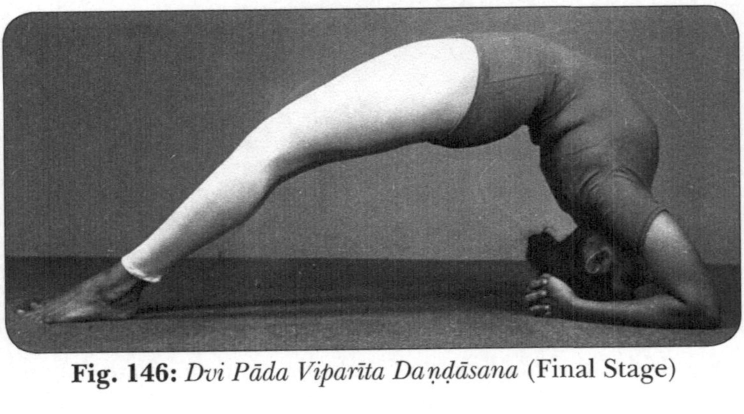

Fig. 146: *Dvi Pāda Viparīta Daṇḍāsana* (Final Stage)

(b) broaden the chest and tighten the buttock muscles;
(c) if the thighs are not properly lifted, the feet go on slipping;
(d) keep the dorsal and the sacral portions of the spine tucked in.

8. Bring the feet in one by one; unlock the fingers and keep your balance by keeping the hips well lifted up. Take the palms nearer the shoulders as in Figure 138.
9. Exhale, lower the trunk to the ground (Figure 137), and lie flat on the back.

Special Instructions

1. If the soles slip on the floor, support them against a wall. Lie 4 to 4½ feet away from the wall and follow all the movements described above until the soles come in contact with the wall.
2. If the elbows slip, do the following: Lie with the head near the wall and the feet away from it. Arch the back and follow the procedure given in the Technique. Come to the position as in Figure 144. In the illustration the elbows are not touching the wall, but if they slip they should be pressed against the wall. This method also gives a better arch of the dorsal area; therefore, both the ways should be practised to improve the final āsana as in Figure 146.
3. Or follow the procedure shown in Figure 147:
   (a) sit on a low stool;
   (b) bend backwards and hold the legs of the stool with both the hands;
   (c) bend further, until the head comes closer towards the floor; if the head does not rest on the floor, it does not matter; the shoulder-blades must be pushed in order to expand and broaden the chest; later, with practice, the head will rest on the floor, or it may be supported with a blanket;

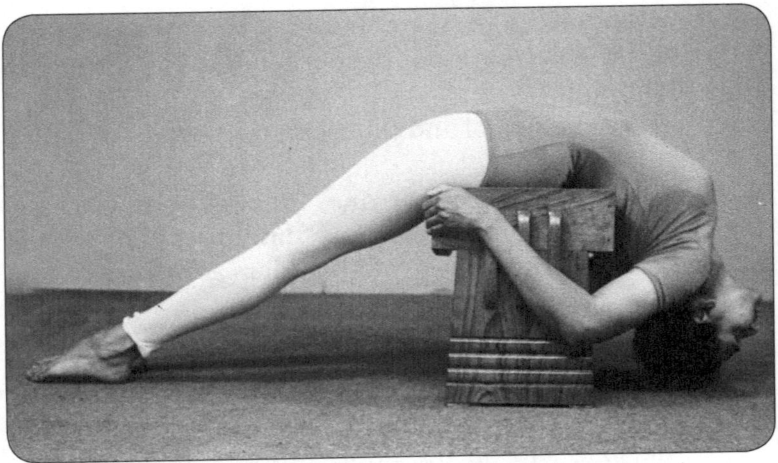

Fig. 147: *Dvi Pāda Viparīta Daṇḍāsana* (Easy Stage)

(d) bend the knees and walk in; raise the head up;
(e) carefully slide the trunk towards the legs until the back of the chest is resting on the bench; wait for a while, taking a few breaths;
(f) raise the whole trunk up, move the buttocks forward off the bench, slide down to the ground and sit.

4. If both these methods are not possible, do as follows:
   (a) lie flat on a bench about 1 to 1½ feet high, or on a low bed;
   (b) place a folded blanket on the edge of the bench so that it will not hurt;
   (c) hold the edges of the bench and slide down until the head reaches the blanket below, or let it remain suspended; broaden the chest (Figure 148);
   (d) if the head is on the floor, entwine the fingers as in *Sālamba Śīrṣāsana* (Figure 149);
   (e) stay in this position for 3 to 5 minutes, release the hands and hold the edges of the bench; bend the knees, slide down towards the head and rest on the floor.

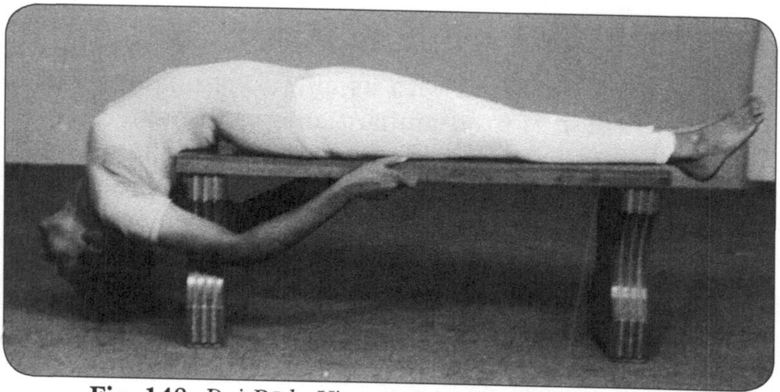

Fig. 148: *Dvi Pāda Viparīta Daṇḍāsana* (Easy Stage)

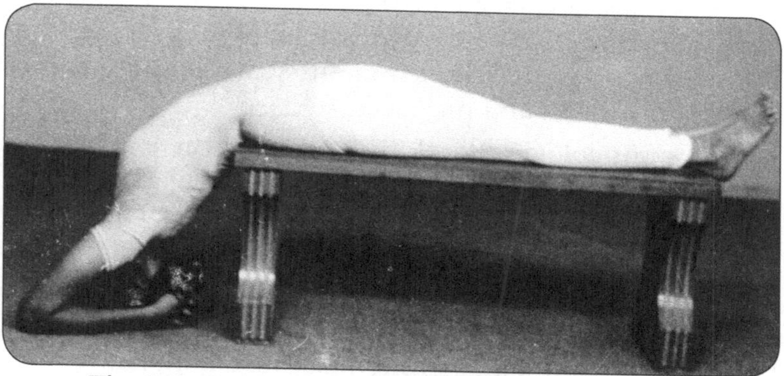

Fig. 149: *Dvi Pāda Viparīta Daṇḍāsana* (Easy Stage)

Note: The methods explained in Special Instructions (3) and (4) are most effective and safe for beginners.

Effects: This exhilarating pose keeps one healthy. The chest expansion gives a feeling of happiness and joy. The modified technique (Figures 147, 149) is intended for those who are depressed, weak, sensitive and emotional. It soothes and relaxes the nerves. It is especially useful at the time of menopause. The method of doing it independently (Figure 146) is useful for girls and adolescents as it brings emotional stability and builds self-confidence by removing fear complexes.

OVERALL EFFECTS ĀSANAS 72 & 73

Weakness of the mind with its attendant anxious states and depression is predominant among women. Even if one makes a show of having a strong mind, one may fall a prey to these conditions, especially after the age of 35. This change is perceptible and results in such symptoms as tremors and coldness of hands and feet.

These two āsanas are excellent for these conditions. They have a magical effect on the mind. When practised with support they relieve tension, relax the nervous system, and rest the brain.

They are advanced in their nature, but once they are mastered they are of great help in keeping the body supple and active, the mind sharp and alert, the conscience clear, and pure.

At a physiological level, they broaden the expanse of the chest and improve respiration and circulation. They relieve pain in the sacrum and the coccyx. The spine becomes elastic, firm and healthy.

They remove dullness and laziness and make women more cheerful and courageous. They have a soothing effect on the mind and strengthen one emotionally.

SECTION-VIII

Āsana: Yoga Kuruṇṭa

Kuraṇṭi is a puppet, a doll made of wood. Puppet-shows are known all over the world, to children as well as to grownups. In Yoga Kuruṇṭa one learns to manipulate oneself in the various Yoga postures by means of a suspended rope as if one were a puppet. Here the puppeteer and the puppet are one, performing their own puppet-show.

Performing Yogāsanas with the aid of a rope has many advantages. Difficult āsanas can be practised with ease. Āsanas in Section VII which are difficult and āsanas such as *Sarvāṅgāsana* and *Halāsana* if found difficult can be practised by the method described in this section. The method is ideal for women who are heavy in the region of the thighs, the buttocks, the stomach and for those who have become flabby after one or two deliveries.

Due to the rope movement the spine becomes supple and even difficult āsanas can be done easily and safely. No jerking is felt, and a sense of direction is developed by regular practice. Old people can do Yoga Kuruṇṭa without injuring themselves.

ARRANGEMENT OF THE ROPE

1. Take a rope 1 inch thick, strong, and convenient to hold, and 16 to 18 feet long. If you are tall, it may need to be a little longer.
2. Make a knot at each end so that the ends do not fray, then knot the two ends firmly together so that a hoop is formed out of the length of the rope. Keep the knot in the centre.
3. Insert this double-thick rope behind two window bars which are about 2 to 2½ feet apart. See that the loops reach your hips evenly on both the sides. Make sure

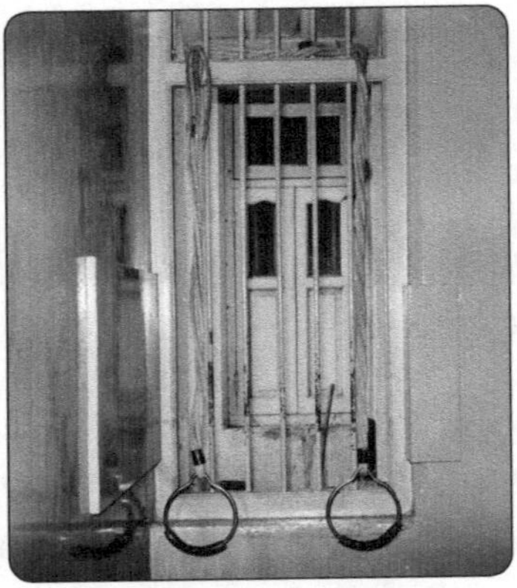

Fig. 150: Rope Arrangement

the window bars are strong enough to support the weight of your body when you pull the ropes in various positions.

4. If there are no window bars suitable to take the rope, two strong hooks or eyes may be screwed into a wall to fix the rope. The space between them should be 2 to 2½ feet; they should be very strong and the frame or the wall into which they are screwed should also be very strong and capable of bearing the pull of a bodyweight, Make sure the double thickness of the rope rests securely in the hook and there is no chance of its coming off the hook during the movements.
5. The window bars or the hooks should be 2 or 3 feet above your head so that when you stand on tip-toe and stretch your arms and fingers up, you are able to touch them. A difference of 1 or 2 inches either way does not matter.
6. Tie a piece of soft cloth round the two loops so that the rope does not cut your hands when you are working.
7. The apparatus is now ready for use (Figure 150).
8. Follow the order of āsanas given below: they are carefully chosen to train the body systematically as each āsana progresses from simple to difficult movements.

74. VARIATION I: *BHUJAṄGĀSANA*

Technique

1. Stand in *Tāḍāsana* (Figure 1), with the back to the wall and two feet away from it, in between the two ends of the suspended rope. Make sure you are standing exactly in the centre. Keep the feet together and extend the toes forward.
2. Turn the arms outwards so that the palms are facing forward. Place the palms on the loops of the rope and grip the rope firmly. Keep the arms straight (Figure 151). Take one or two breaths.
3. Exhale, bend the elbows and bend the trunk down in half *Uttānāsana*. Keep the knees straight and the elbows facing the ceiling (Figure 152a).

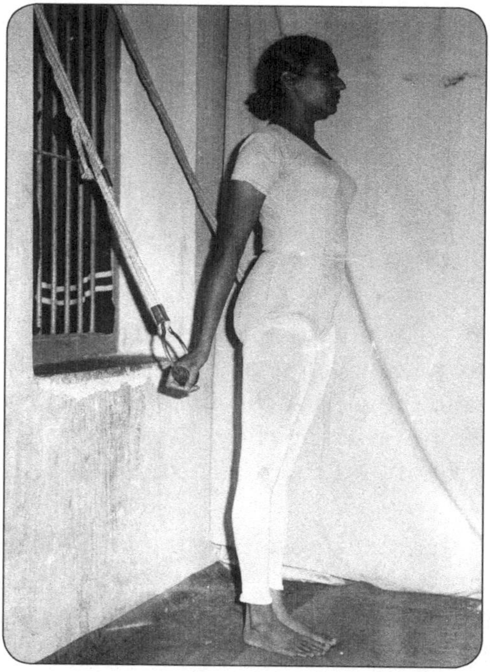

Fig. 151: Variation I: *Bhujaṅgāsana* (Intermediate Stage)

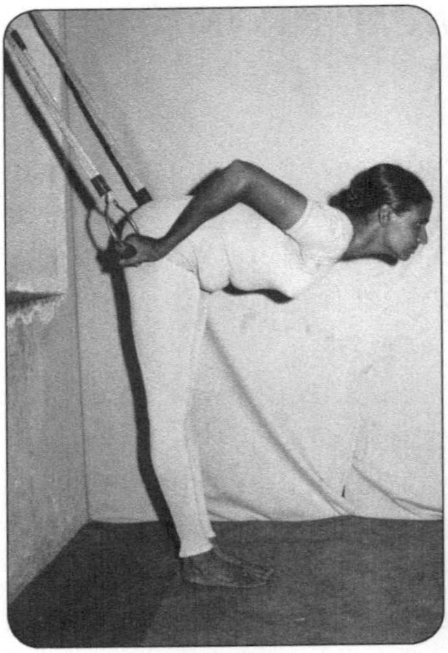

Fig. 152(a): Variation I: *Bhujaṅgāsana* (Intermediate Stage)

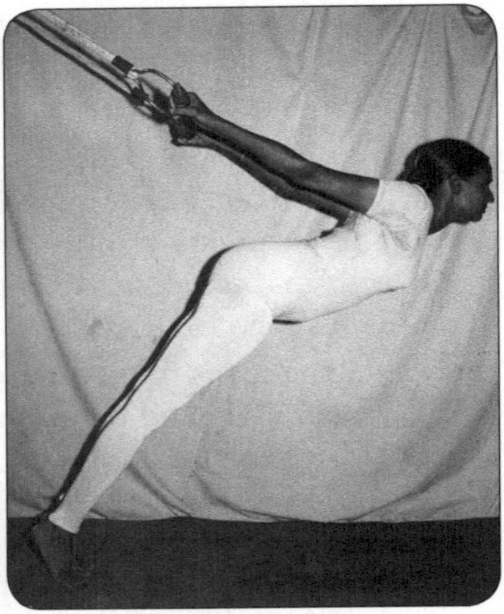

Fig. 152(b): Variation I: *Bhujaṅgāsana* (Intermediate Stage)

4. Inhale, raise the head, make the spine concave and take the body forward as far as it will go. Raise the heels and come onto the mounts of the toes by straightening the arms (Figure 152b). Keep the knees and the elbows straight; let the palms face the ground; press the front of the feet firmly into the floor.
5. Exhale, tighten the buttocks and pull them towards the floor. Extend the trunk further down to get a complete concave movement and look up. Tuck in the coccyx and the sacrum, broaden the chest, and pull the abdomen towards the chest. Keep a strong pull on the arms throughout; the thighs should stay firm (Figure 153).
6. Stay in this final position for 5 to 10 seconds with normal breathing.
7. Exhale, lift the thighs and the buttocks up, press the toes firmly into the floor, raise the trunk and come to the position as in Figure 152b.

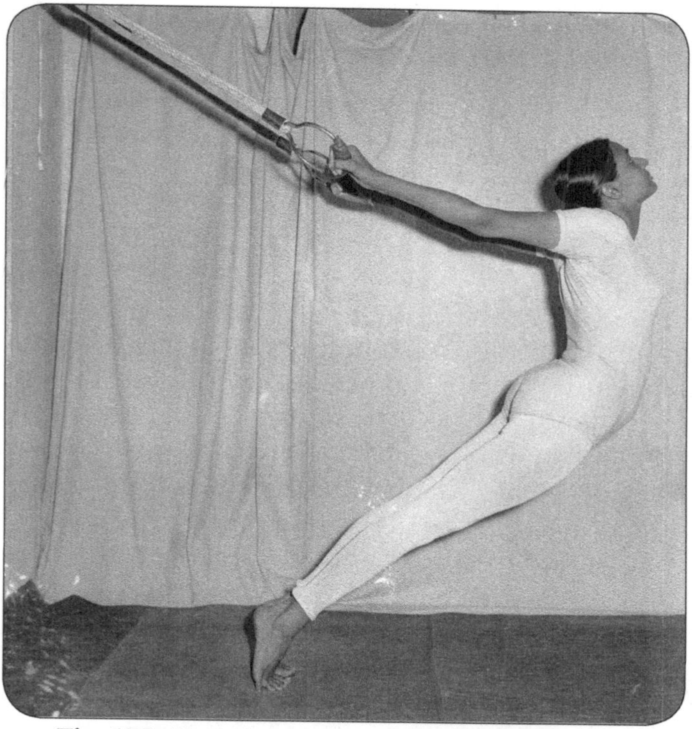

Fig. 153: Variation I: *Bhujaṅgāsana* (Final Stage)

8. Bend the elbows and bring the trunk back to half *Uttānāsana* (Figure 152a). Lift the trunk up to come to *Tāḍāsana* (Figure 151).
9. These movements form one cycle. Repeat 4 to 6 cycles at a stretch.

Notes:

1. If it is difficult to do the movements with the feet together, keep them about 8 to 12 inches apart and do the cycle.
2. Make sure that both the arms are pulled with even action.
3. The movements should not be too fast or too slow.

75. VARIATION II: *BHUJAṄGĀSANA* AND *ŪRDHVA MUKHA PAŚCIMOTTĀNĀSANA II*

This variation is more intensive than the previous one. The lower portion of the spine is stretched more as the body is closer to the wall. Two āsanas are performed here forming one cycle.

Technique

1. Stand in *Tāḍāsana* (Figure 1), with your back to the wall. Turn the arms outwards so that the palms face forward. Place the palms face down on the loops of the rope and grip the rope firmly. Let the heels and the buttocks touch the wall. Take one or two breaths.
2. Exhale, bend the trunk forwards and come to *Uttānāsana* (Figure 154). Bring the head near the knees and keep the legs straight.
3. Inhale, raise the head up, make the spine concave, and push the trunk forward as far as it will go straightening the arms. Raise the heels slightly but support them

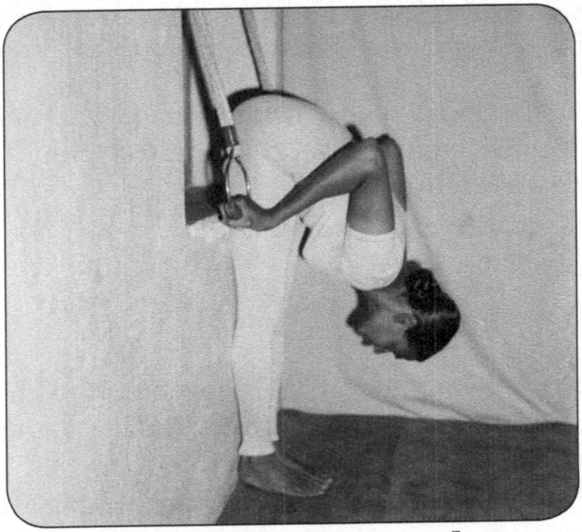

Fig. 154: Variation II: *Bhujaṅgāsana, Ūrdhva Mukha Paścimottānāsana I* (Intermediate Stage)

on the wall. Stand firmly with the mounts of the toes pressing the floor and incline the sides of the trunk towards the armpits. Keep the knees and the elbows straight (Figure 155).

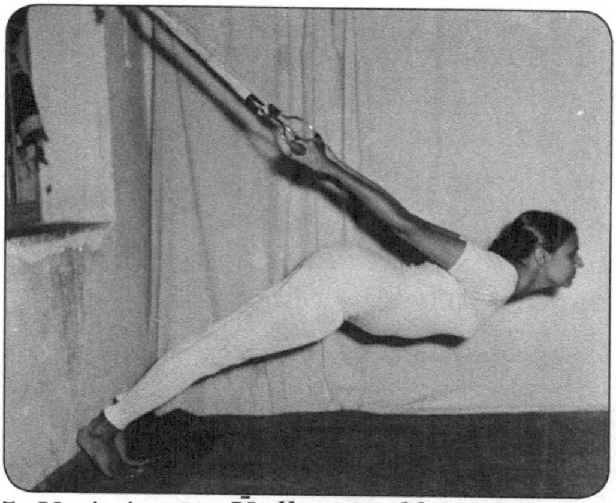

Fig. 155: Variation II: *Ūrdhva Mukha Paścimottānāsana* (Final Stage)

4. Exhale, tighten the buttocks and push them towards the floor so that the hip joints and the abdomen are stretched. Raise the head and look up (Figure 156). Observe the following points:
   (a) keep the knees and the thighs tight;
   (b) broaden the chest and push the shoulder-blades in;

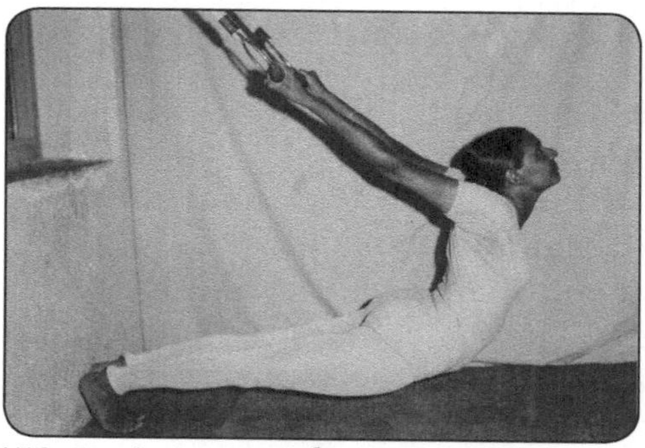

Fig. 156: Variation II: *Bhujaṅgāsana* (Final Stage)

(c) tuck in the sacrum and the coccyx;

(d) keep the arms straight and the elbows locked.

5. Stay in this final position for 5 seconds, breathing normally.
6. Exhale, pull the buttocks and the hip-joints up (Figure 155), and take the head down. Bend the trunk towards the legs, straighten the arms and turn the wrists inwards so that they face each other.
7. Pull the buttocks down towards the floor. This is *Ūrdhva Mukha Paścimottānāsana II* (Figure 157). Stay in this final position for 5 seconds, breathing normally, observing the following points:

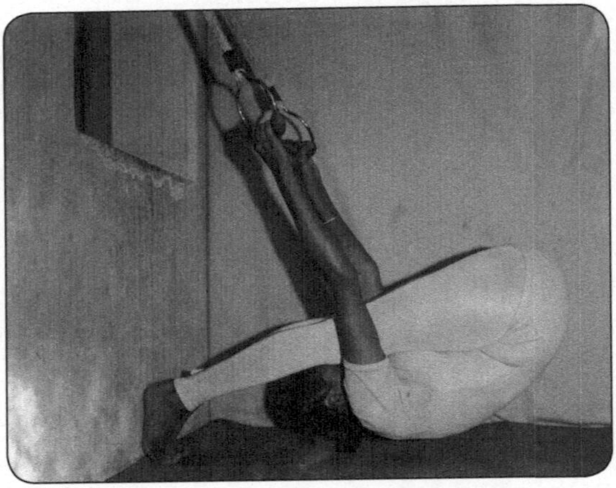

Fig. 157: Variation II: *Ūrdhva Mukha Paścimottānāsana* (Final Stage)

(a) press the feet firmly against the wall to lower the buttocks down;

(b) let the head, the chest and the abdomen come closer towards the thighs.

8. Exhale, pull the ropes with the hands and raise the head up (Figure 156). Push the buttocks and the thighs backwards towards the wall (Figure 155), then come to the position in Figure 154 and then to *Tāḍāsana*, Repeat all these movements 3 to 4 times.

76. VARIATION III: *PŪRVOTTĀNĀSANA*

Technique

1. Stand facing the wall. Hold the loops of the rope. Keep the toes touching the wall and the heels on the floor.
2. Take the head back, straighten the knees, exhale and swing the whole body backwards by pressing the wall with the toes and stretching the arms fully (Figure 158).
3. Remain in this final position for 5 to 10 seconds, breathing normally and observing the following points:
   (a) raise the sternum and bend the head backwards;
   (b) make the spine concave;
   (c) tighten the buttocks and stretch the thighs;
   (d) stretch the abdomen;
   (e) keep the elbows straight and pull evenly with both the arms.
4. Maintain the curvature of the spine and raise the arch of the body by bending the elbows. Inhale, raise the trunk with a swing and stand in *Tāḍāsana*. Repeat all these movements 3 to 4 times.

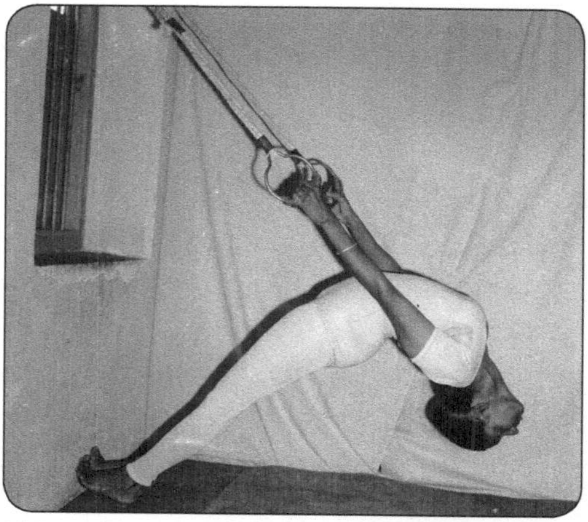

Fig. 158: Variation III: *Pūrvottānāsana* (Final Stage)

Special Instruction

Those who are unable to do this āsana while standing close to the wall may stand 1½ feet away from the wall facing it. Bend the knees and curve the spine; stretch the legs one after another to touch the wall (Figure 159) and then come to the position as in Figure 158. While getting up, take the feet back one after another and stand straight.

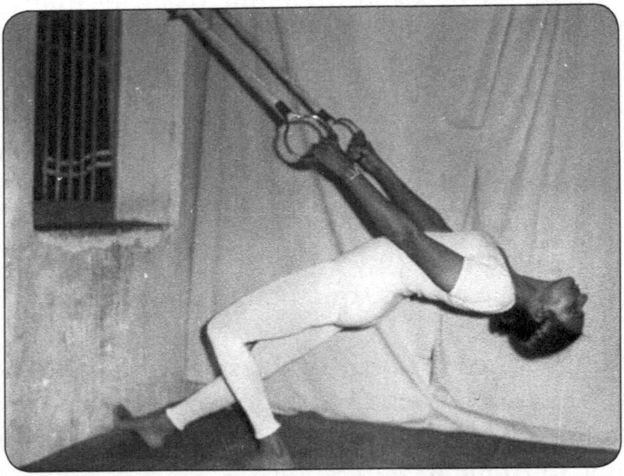

Fig. 159: Variation III: *Pūrvottānāsana* (Intermediate Stage)

77. VARIATION IV: *ŪRDHVA HASTA DHANURĀSANA*

This is a more intensive stretch than that of *Bhujaṅgāsana*.

Technique

1. Stand in *Tāḍāsana* (Figure 1) with the back to the wall, keeping the toes on the floor and the heels slightly up on the wall.
2. Raise the arms over the head as in *Vṛkṣāsana* (Figure 2). Release the interlock and hold the ropes. Take one or two breaths.
3. Exhale, straighten the arms and the legs; take the head back and look back; arch the body by sliding the hands

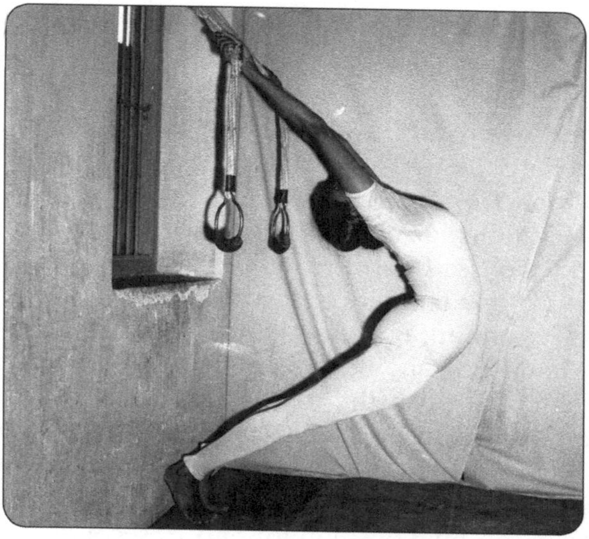

Fig. 160: Variation IV: *Ūrdhva Hasta Dhanurāsana* (Final Stage)

down the rope while taking the body forwards. Keep the hand grip on the ropes firm (Figure 160).

4. Stay in this final position for 5 to 10 seconds, breathing normally. This variation is more intense than variation II. Observe the following points:
   (a) stretch both the arms so that the armpits open;
   (b) press the feet firmly against the wall;
   (c) if the knees start to bend, stop arching the body;
   (d) tighten the buttocks, take the spine into the body, extend the front of the body from the groins to the top of the chest;
   (e) tuck in the shoulder-blades and broaden the chest;
   (f) raise the sternum up, to take the head further back.
5. Exhale, hold the rope firmly, bend the elbows, raise the head up. Pull on the rope and push the body back; the initiative to come up should be from the sides of the lower abdomen. Come to *Tāḍāsana*.
6. Repeat these movements 3 to 4 times.

78. VARIATION V: *UṢṬRĀSANA*

Technique

1. Kneel against the wall with the thighs and the knees touching the wall as for *Uṣṭrāsana* (Figure 133). This is position 1.
2. Raise the hands and hold the rope firmly. Exhale and bend the head and the trunk backwards, curving the spine and making it concave.
3. While bending back the hands slide on the rope, but the hand-grip should be kept firm. Take a few breaths.
4. Exhale and push the thighs against the wall; tighten the buttocks, raise the sternum, and throw the head back (Figure 161). This is the final position, similar to *Uṣṭrāsana*.
5. Stay in this final position for 5 to 10 seconds, breathing normally.
6. Inhale, raise the head up, bend the elbows and use them as levers to raise the trunk up. Come to position 1.
7. Repeat all movements 3 to 4 times.

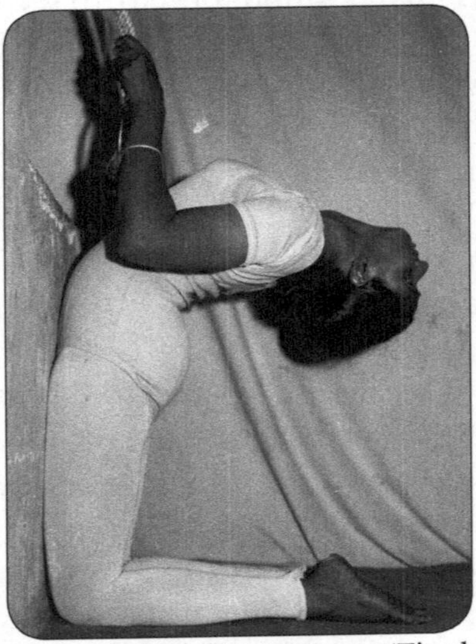

Fig. 161: Variation V: *Uṣṭrāsana* (Final Stage)

OVERALL EFFECTS OF ĀSANAS 74 to 78

These āsanas are safe to perform; because of the rope there is no jerk on the spinal vertebrae during movement. The āsanas are beneficial for those affected by slipped disc, backache, pain in the shoulders, the neck, and the waist; rheumatism of the shoulders and the spine, pain in the elbows and the wrists; stiffness of the body, hunchback; weakness in the waist and the buttocks; contraction of the chest muscles, pain in the breast, heaviness or insufficient growth of the breasts.

As the chest expands in these āsanas, the intake of oxygen increases. The breast muscles and thigh muscles are toned and the abdomen is strengthened.

79. VARIATION VI: *SĀLAMBA SARVĀṄGĀSANA, HALĀSANA* AND VARIATIONS

Those who cannot practise *Sālamba Sarvāṅgāsana* and *Halāsana* due to overweight, sprain in the back, or in the absence of an assistant, should follow the technique given below. The ropes help lift the body so that it does not collapse; the weight of the body is not felt on the neck and the shoulders; no jerk is experienced while lifting the trunk. These āsanas can be done easily with the aid of ropes.

Technique

1. Bend the knees, draw the legs towards the stomach, and sit as close as possible to the wall, facing it, as in *Malsana* (Figure 45).
2. Raise the hands and hold the rope.
3. Exhale, drop the buttocks down onto the floor, raise the legs up and place the feet on the wall; slide down until the back of the body and the back of the head are on the floor (Figure 162). Breathe normally.

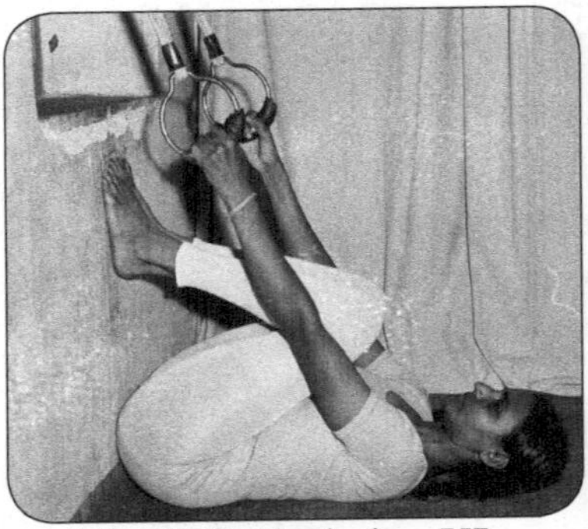

Fig. 162: Variation VI: *Sālamba Sarvāṅgāsana* (Intermediate Stage)

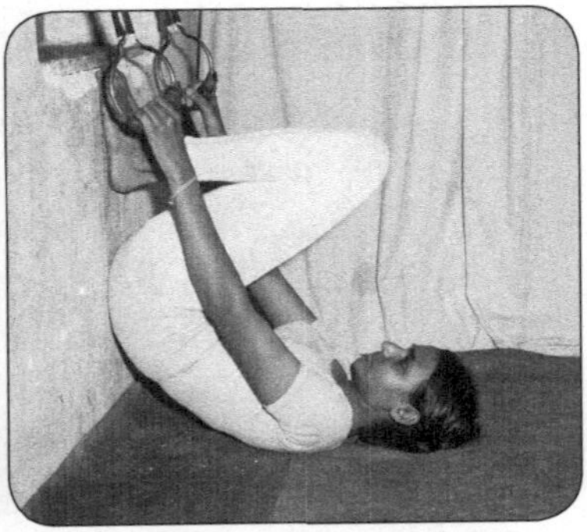

Fig. 162(a): Variation VI: *Sālamba Sarvāṅgāsana* (Intermediate Stage)

4. Exhale and raise the trunk and the buttocks up towards the wall by pulling hard on the rope (Figure 162a).
5. Climb the feet further up and pull on the rope to bring the trunk closer to the wall (Figure 163).
6. Straighten the legs on the wall, pull on the rope and come to *Sarvāṅgāsana* (Figure 164 side view, 164a front view).
7. Stay in this final position for 3 to 5 minutes, breathing normally, and come to *Halāsana* (Figure 167).

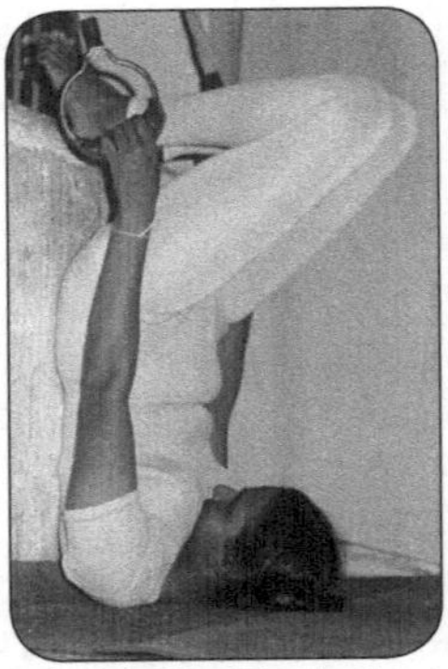

Fig. 163: Variation VI: *Sālamba Sarvāṅgāsana* (Intermediate Stage)

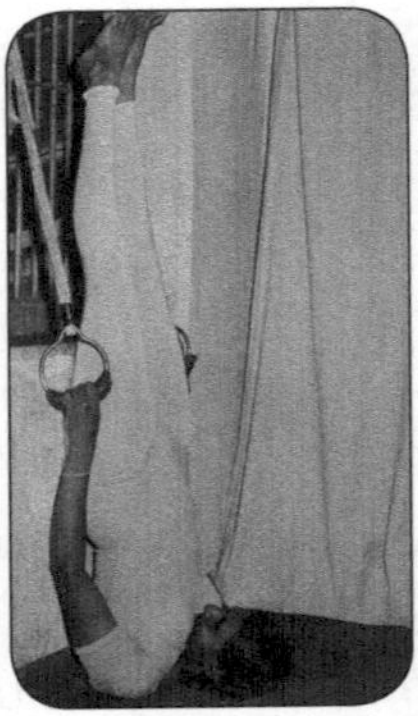

Fig. 164: Variation VI: *Sālamba Sarvāṅgāsana* (Final Stage)

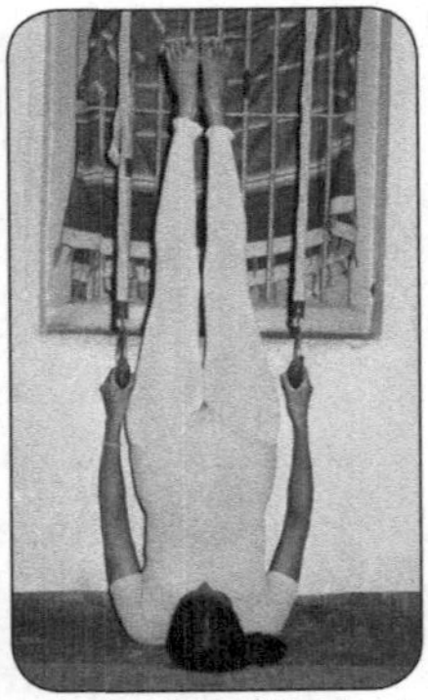

Fig. 164(a): Variation VI: *Sālamba Sarvāṅgāsana* (Final Stage)

Technique

1. Rest the buttocks against the wall and bend both the legs at the knees (Figure 165).
2. Bring both the feet to the floor (Figure 166).
3. Stretch your legs; if possible, release the grip on the ropes and let the hands be free. As the back, the waist, and the buttocks are supported on the wall, they will remain lifted up without any special efforts (Figure 167). Breathe normally.

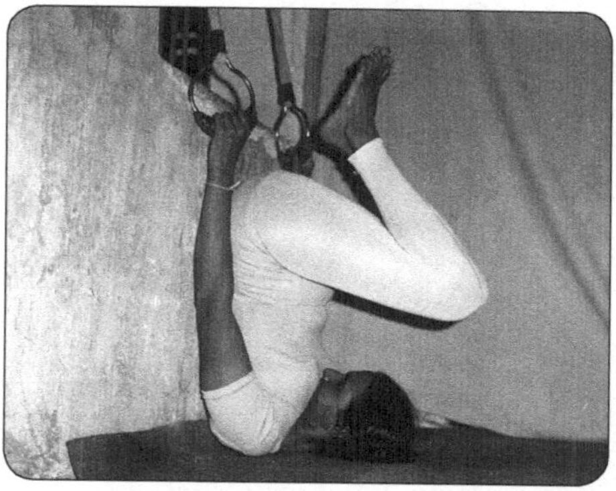

Fig. 165: Variation VI: *Halāsana* (Intermediate Stage)

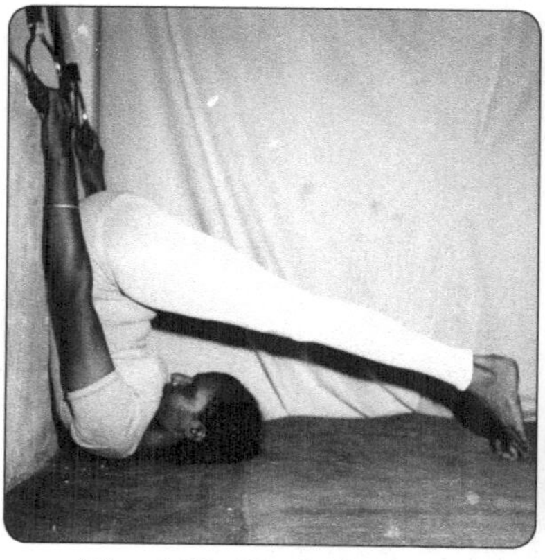

Fig. 166: Variation VI: *Halāsana* (Intermediate Stage)

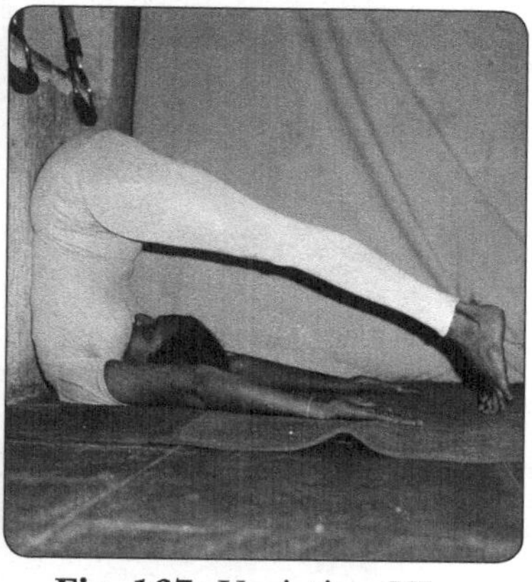

Fig. 167: Variation VI: *Halāsana* (Final Stage)

4. From this position hold the rope and come to *Karṇapīḍāsana* (Figure 168), *Supta Koṇāsana* (Figure 169), *Pārśva Halāsana* (Figure 170), *Eka Pāda Sarvāṅgāsana* (Figure 171), and *Pārśvaika Pāda Sarvāṅgāsana* (Figure 172), in succession. All these āsanas can also be done without holding the rope.

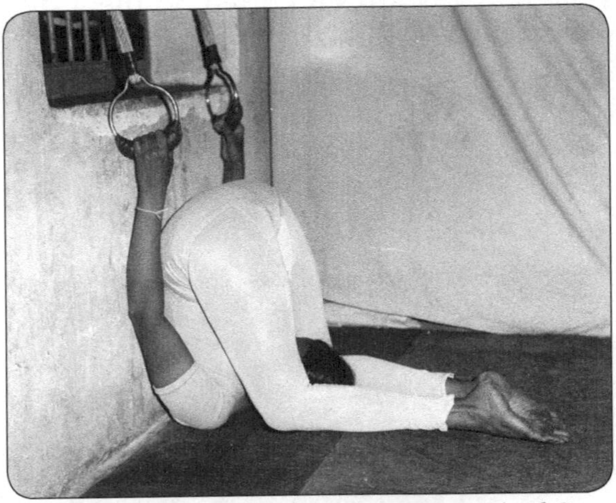

Fig. 168: Variation VI: *Karṇapīḍāsana* (Final Stage)

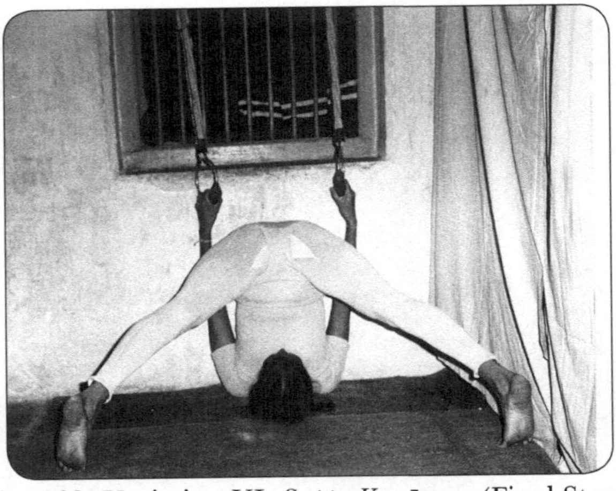

Fig. 169: Variation VI: *Supta Koṇāsana* (Final Stage)

5. Now, hold the rope, bend the knees (Figure 165), and slide down (Figures 162a, then 162).

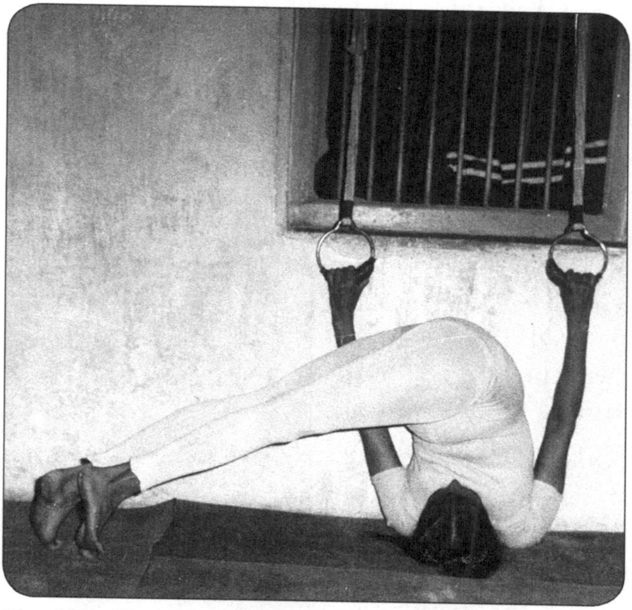

Fig. 170: Variation VI: *Pārśva Halāsana* (Final Stage)

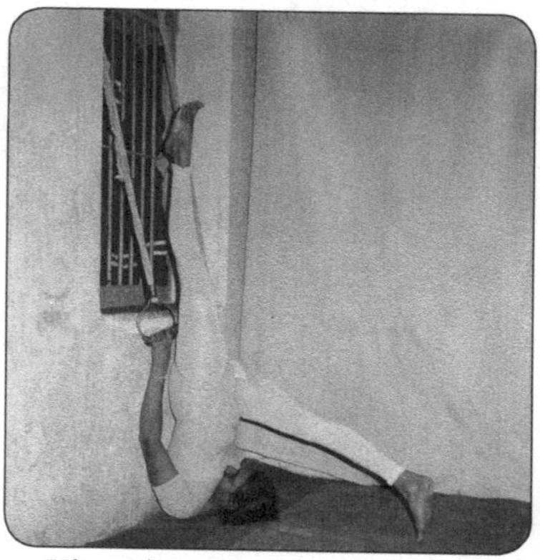

Fig. 171: Variation VI: *Eka Pāda Sarvāṅgāsana* (Final Stage)

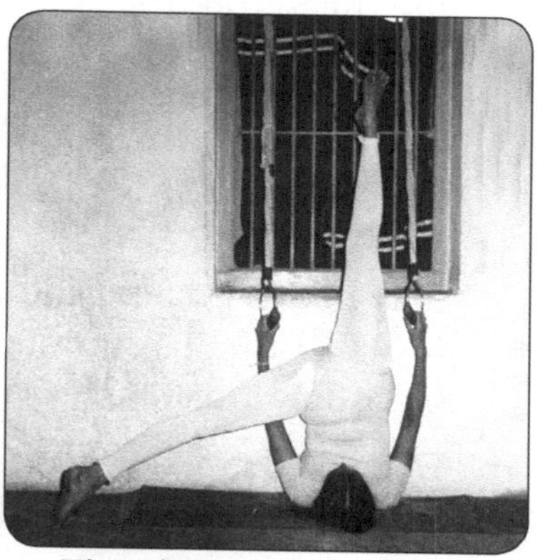

Fig. 172: Variation VI: *Pārśvaika Pāda Sarvāṅgāsana* (Final Stage)

80. VARIATION VII: *ŪRDHVA MUKHA PAŚCIMOTTĀNĀSANA I*

In Section V a variation of the above āsana is described, lying flat on the back. Those who are unable to do that may follow the variation given here:

Technique

1. Bend the knees and sit as in *Mālāsana* (Figure 45) 1 to 1½ feet away from the wall, facing it. Hold the rope and lower the buttocks to the ground.
2. Exhale, take the legs up, stretch them and place the heels on the wall.
3. Pull the rope, exhale, extend the trunk, and bend forward; place the head on the shins (Figure 173).
4. Tighten the hamstring muscles and extend the trunk towards the feet.
5. Stay in this final position for ½ to 1 minute, breathing normally.
6. Exhale, bend the knees and bring the legs down. Release the rope.

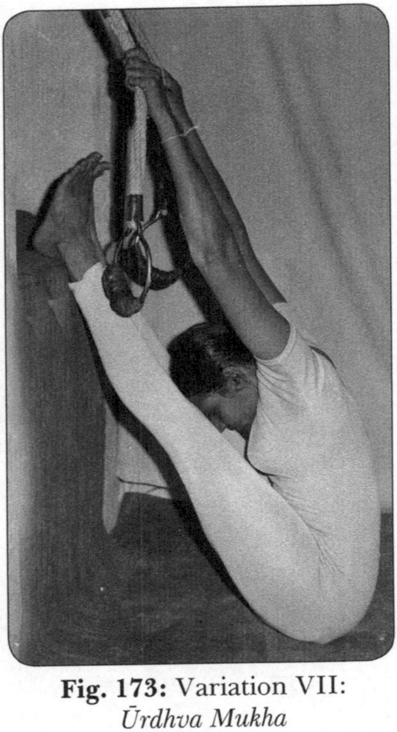

Fig. 173: Variation VII: *Ūrdhva Mukha Paścimottānāsana* (Final Stage)

Effects: This āsana is very helpful to those who suffer from umbilical hernia and protruded abdomen.

OVERALL EFFECTS OF *YOGA KURUṆṬA*

All these āsanas performed with different variations of movement help bring freedom of movement in the joints. The concave curvatures of the back help circulate the blood in that area.

Sālamba Sarvāṅgāsana and its variations performed in this way have the same effects as those mentioned in Section IV. One can perform them accurately with the support of the wall and the help of the rope. They are especially helpful to women as they ease the tension in the pelvic area and stretch the pelvic organs more effectively than when done independently.

By the practice of *Yoga Kuruṇṭa* one gains agility, lightness of the body, speed in movements, and alertness in the brain.

Caution: People suffering from dislocation of the arms should avoid these āsanas.

SECTION-IX

Āsanas and Prāṇāyāma during Pregnancy

Normally women are afraid or nervous to do āsanas and prāṇāyāma during pregnancy. This section has been specially written to give women the courage to do Yoga at this time and to show them which āsanas they can safely practise to ensure better health during pregnancy and delivery, as well as in the post-natal period.

The āsanas mentioned here are simple to perform. They are not complicated, nor in any way dangerous. They are designed to keep the expectant mother healthy so that she can avoid the usual warning signals such as vomiting, morning sickness, constipation, swelling, headache, toxaemia, and so on. They aid proper digestion, circulation and easy breathing. The prāṇāyāma that is given is mainly intended to remove fatigue, nervous tension and to eliminate toxins so that the mental and the physical states remain healthier and happier. Also, the āsanas have been carefully chosen to ensure that the foetus is given maximum room for its free movement and growth in the mother's womb. They have also been chosen with a view to facilitating a natural and easy delivery.

Most of the illustrations given here were taken during the 7th and the 9th month of pregnancy. In performing the āsanas one should refer to the hints and techniques as well as to the illustrations.

The sādhaka must use her discretion and judgement in her Yoga practice. Some may not be able to follow the entire programme given in this book, but may select the āsanas that maintain physical and mental well-being and ensure comfortable delivery. A feeling of radiant health after practice is a sign that one is working correctly; if one feels tired or exhausted, either the practice is faulty or one has over-done it. It is wrong to over-strain.

The same āsanas and prāṇāyāma which are practised during the course of normal life are done during pregnancy, but with some modifications. To avoid repetition, only the specially modified techniques are described in this section. Hence, to perform an āsana one has to refer to the relevant section for general details, but the hints and the modified techniques given in this section should be carefully studied and then followed.

CAUTIONS

1. First read Nos. 55, 56 and 58 from Chapter X (Part II). Avoid standing āsanas from Section I if you have a tendency to repeated miscarriage.
2. During pregnancy, avoid jumping to spread the legs apart while doing the postures from Section I. However, all these postures may be done up to six months according to one's capacity and constitution; later, one has to use one's discretion as to how much one should do.
3. Do not bend or extend beyond your capacity.
4. Your efforts should be directed towards extending your spine (Figures 179, 180, 181).
5. Shorten the duration of your stay in the āsanas to avoid fatigue.
6. You should not feel any restriction or interruption in your respiration while performing āsanas. In every pose see that the diaphragm is kept soft and free so that breathing becomes easier.
7. In the forward bending āsanas of Section II you must not bend forward and compress the foetus. Instead, you should keep the spine concave and the chest well lifted so that the foetus remains free to move within.
8. Do not constrict or compress the uterine system while doing the āsanas.
9. Do the āsanas with comfort and protect the life that is within.
10. After the first three months practise the āsanas and prāṇāyāma according to the instructions given in this section.

ĀSANAS FROM SECTION I

3. *UTTHITA TRIKOṆĀSANA*

(right side, Figure 4; left side, Figure 174)

Hints

1. Follow the techniques given in Section I, Āsana 3, but do not jump to spread the legs apart.

2. Those who have practised Yoga before pregnancy can bend the trunk sideways to reach the ankle.

3. For those who are new to Yoga, if the palm cannot reach the ankle, or if in attempting to do so the side of the pelvis gets compressed, keep the palm on the middle of the shin bone.

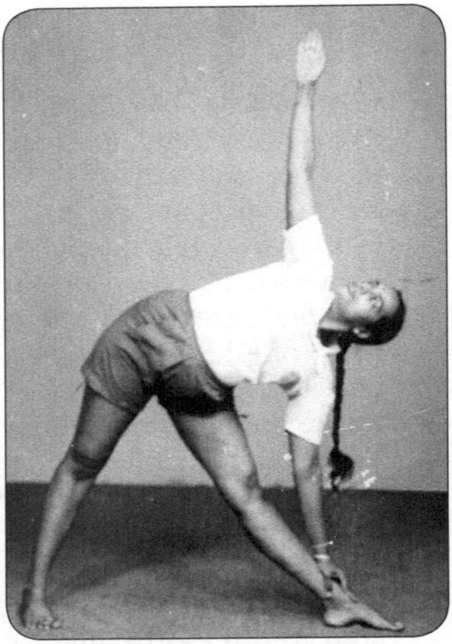

Fig. 174: *Utthita Trikoṇāsana* (Final Stage)

4. Extend the anterior portion of the trunk from the pelvis to the chest, in the direction of the head. Keep the two sides of the trunk parallel to each other.

5. Do not hold your breath while doing any movement.

6. In the early stages of pregnancy one can stay from 30 to 60 seconds on each side. Later, decrease the duration to 15 or 20 seconds.

4. *UTTHITA PĀRŚVAKOṆĀSANA*

(right side, Figure 5; left side, Figure 175)

Hints

1. Follow the techniques given in Section I, Āsana 4, but do not jump into the posture.
2. Those who have practised before may reach the floor easily (Figure 175), but those who cannot, should follow Hints 3 and 4 given below.

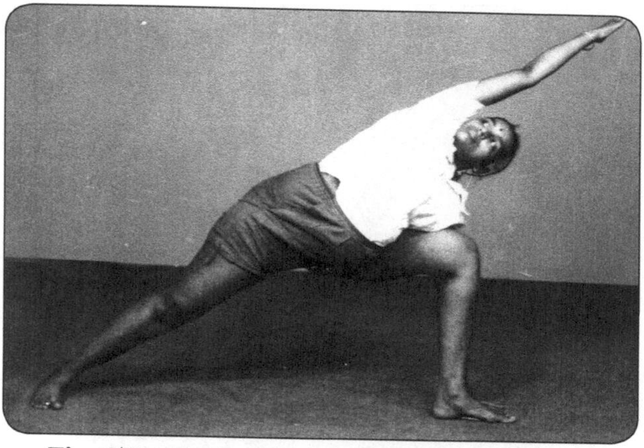

Fig. 175: *Utthita Pārśvakoṇāsana* (Final Stage)

3. Take a wooden block (as shown in Figure 177) and place it by the outer edge of the left foot. Place your left palm on the block; this creates space between the left thigh and the left side of the trunk and ensures that the left side of the pelvis and the abdomen do not press against the thigh. The chest also remains free to breathe easily.
4. While doing the posture on the right side, the block should be placed by the side of the right foot for the right palm to be placed on it.
5. Stay in the final āsana for 15 to 20 seconds, breathing normally.

5. *VĪRABHADRĀSANA I*

(right side, Figure 7; left side, Figure 176)

Hints

1. Follow the techniques given in Section I, Āsana 5, without jumping.
2. If it is difficult to bend the left knee to 90° as in Figure 176, keep the thigh slightly up. Do not press the abdomen against the thigh.

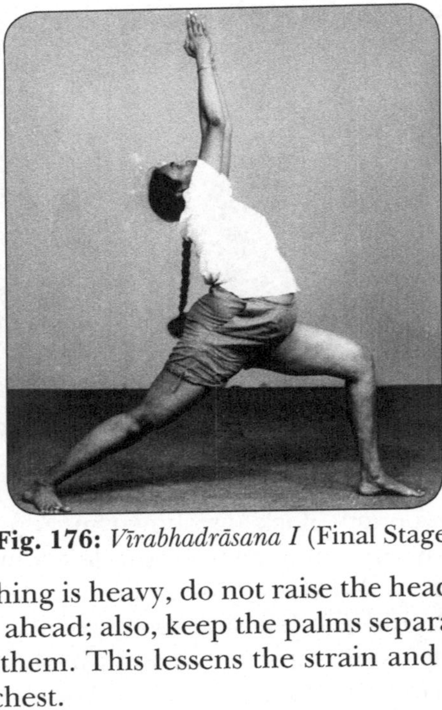

Fig. 176: *Vīrabhadrāsana I* (Final Stage)

3. If breathing is heavy, do not raise the head up but look straight ahead; also, keep the palms separate instead of joining them. This lessens the strain and the pressure on the chest.
4. Stretch the spine towards the head to avoid pressure on the uterus.
5. If breathing is difficult, do not stay longer than 10 seconds.
6. If you suffer from high blood pressure or have a tendency towards it, avoid doing this āsana.

6. *VĪRABHADRĀSANA II* (*Figure 8*)

Hints

1. Follow the techniques given in Section I, Āsana 6, but do not jump into the posture.
2. Keep the pelvic region widening sideways, to give the foetus more room in which to move.
3. Breathe normally, staying for 15 to 20 seconds on each side.

8. *ARDHA CANDRĀSANA*
(*right side, Figure 10; left side, Figure 177*)

Hints

1. Follow the techniques given in Section I, Āsana 8, but instead of keeping the palm on the floor, keep it on a wooden block (Figure 177).
2. If the palm is kept on the floor, the spine remains in a slanting position and the sides of the pelvis become narrow, which is harmful for the foetus. Therefore, the hand should be kept on a block.

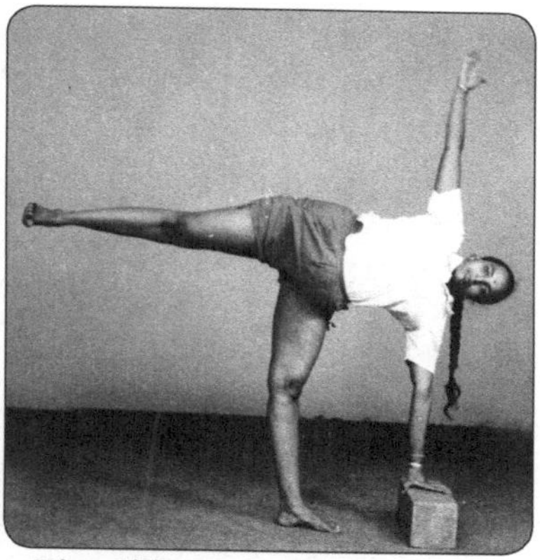

Fig. 177: *Ardha Candrāsana* (Final Stage)

3. When the pose is done in this way, as shown in Figure 177, the pelvis is broadened, breathing becomes easier for the mother, and room is created for the foetus.
4. If you find this posture difficult to perform, follow Special instructions 3 and 4 in Section I, Āsana 8.

10. *PĀRŚVOTTĀNĀSANA* (*Figures 178, 179*)

Hints

1. Follow techniques 1 to 5 in Section I, Āsana 10 (Figures 14, 178). Do not jump into the posture.
2. Raise the pelvis, extend and expand the chest.
3. Stay in this position for 10 to 15 seconds.
4. While bending the trunk to the side it should remain parallel to the floor so that there is no pressure on the abdomen. The spine, from the tail-bone towards the cervical area, should extend towards the head. Do not attempt to touch your knee.
5. Do not cave in the chest.
6. Stay in this position for 5 to 10 seconds, breathing normally.
7. Then raise the trunk up and repeat the posture on the other side.
8. Follow the breathing instructions given in Section I.

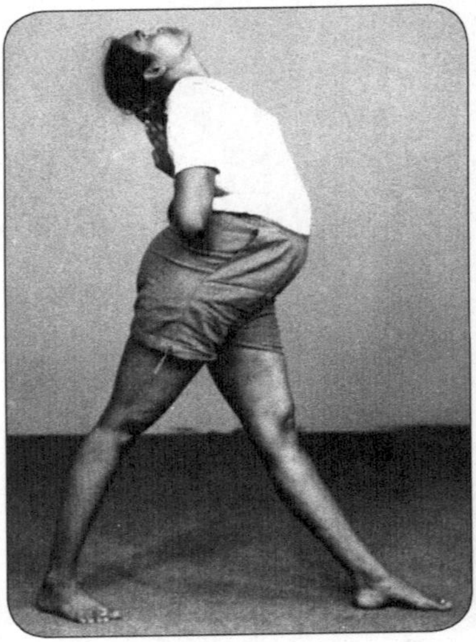

Fig. 178: *Pārśvottānāsana* (Intermediate Stage)

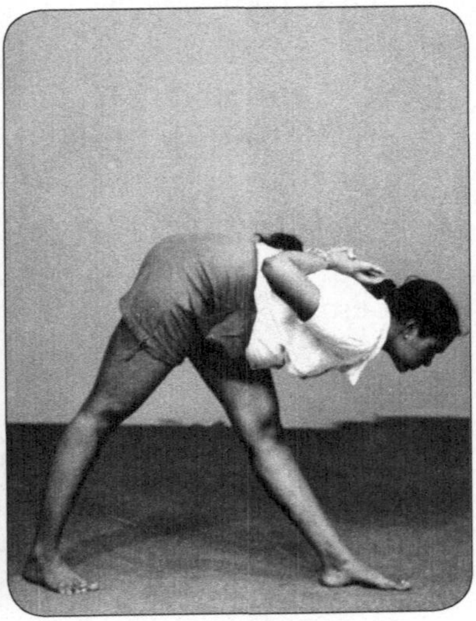

Fig. 179: *Pārśvottānāsana* (Final Stage)

11. *PRASĀRITA PĀDOTTĀNĀSANA*

(Figures 16, 17, 180, 181)

Hints

1. Follow techniques 1 to 5 in Section I. Do not jump into the posture.
2. Do not bend down as in Figure 18, but extend the spine towards the head, making it concave, with the palms on the floor (Figures 16, 17).
3. Stay for 15 to 20 seconds, breathing normally.
4. If you find it difficult to place the palms on the floor, try the following method.
5. Place a wooden block or a box on the floor, 5 to 6 inches high or even higher.
6. Keep it 1½ to 2 ft. forward and not in line with the feet. In Figure 18 the palms and the feet are in line with each other, whereas in Figure 180 the hands are 6 inches forward. In this method the block may be kept even further forward to avoid contraction of the abdomen.

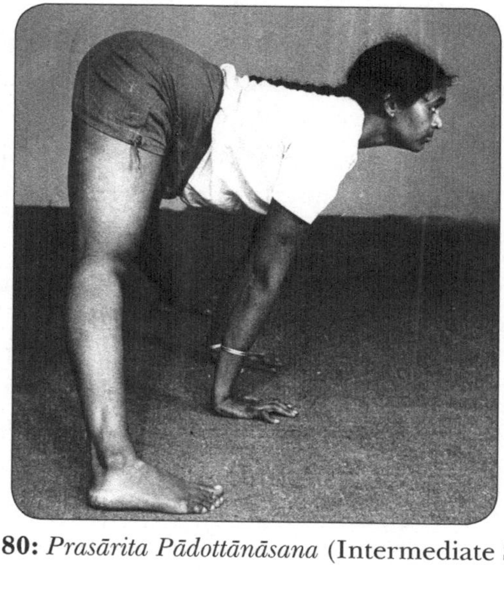

Fig. 180: *Prasārita Pādottānāsana* (Intermediate Stage)

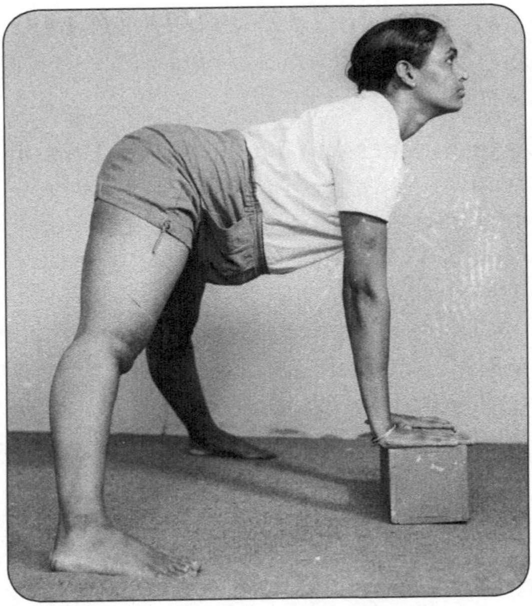

Fig. 181: *Prasārita Pādottānāsana* (Easy Stage)

7. Rest the palms on the block and make the spine concave (Figure 181).
8. Adjust the distance between the palms and the feet according to the height of the trunk to make extension of the spine and breathing easier.
9. Stay for 15 to 20 seconds, breathing normally.
10. Raise the trunk up, and bring the feet together without jumping.

Effects: These āsanas keep the body movements free and improve breathing. They remove tautness of the body, backaches, and heaviness in the abdomen. *Ardha Candrāsana* (Figure 177), *Pārśvottānāsana* (Figure 178), and *Prasārita Pādottānāsana* (Figure 181) are useful in relieving morning sickness.

Caution: Avoid the standing poses if symptoms of toxaemia are traced or if there is undue physical fatigue.

ĀSANAS FROM SECTION II

16. *JĀNU ŚĪRṢĀSANA* (*Figure 182*)

Hints

1. Sit in *Daṇḍāsana* (Fig. 23), but keep a folded blanket, 3 to 4 inches thick, under the buttocks so that the buttocks are up and the feet are below.
2. Bend the right knee, place the right heel near the right groin, and pull the knee back so that the angle between the two legs is an obtuse one.

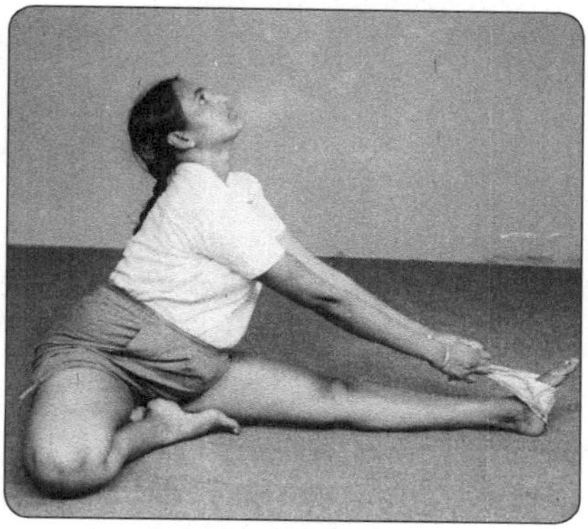

Fig. 182: *Jānu Śīrṣāsana* (Intermediate Stage)

3. Take a handkerchief, a cloth, or a rope, put it round the left foot and hold both the ends of the cloth with hands.
4. Inhale, extend the spine and lift it up. Make it as concave as possible and take the head back.
5. Stay for 10 to 15 seconds, breathing normally, observing the following points:
   (a) keep the trunk facing forward;
   (b) extend the spine from the base of the trunk upwards.
6. Inhale and raise the head up.
7. Release the arms without dropping the extended spine.

Now, extend the right leg to *Daṇḍāsana* (Figure 23) and bend the left leg. Follow techniques 2 to 5 on the other side, reversing the instructions for right and left. Remain for the same length of time and come back to *Daṇḍāsana* (Figure 23).

Effects: This āsana strengthens the spine and the muscles of the back and the waist so that the foetus remains well supported. The heaviness felt in the tail-bone can be lessened by the practice of this āsana.

23. *BADDHA KOṆĀSANA* (*Figure 183*)

Hints

1. Sit in *Daṇḍāsana* (Figure 23), keeping a folded blanket 3 to 4 inches thick under the buttocks so that they are up and the feet are below.
2. Follow techniques 2 to 9 in Section II, Āsana 23.
3. In this position, as the buttocks are higher than the feet, the heels will not come close to the perineum (Figure 183).
4. One can rest the palms by the sides of the buttocks as in *Daṇḍāsana*, instead of holding the feet.
5. To sit longer in this position, keep the back against the wall so that it is supported throughout and no strain is felt on the back.

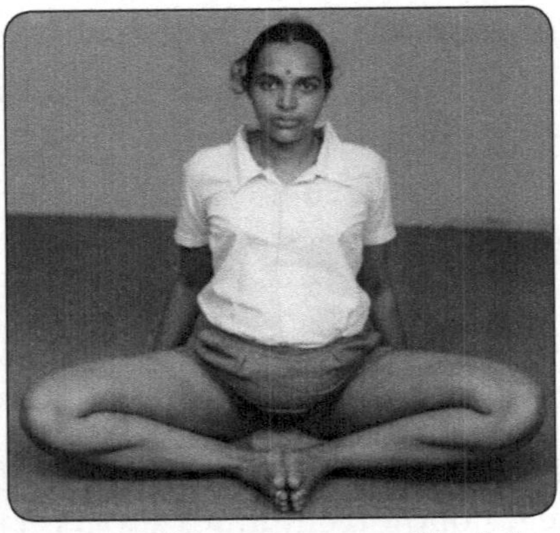

Fig. 183: *Baddha Koṇāsana* (Final Stage)

24. *SUPTA BADDHA KOṆĀSANA (Figures 38, 39)*

Hints

1. Follow techniques 1 to 5 (Figure 38) in Section II, Āsana 24.
2. In advanced pregnancy, one may find it difficult to keep the whole trunk down. In that case, keep two pillows under the chest and the waist as shown in Figure 186. The bottom one is placed lengthwise and the top one across it (Figure 186). A pillow may be kept under the head.
3. Follow techniques 6 to 8 in Section II, Āsana 26 (Figure 39).
4. One can stay in these two positions for any length of time, as they are restful.

25. *UPAVIṢṬHA KOṆĀSANA (Figure 184)*

Hints

1. Sit in *Daṇḍāsana* (Figure 23), but on a folded blanket 3 or 4 inches high.
2. Follow techniques 2 and 3 given in Section II, Āsana 25.
3. Keep the palms as in *Daṇḍāsana* and lift the spine upwards.
4. Do not hold the toes and do not bend forward.
5. This āsana may be done while resting the trunk against the wall so that the spine remains supported throughout.
6. Sit as long as possible, without straining. Breathe normally.
7. To come back to *Daṇḍāsana* do not bring the legs forward while keeping them straight, but bend the knees one at a time and bring the legs to the centre one after the other so that there is no strain on the groins.

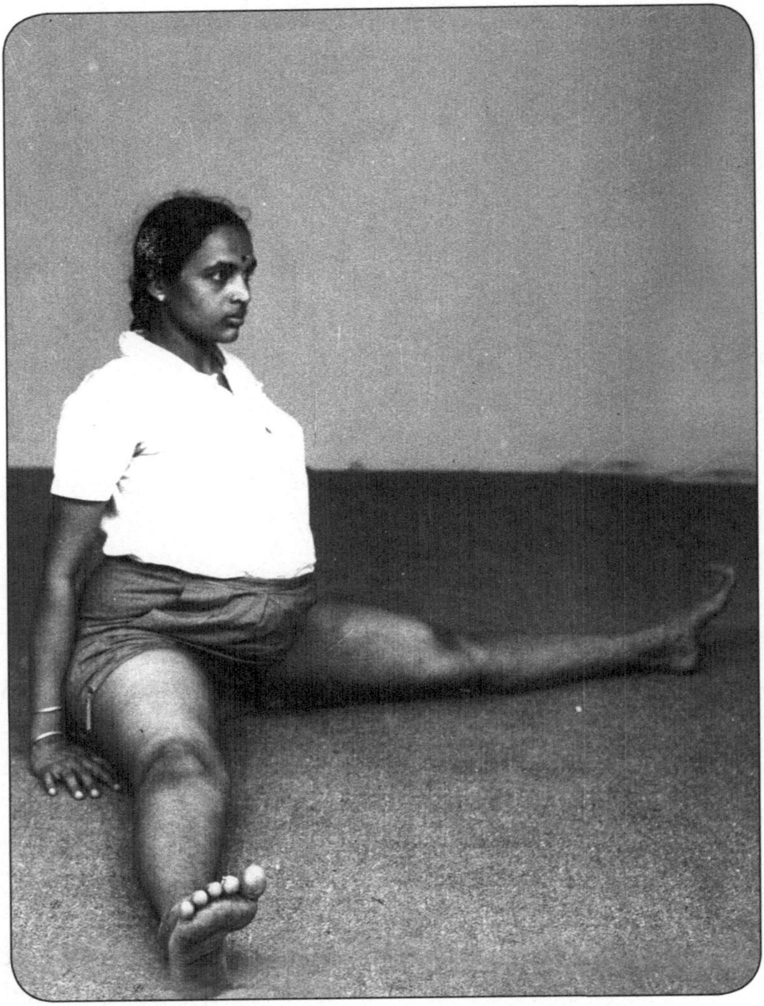

Fig. 184: *Upaviṣṭha Koṇāsana* (Easy Stage)

Effects: These āsanas from Section II are helpful for easy delivery and labour pains can be minimised by their regular practice. The passing of urine is made easy and discharge from the vagina is checked. The pelvic region remains broad, giving room for the movement of the foetus. The spine is strengthened.

ĀSANAS FROM SECTION III

30. *VĪRĀSANA* *(Figure 49)* and
32. *VĪRĀSANA* CYCLE *(Figures 54, 185)*

Hints

1. Follow techniques 1 to 3 in Section III, Āsana 30. Keep a folded blanket 3 to 4 inches high under the buttocks so that they are higher than the feet.
2. If it is difficult to keep the knees together, keep them apart to avoid compression of the abdomen.
3. Stay in this position as long as possible, breathing normally.
4. Now follow techniques 2 to 5 in Section III, Āsana 32 (Figure 185).

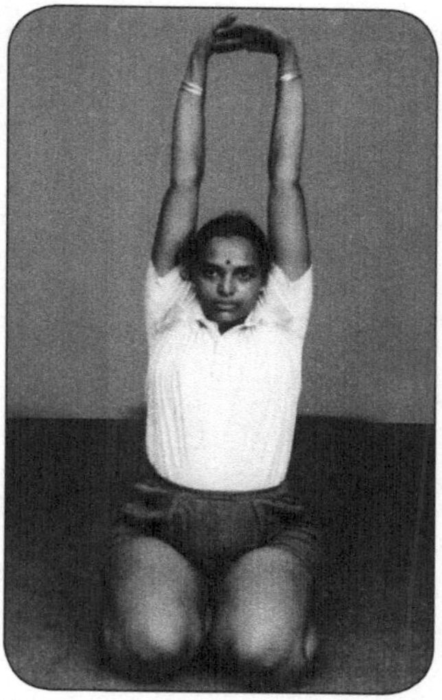

Fig. 185: *Vīrāsana* Cycle (Final Stage)

Effects: *Vīrāsana* removes the swelling of the legs during pregnancy and prevents varicose veins. A folded blanket raises the height of the trunk so that the uterus is not pressed downwards. Raising of the arms makes breathing easy and releases wind.

33. *SUPTA VĪRĀSANA* (*Figure 186*)

Hints

1. Sit in *Vīrāsana* (Figure 49).
2. Keep two pillows behind the buttocks, the bottom one lengthwise and the top one across.
3. Now, follow techniques 2 to 7 in Section III, Āsana 33.
4. In this āsana the trunk remains on the pillows so that the level of the trunk and the head is higher than the thighs. Keep the arms alongside the trunk (Figure 57), or stretch them over the head as in Figure 186.

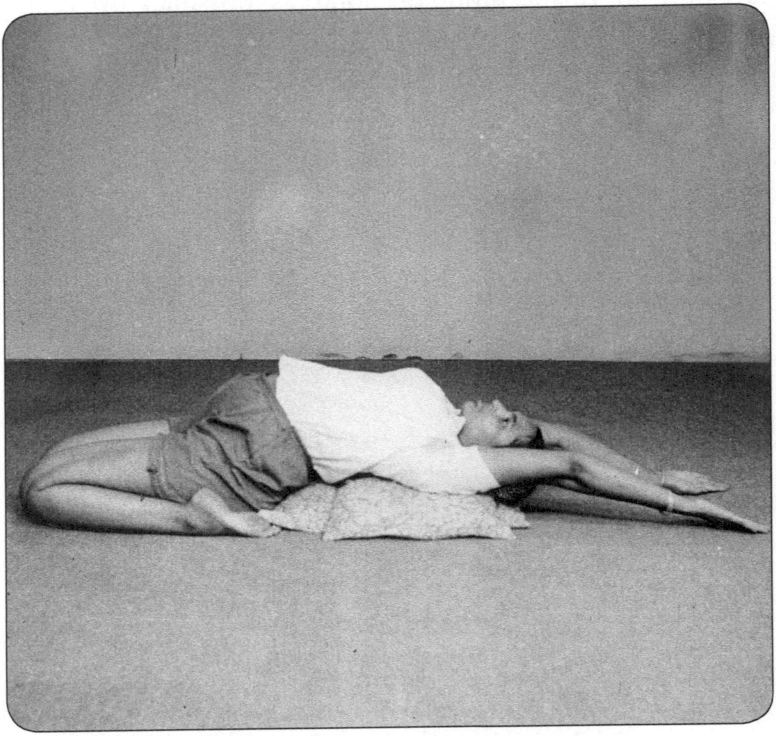

Fig. 186: *Supta Vīrāsana* (Final Stage)

Effects: This āsana relieves morning sickness, constipation and flatulence.

34. *PARVATĀSANA* (*Figure 187*)

Hints

1. Sit in *Daṇḍāsana* (Figure 23) on a folded blanket 3 to 4 inches high, as described in *Vīrāsana* (Figure 185).
2. Follow techniques 2 to 6 in Section III, Āsana 34.

Effects: This āsana improves the functioning of the kidneys. The āsanas from this section make breathing easier and are of great help in relieving morning sickness and constipation. They remove the swelling of the hands, legs and face.

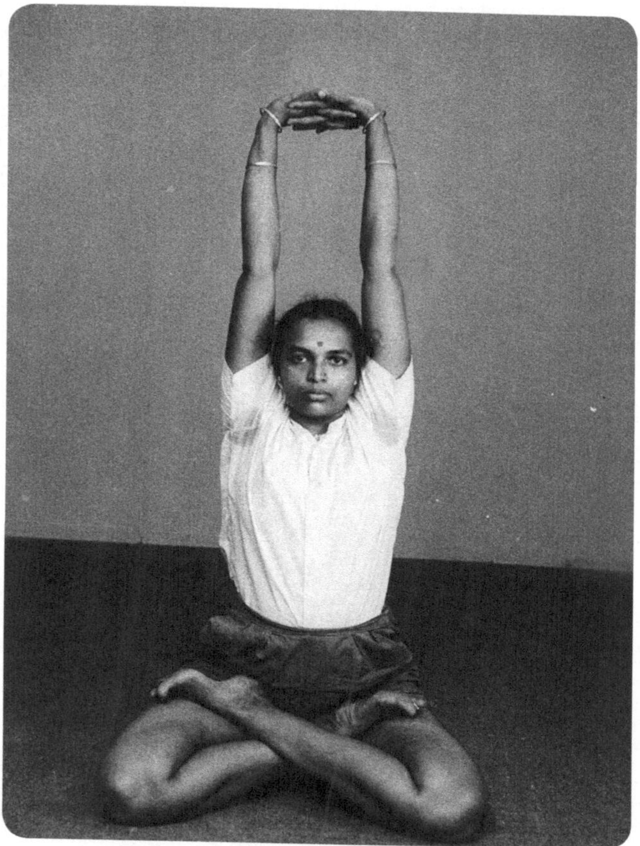

Fig. 187: *Parvatāsana* (Final Stage)

ĀSANAS FROM SECTION IV

38. *SĀLAMBA ŚĪRṢĀSANA* (*Figures 70A, 188, 189*)

Hints

1. Those who are accustomed to doing *Sālamba Śīrṣāsana* may continue with it after conception has taken place and may do it independently, without support (Figures 188, 189), as described in Techniques B and C.
2. Those who are starting after becoming pregnant must do *Śīrṣāsana* either with the support of a wall (Figure 65), or must ask a helper to assist, as mentioned in Technique A (Point 11), Section IV, Āsana 38.
3. Normally *Śīrṣāsana* can be comfortably practised up to 7 months of pregnancy, but slim women and those who are accustomed to practising it can continue until the last day of pregnancy, so long as there is no difficulty

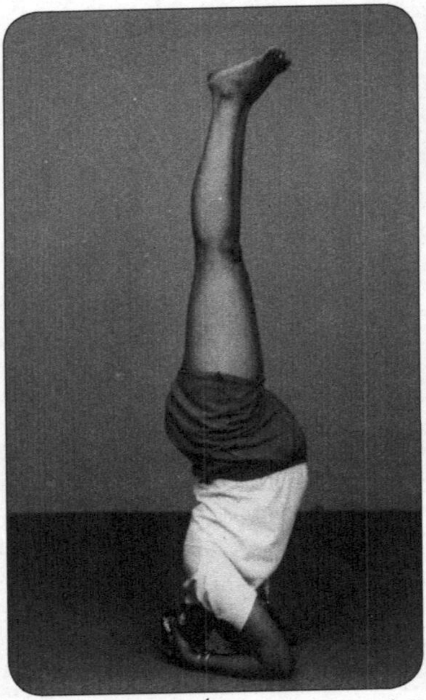

Fig. 188: *Sālamba Śīrsāsana* (Final Stage)

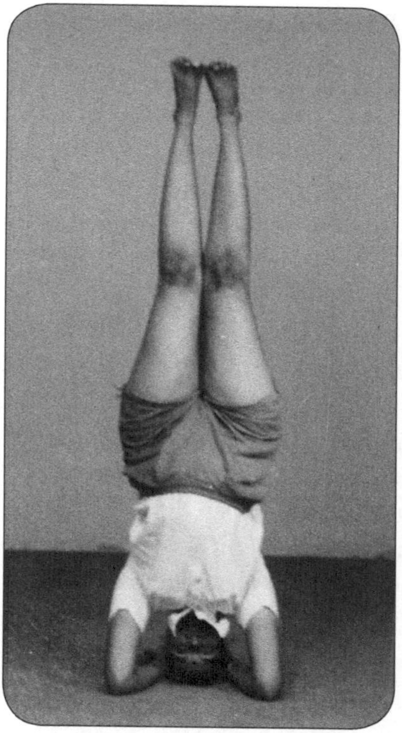

Fig. 189: *Sālamba Śīrsāsana* (Final Stage)

or jerking in going up or coming down. Do not jump heavily.

4. Do not keep the feet together. Keep the tips of the big toes joined and the heels apart as in Figures 188, 189. You may find it difficult even to keep the thighs together, in which case they should be kept apart as in Figure 70a.
5. The duration may vary from 3 to 5 minutes. Breathing should be normal.
6. If heaviness is felt in the chest and the heart and if the heart beats are fast, *Śīrṣāsana* should be avoided.
7. If you have high blood pressure or a tendency towards it, avoid *Śīrṣāsana* and variations.

39. *PĀRŚVA ŚĪRṢĀSANA* (*Figure 190*)

Hints

1. Beginners who have started the practice of Yoga after becoming pregnant should avoid this āsana.
2. Those who are accustomed to practising and have mastered this āsana before conception took place may comfortably continue with its practice up to the 7th month of pregnancy.
3. Keep the big toes together and the heels apart.
4. Follow techniques 1 to 5 from Section IV, Āsana 39.

   While turning the trunk to the side, do not compress the abdomen by turning more and more. All attention should be paid to the extension of the spine rather than to rotation (Figure 190).
5. If breathing becomes difficult, it means one has turned too far and the abdomen is being compressed.
6. Stay in this āsana for 5 to 10 seconds, breathing normally.

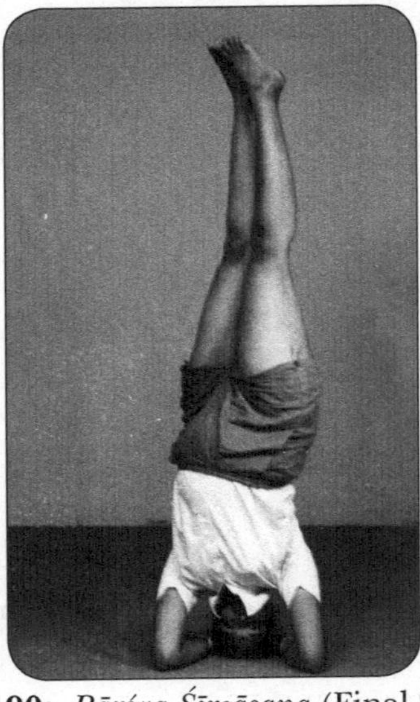

Fig. 190: *Pārśva Śīrṣāsana* (Final Stage)

40. *PARIVṚTTAIKAPĀDA ŚĪRṢĀSANA* (*Figure 191*)

Hints

1. Beginners who have started practice after pregnancy should avoid this āsana as it requires perfect balance.
2. Those who have mastered this āsana before pregnancy may continue practising it up to the 7th month.
3. Do not spread the legs too wide apart.
4. More than rotating the spine, it is important to keep the spine firm (Figure 191). The front thigh should not press the abdomen.

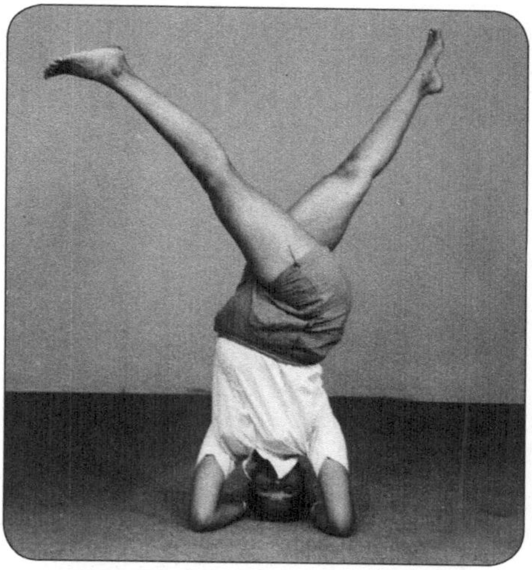

Fig. 191: *Parivṛttaikapāda Śīrṣāsana* (Final Stage)

5. Follow techniques 1 to 6 from Section IV, Āsana 40.
6. If breathing is difficult, it means one has turned too much.
7. Stay in this āsana for 5 to 10 seconds with normal breathing.

Effects: These āsanas are good in cases of severe vomiting, blurred vision, bleeding, white discharge, swellings, varicose veins and cramps. They bring freshness to the mind.

47. *SĀLAMBA SARVĀṄGĀSANA* (*Figures 192, 193*)

Hints

1. Those who have practised before pregnancy may find it easier to do this posture without any support, as in Figure 192.
2. Follow Technique A, Section IV, Āsana 47, to raise the trunk up. Do not join the legs together, but keep them 5 to 6 inches apart.
3. Keep the folded blanket 2 to 3 inches higher than the level of the head. (See Section IV, Āsana 47, Special Instruction 4.)
4. The posture can also be done with support. Ask a helper to raise your trunk and support your back against a bench (Figure 193).

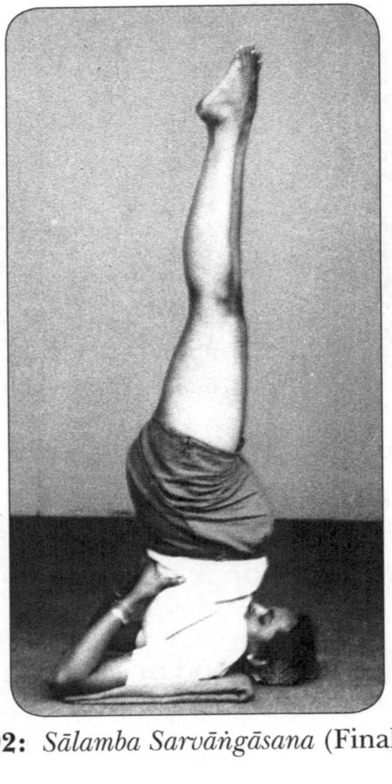

Fig. 192: *Sālamba Sarvāṅgāsana* (Final Stage)

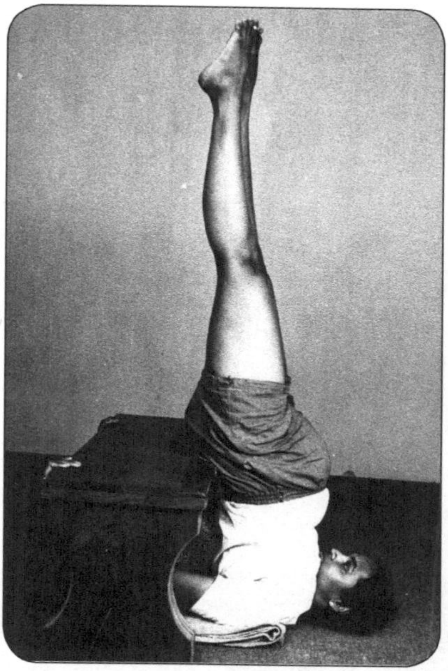

Fig. 193: *Sālamba Sarvāṅgāsana* (Easy Stage)

5. Keep the toes together and the heels apart, as in *Śīrṣāsana*.
6. Stay in this āsana for 3 to 5 minutes or longer, if you are comfortable. Breathe normally.
7. This pose can comfortably be done up to the 7th month. Later, if heaviness is felt in the chest or the abdomen, it should be avoided. If one can stay comfortably, there is no harm in doing so. The āsana in Figure 193 is taken at the 9th month of pregnancy.
8. While coming down from the pose do not jerk and do not come down with a bang. One has to come down skillfully, without disturbing the foetus inside.

Effects: This āsana keeps the brain calm and quiet. It soothes the nerves and improves the circulation in the chest area. It is good for relief from toxaemia of pregnancy and for varicose veins.

48. *HALĀSANA* *(Figures 88, 194, 195)*

Hints

1. Up to the 3rd month one can practise with the feet on the floor (Figure 88).
2. Later the posture has to be modified as shown in Figure 194 or 195; the position shown in Figure 195 is more comfortable and restful of the two.
3. The legs should be either parallel to the floor as in Figures 194 and 195 or they should be kept even higher to avoid pressure on the abdomen. (Figures 194a and 195a).
4. Keep the legs 6 to 8 inches apart if the uterus is being compressed.

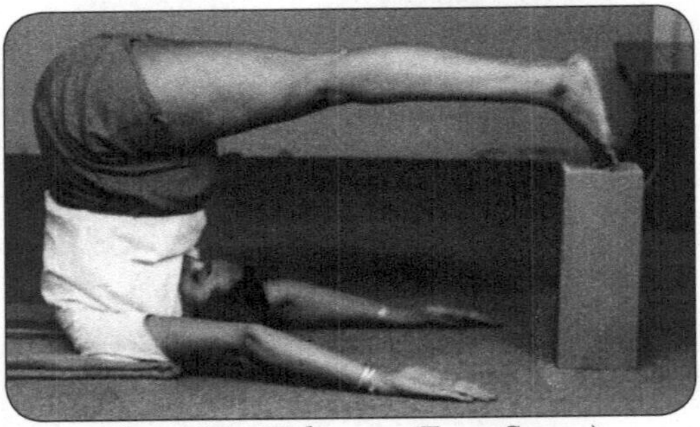

Fig. 194: *Halāsana* (Easy Stage)

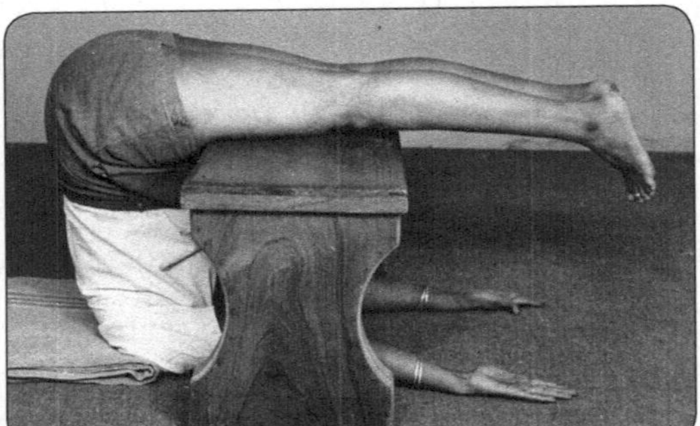

Fig. 195: *Halāsana* (Easy Stage)

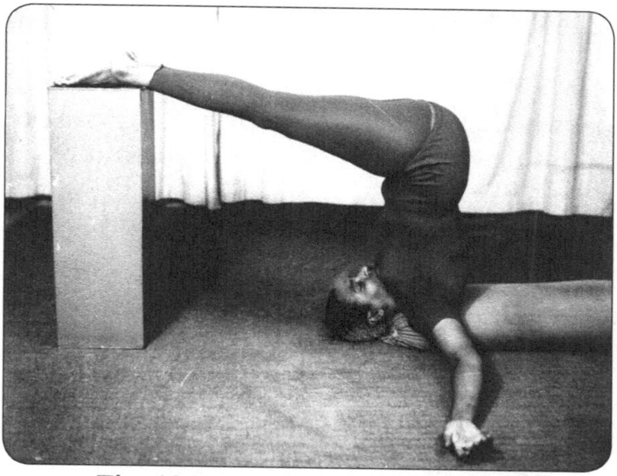

Fig. 194(a): *Halāsana* (Easy Stage)

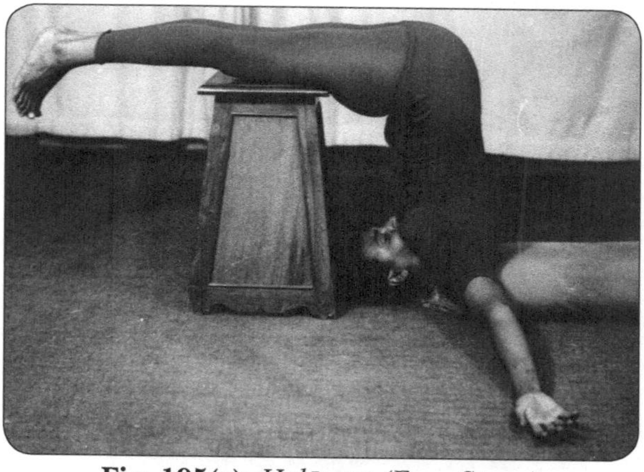

Fig. 195(a): *Halāsana* (Easy Stage)

5. Follow techniques 1 to 5 from Section IV, Āsana 48.
6. This posture can comfortably be done up to the 7th month, but later, if pressure is felt on the chest or if the womb starts feeling compressed, it should be avoided.

Effects: This posture soothes the nerves and keeps the spine firm. Both the āsanas help keep the mother's health in perfect condition.

52. *EKA PĀDA SARVĀṄGĀSANA* (*Figure 196*)

Hints

1. Those who have started Yoga practice before pregnancy may do this variation, otherwise it should be avoided.
2. Follow the techniques in Section IV, Āsana 52, but do not lower the leg down to the ground. Keep a bench or a stool 2 to 2½ feet high and place the foot on it.
3. The leg should remain parallel to the ground and should not come down too far (Figure 196).

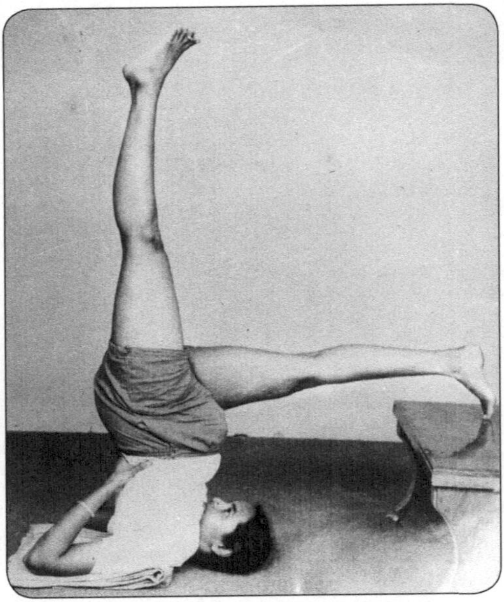

Fig. 196: *Eka Pāda Sarvāṅgāsana* (Easy Stage)

4. Keep the left leg perpendicular and raise the spine up. The groin of the leg which is down should not be pressed against the abdomen.
5. Stay for 5 to 10 seconds, breathing normally.

Effects: This āsana strengthens the spine and blood is circulated in the groins and in the pelvic region.

55. *ŪRDHVA PADMĀSANA IN SARVĀṄGĀSANA*

(Figure 197)

Hints

1. This is an advanced pose; it should only be practised by those who have already mastered it and not by a beginner.

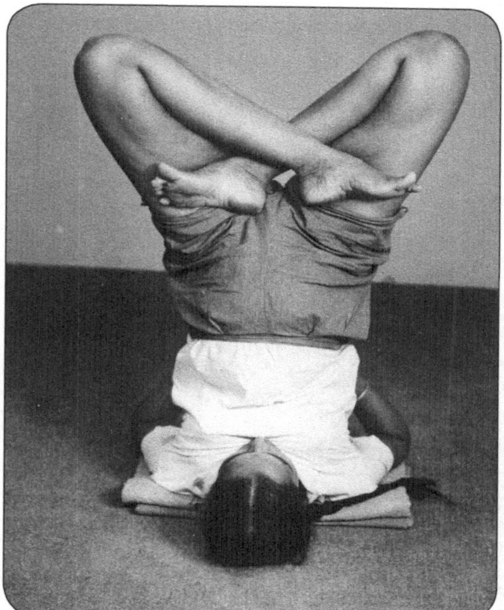

Fig. 197: *Ūrdhva Padmāsana* in *Sarvāṅgāsanaa* (Final Stage)

2. It can safely be done up to the 7th month. Later, one has to omit it.
3. This āsana can also be done with support. Do *Sarvāṅgāsana* with support, as in Figure 193, and then cross the legs in *Padmāsana*.
4. One need not stay too long in this pose. It depends on one's strength.

Effects: This pose strengthens the back and widens the pelvic region.

ĀSANAS FROM SECTION VI

64. *BHĀRADVĀJĀSANA I* (*Figure 198*)

Hints

1. Keep a folded blanket 2 to 2½ inches thick under the buttocks.
2. The feet should be lower than the buttocks.
3. Follow techniques 1 to 6 from Section VI, Āsana 64. Do not take the left arm backwards to clasp the right upper arm, but do as in Figure 198.

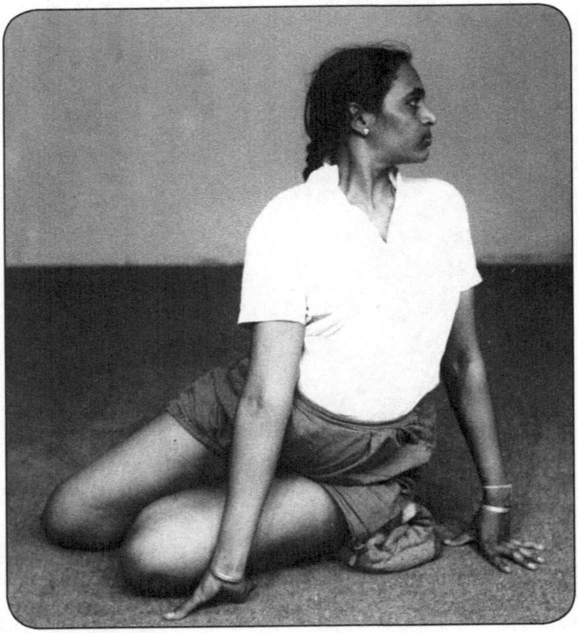

Fig. 198: *Bhāradvājāsana I* (Intermediate Stage)

4. Lift up the trunk instead of twisting it more.
5. This āsana may be done up to the 7th month.

Effects: This āsana strengthens the lower spine and keeps the waist muscles firm.

ĀSANAS FROM SECTIONS XI AND XII

MUDRĀ, *ŚAVĀSANA*, *PRĀṆĀYĀMA* AND *DHYĀNA*

Hints

1. As regards mudrā (Figures 210, 211), *Śavāsana* (Figure 199), prāṇāyāma (Figures 200, 201), and dhyāna (Figure 215), they should be done till the end of pregnancy. They make the body physically strong and healthy, and they soothe the nerves of the mother and make her calm and quiet. They bring mental health and happiness and make the mind pure.

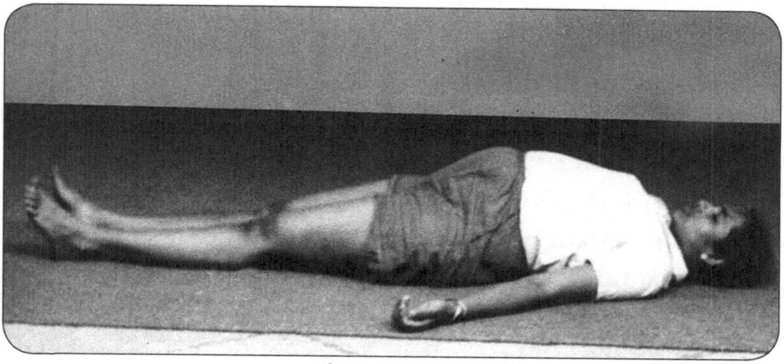

Fig. 199: *Śavāsana* (Final Stage)

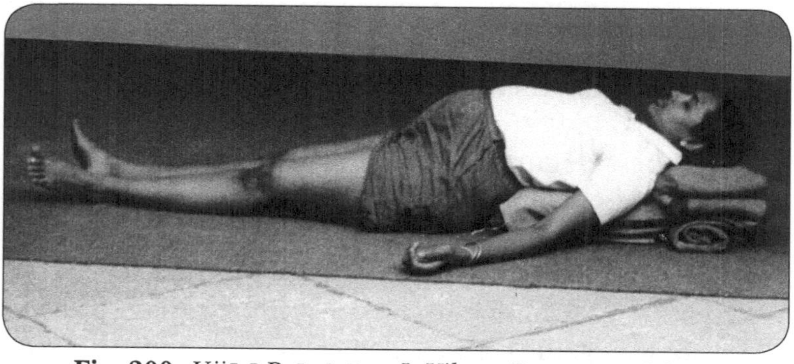

Fig. 200: *Ujjāyī Prāṇāyāma I; Viloma Prāṇāyāma I & II*; Preparation for Deep Breathing I & II (Final Stage)

2. It is considered that not only the mother's physical health but her state of mind has a profound effect on the unborn child. The foundation is laid in the womb itself for the child to develop on a morally and spiritually higher plane.
3. Although all these practices are useful throughout pregnancy, particular stress should be laid on the practice of *Śavāsana*, *Ujjāyī Prāṇāyāma I*, and *Viloma Prāṇāyāma I* & *II* in *Śavāsana* (Figure 200), for they soothe and relax the nerves and keep the blood pressure under control.
4. The practice of these prāṇāyāma minimises the spasms and strains during labour and facilitates the easy expulsion of the child. It makes delivery easy as the mother knows the right type of relaxation. It restores the mother's energy soon after delivery.
5. Do preparation for Deep Breathing I and II and *Ujjāyī Prāṇāyāma I* in *Śavāsana* as often as possible for overcoming tiredness and fatigue and also for normal movement of the foetus.
6. Hint 5 should be performed in the following manner:
   (a) place a pillow lengthwise from the waist to the head so that the chest remains at the same level as the abdomen, or a little higher;
   (b) place another pillow or a folded blanket under the head to keep the level of the head higher than the chest (Figure 200). In this position the body is in a descending plane from the head to the pelvis, avoiding tension in the head and heaviness in the chest, and facilitating breathing.
7. When performing prāṇāyāma in a sitting position a folded blanket 3 to 4 inches high should be placed under the buttocks to keep the spine lifted up and

to prevent the uterus from being compressed. *Ujjāyī Prāṇāyāma II*, *Sūrya Bhedana Prāṇāyāma*, *Nāḍi Śodhana Prāṇāyāma* and *Dhyāna* should all be performed in this manner.

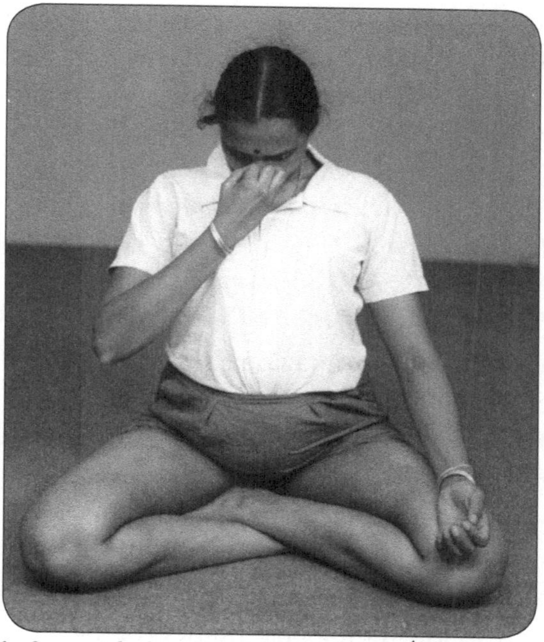

Fig. 201: *Sūrya Bhedana Prāṇāyāma, Nāḍi Śodhana Prāṇāyāma* (Final Stage)

ORDER OF PRACTICE DURING PREGNANCY

1. Up to three months all āsanas can be done except these in Section V. After this period, as the size of the foetus increases, attention should be paid to strengthening the muscles of the back and the spine, avoiding pressure on the abdomen (see Chapter X, No. 56).

2. (A) *Sālamba Śīrṣāsana* (Figures 70a, 188, 189); *Pārśva Śīrṣāsana* (Figure 190); *Parivṛttaikapāda Śīrṣāsana* (Figure 191); *Utthita Trikoṇāsana* (Figures 4, 174); *Utthita Pārśvakoṇāsana* (Figures 5, 175);

Vīrabhadrāsana I (Figures 7, 176); *Vīrabhadrāsana II* (Figure 8); *Ardha Candrāsana* (Figures 10, 177); *Pārśvottānāsana* (Figures 178, 179); *Prasārita Pādottānāsana* (Figures 18, 180, 181); *Sālamba Sarvāṅgāsana* (Figures 192, 193); *Halāsana* (Figures 194, 195); *Eka Pāda Sarvāṅgāsana* (Figure 196); *Ūrdhva Padmāsana* in *Sarvāṅgāsana* (Figure 197); *Jānu Śīrṣāsana* (Figure 182); *Baddha Koṇāsana* (Figure 183); *Supta Baddha Koṇāsana* (Figures 38, 39); *Upaviṣṭha Koṇāsana* (Figure 184); *Bhāradvājāsana* (Figure 198); *Vīrāsana* and Cycle (Figures 49, 54,185); *Supta Vīrāsana* (Figure 186); *Parvatāsana* (Figure 187); *Śavāsana* (Figure 199).

(B) Dhyāna and prāṇāyāma (Figures 215, 200, 201); *Śavāsana* (Figure 199).

Practice B should preferably be done separately from practice A. If they are done at a stretch, a minimum of 15 minutes should elapse between the end of practice A and the beginning of practice B.

3. If it is difficult to do all the āsanas in Practice 2 every day, the following may be omitted on alternate days:

   Pārśva Śīrṣāsana (Figure 190); *Parivṛttaikapāda Śīrṣāsana* (Figure 191); *Vīrabhadrāsana I* (Figures 7, 176); *Eka Pāda Sarvāṅgāsana* (Figure 196); *Ūrdhva Padmāsana* in *Sarvāṅgāsana* (Figure 197); *Bhāradvājāsana I* (Figure 198).

4. Those who start Yoga after becoming pregnant may adopt the following order if they find it difficult to master all the above mentioned āsanas during pregnancy:

   (A) *Sālamba Śīrṣāsana* (Figure 65); *Utthita Trikoṇāsana* (Figures 4, 174); *Utthita Pārśvakoṇāsana* (Figures 5, 175); *Vīrabhadrāsana II* (Figure 8); *Pārśvottānāsana*

(Figures 178, 179); *Prasārita Pādottānāsana* (Figure 181); *Sālamba Sarvāṅgāsana* (Figure 193); *Halāsana* (Figure 195); *Jānu Śīrṣāsana* (Figure 182); *Baddha Koṇāsana* (Figure 183); *Upaviṣṭha Koṇāsana* (Figure 184); *Vīrāsana* and Cycle (Figures 49, 54, 185); *Śavāsana* (Figure 199).

(B) Preparation for Deep Breathing I and II; *Ujjāyī Prāṇāyāma I*; *Viloma Prāṇāyāma I* and *II* (Figure 200): *Śavāsana* (Figure 199).

As mentioned in No. 2 above, practice A and B should, if possible, be done separately; if this is not possible, an interval of a minimum of 15 minutes should elapse between the two.

Sālamba Śīrṣāsana, *Sālamba Sarvāṅgāsana* and *Halāsana* may be omitted if one finds difficulty in doing them or if there is no assistant to help. The other āsanas can be performed safely.

5. Two types of prāṇāyāma may be done every day:

   First day of the week: Preparation for Deep Breathing I and II (Figure 200); *Ujjāyī Prāṇāyāma II* (Figure 213); Second day of the week: *Viloma Prāṇāyāma I* and *II* (Figure 200); *Sūrya Bhedana Prāṇāyāma* (Figure 201); Third day of the week: *Ujjāyī Prāṇāyāma I* (Figure 200); *Nāḍi Śodhana Prāṇāyāma* (Figure 201).

   Repeat this programme on the other three days. Every prāṇāyāma practice must end in *Śavāsana*.

6. *Śavāsana* should be done at least twice a day—in the morning and in the evening. It should preferably be practised as often as possible, whenever one feels the need for resting.

7. It is advisable to do dhyāna early in the morning, or before any prāṇāyāma practice (see Chapter XVI).

SECTION-X

Āsanas: Advanced

This section is included to show that even the most complicated and advanced postures are within the reach of women and can be performed by them without detracting from their femininity. Many a time it is claimed that complicated postures should not be done after marriage, or that they should be discontinued as age advances. However, let me assure you that these postures have no ill effects whatsoever. On the contrary, not only are they helpful in making the inner organs stronger and healthier, but they help develop strength of character, stability, intellectual clarity, and a poised personality as well.

The postures chosen here are based on various types of movements to show the range of movement that the body can perform, such as knotting oneself in a posture where the abdominal organs are contracted, balancing on the arms, intensive backward stretches. Again one should understand that the more intensive movements have a better and a more intensive effect on the entire system than do the milder ones.

As this book is specifically intended for women of all ages to help them generally, I have not given the techniques of these postures but have presented them for the benefit of those who wish to know and study further.

They may do so, after mastering all the āsanas given in this book through my father's book *Light on Yoga.*

The following are the āsanas that have been illustrated:

81. *Yoganidrāsana* *(Figure 202)*

Yoganidrā is a state of being between sleep and wakefulness. In this pose one lies on the floor and interlocks the feet behind the head. The spine is given maximum extension.

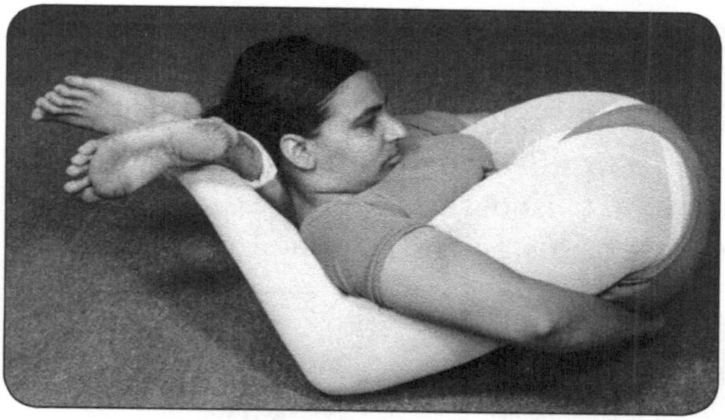

Fig. 202: *Yoganidrāsana* (Final Stage)

All the internal organs of the abdomen are contracted, toned and massaged. The body gets rested and revitalised.

82. *Ūrdhva Kukkutāsana* *(Figure 203)*

Kukkuta means cock, and this posture imitates the shape of a strutting cock. The lotus posture is performed while balancing on the arms. Here again the spine is stretched intensely. This āsana develops strong arms and healthy abdominal organs.

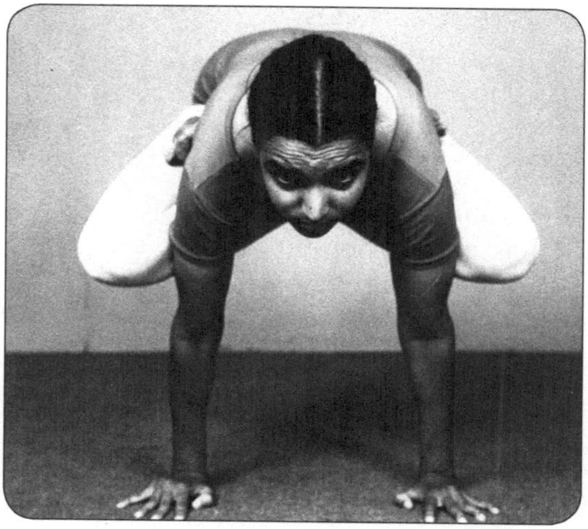

Fig. 203: *Ūrdhva Kukkutāsana* (Final Stage)

83. *Pārśva Kukkuṭāsana* *(Figure 204)*

Pārśva means side or flank, and the same posture is performed while taking the *Padmāsana* to both the sides alternately. The effects of the previous āsana are intensified and the lateral twist of the spine gives additional massage to the internal organs, thus strengthening them.

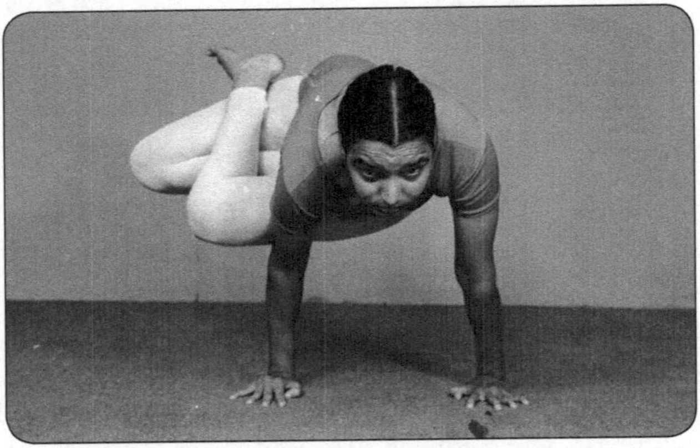

Fig. 204: *Pārśva Kukkuṭāsana* (Final Stage)

84. *Pīñcha Mayūrāsana*
(Figure 205)

Pīñcha means feather, mayūra is peacock. This āsana imitates a peacock showing its feathers. It removes stiffness in the neck, the shoulders, and the shoulder-blades and has all the benefits of the inverted poses.

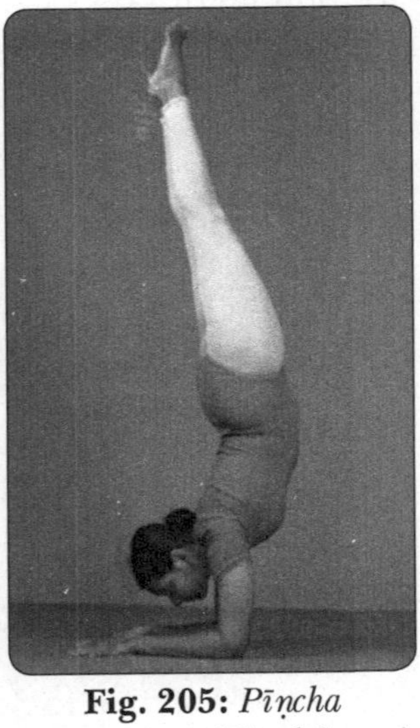

Fig. 205: *Pīṇcha Mayūrāsana* (Final Stage)

85. *Kapotāsana* *(Figure 206)*

Kapota means pigeon. In this āsana the Yogi imitates the shape of a pigeon. It is a difficult back-bending posture in a kneeling position. It tones the entire spine, expands the chest, strengthens the heart, the abdomen and the genital organs.

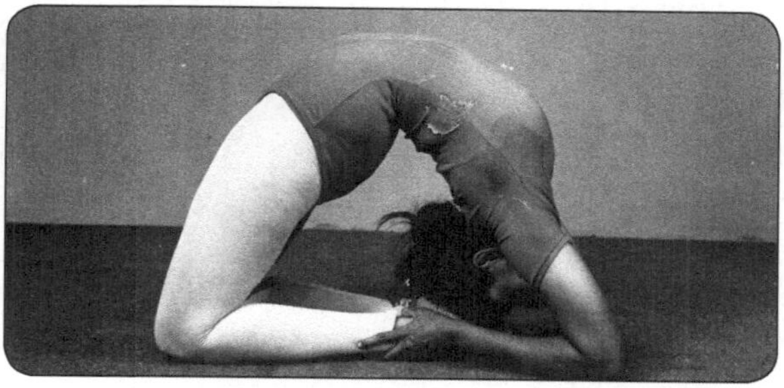

Fig. 206: *Kapotāsana* (Final Stage)

86. *Eka Pāda Rājakapotāsana* *(Figure 207)*

This is a difficult back-bending posture imitating the king pigeon's puffed chest. One leg kneels behind and the other is bent in front. The pose is beneficial to the lower spine, the pubic region and the urinary system. The endocrine glands receive a fresh supply of blood and the neck and the shoulders are made to work to their maximum, removing any stiffness.

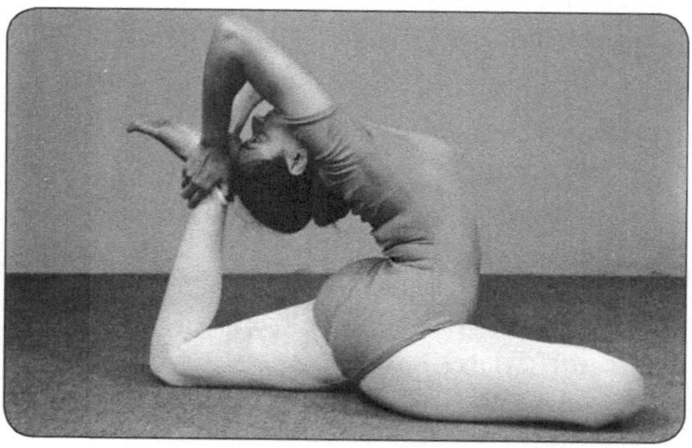

Fig. 207: *Eka Pāda Rājakapotāsana* (Final Stage)

87. *Vṛścikāsana* *(Figure 208)*

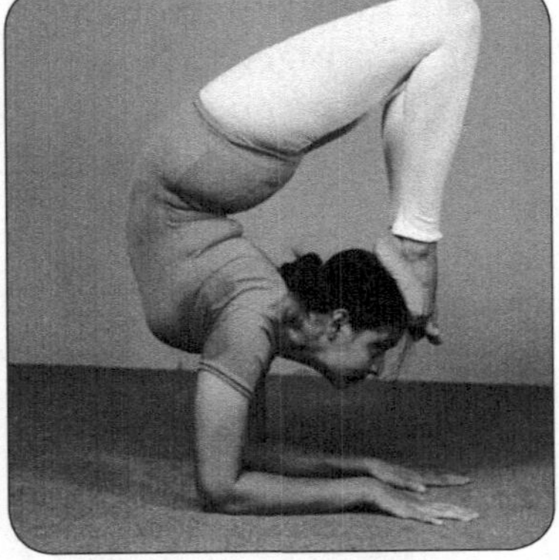

Fig. 208: *Vṛścikāsana* (Final Stage)

Vṛścika means scorpion. This pose resembles a scorpion with its tail up. In this āsana the body is balanced on the forearms and the spine is curved backwards so that it bends and the feet reach the head. The lungs expand and the abdominal muscles are stretched. The head is the seat of knowledge and also of emotions such as anger, hatred, pride and intolerance. The sādhaka stamps the feet on the head to learn that there is no difference between the head and the foot as the Self exists all over the body. This helps to develop humility and calmness.

88. *Naṭarājāsana* *(Figure 209)*

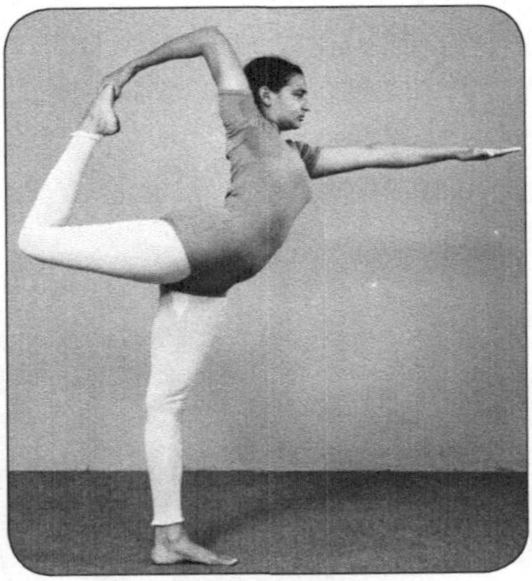

Fig. 209: *Naṭarājāsana* (Final Stage)

Naṭa means dance and Rāja means King. Natarāja is the Lord of Dance. It is another name for Lord Śiva. This beautiful āsana is dedicated to Śiva who is the source of Yoga. The posture is done by balancing on one leg and holding the toes of the other leg from behind, forming a circular shape. The expansion of the chest and the rotation of the shoulders do not allow calcium to form around the shoulders.

PART–III

Experience

CHAPTER XIII

On the Threshold of Peace

SECTION-XI

Mudrā and *Śavāsana*

Although most of the sections have been divided according to āsana and prāṇāyāma, this section is devoted to *Mahā Mudrā, Ṣaṇmukhī Mudrā* and *Śavāsana. Śavāsana* is the common denominator for both āsana and prāṇāyāma. In *Śavāsana* one achieves relaxation of the body, quiet respiration, tranquility of the nervous system, mental poise and peace of mind. All these are essential to prāṇāyāma and dhyāna.

Mahā Mudrā aims at practice in lifting the spine with support and at control over contraction of the abdominal organs. *Ṣaṇmukhī Mudrā* teaches withdrawal of the senses; the eyes and the ears are closed outwardly, but they are kept attentive and watchful inwardly—this draws one away from the world and takes one deep into the Inner Self.

All these three practices are preparatory for prāṇāyāma. The sādhakā learns to relax, to gain mastery of the elementary bandhas, and to control the sense organs. She learns to look inwards.

Ṣaṇmukhī Mudrā and *Śavāsana* may be practised at any time. If practised before going into bed, they are ideal for sound sleep.

89. *MAHĀ MUDRĀ*

Mahā means great or noble; mudrā means lock or seal, or the act of sealing. In this sitting posture the main apertures of the body are sealed. The spine is lifted by gripping the toes with the fingers and pulling them; this gives a firm support to the spine in its upward stretch. This mudrā may be practised before *Jānu Śīrṣāsana* (Figure 26).

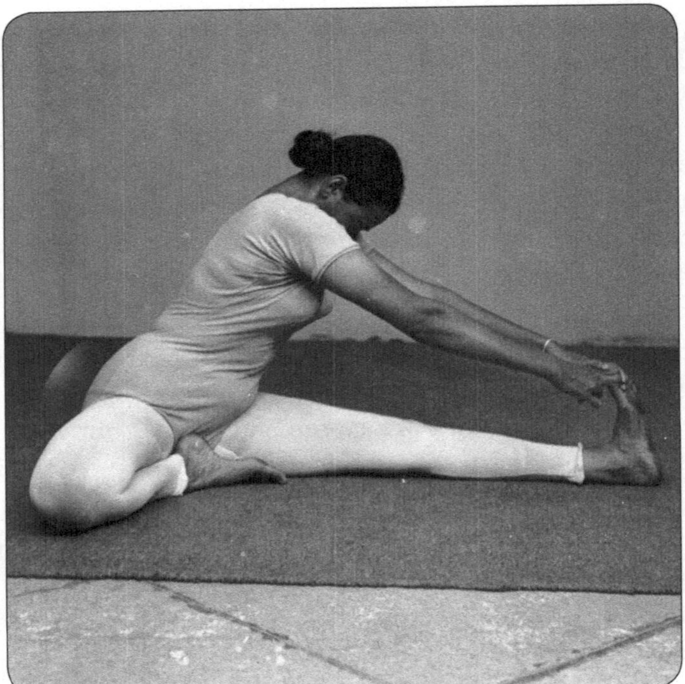

Fig. 210: *Mahā Mudrā* (Final Stage)

Technique

1. Sit in *Daṇḍāsana* (Figure 23).
2. Keep the left leg straight and bend the right knee, placing the outer sides of the thigh and the calf on the floor; take the heel close to the perineum. The bent leg should be at a right angle to the extended one.

3. Extend the arms and hook the big toe of the left foot with the thumbs, the index and the middle fingers of both the hands.
4. Straighten both the arms at the elbows.
5. Grip the toes well to lift up the trunk and to extend the spine. Raise the trunk more by maintaining the grip and pressing the thighs to the floor.
6. Lower the head from the nape of the neck until the chin rests in the hollow of the collar bone.
7. Relax the head and the forehead. Do not constrict the throat. (See Chapter XIV, *Jālandhara Bandha,* Nos. 29 to 31). Close the eyes.
8. Exhale whatever breath is in the lungs and then inhale fully. Tighten the abdomen from the anus to the diaphragm and stretch the spine upwards. Remain in this final position for 3 to 5 seconds (Figure 210), hold the breath, and observe the following points:
   (a) keep the chest expanded;
   (b) relax the eyes, the forehead, the tongue, and the facial muscles;
   (c) see that the body does not tilt to the right;
   (d) increase the grip on the toes to extend the spine.
9. Exhale, and while exhaling relax the abdominal tension without dropping the spine. Inhalation, retention and exhalation complete one cycle. Perform 5 to 8 cycles.
10. After completing the cycles, raise the head, open the eyes, straighten the right leg and come to *Daṇḍāsana* (Figure 23).
11. Now, keep the right leg straight and bend the left knee.

    Repeat the techniques 2 to 10, substituting the word right for left and vice versa.
12. Retention of breath must be equal on both the sides.

Effects: By the practice of *Mahā Mudrā* the three bandhas, namely, *Jālandhara Bandha, Uḍḍīyāna Bandha* and *Mūla Bandha*, are achieved to some extent.

Bandha means bound. It is an action whereby certain organs or parts of the body are contracted and controlled. In *Jalandhara Bandha* the neck and the throat are contracted by locking the chin in the notch between the collar-bones and the top of the sternum bone. In *Uḍḍīyāna Bandha* the abdominal organs are drawn towards the spine with the diaphragm lifted up. In *Mūla Bandha* the lower abdomen between the navel and the anus is contracted and pulled towards the diaphragm so that the region between the vagina and the anal mouth is locked upwards. These three bandhas help the sādhaka master the methods of prāṇāyāma as described in this book.

Mahā Mudrā helps correct displacement of the uterus, cures leucorrhoea and tones the abdominal organs. It relieves headaches, heaviness, and burning in the chest, dizziness, and blackout.

na hi pathyamapathyam vā rasāḥ sarvépt nīrasāḥ
api bhuktam viṣam ghoram pīyūṣamiva jīryati
kṣayakuṣṭagudāvartagulmājirṇapurogamāḥ
tasya dośāḥ kṣayam yānti mahāmudram tu yo'bhyaset
H.P. III, 16, 17

[One who practises the *Mahā Mudrā* need not have any restrictions in diet; whether or not she has a taste for food, her digestion is excellent; she can drink poison and digest it as though it were nectar; wasting disease (consumption - tuberculosis), leprosy, indigestion, enlargement of the liver and spleen run away from him.]

Thus says the Haṭha Yoga Pradīpikā in praise of *Mahā Mudrā*.

90. ṢAṆMUKHĪ MUDRĀ

This Mudrā is dedicated to the six-headed Kārtikeya, the leader of the divine army.

This Mudrā is also known as Parāngmukhī, Sāmbhavī and Yoni Mudrā. The Yogi here seals the organs of sense and looks within himself. This Mudrā may be practised at any time, whenever convenient.

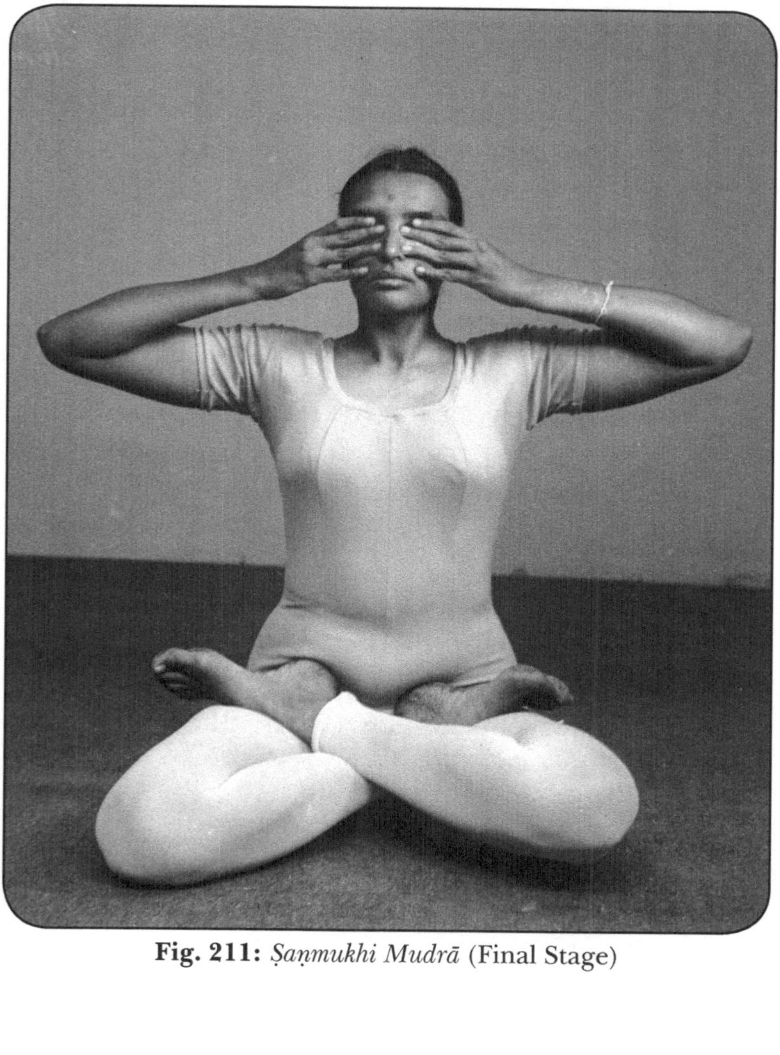

Fig. 211: *Ṣaṇmukhi Mudrā* (Final Stage)

Technique

1. Sit in *Padmāsana* (Figure 52). Keep the spine erect and the head as if floating on it. Relax the skin of the forehead.
2. Bend the elbows, bring the hands towards the eyes. Keep the elbows in line with the shoulders. Insert the thumbs in the ears to shut off all external sound. If the thumbs cause ear pain, press the tragi (the projections at the entrance to the ears) over the ears with the thumbs.
3. Bring the upper lids downwards and close the eyelids lightly. Keep the pupils of the eyes exactly in the middle and do not disturb them.
4. Extend the index and the middle fingers and place them on the closed eyes so that the first two phalanges only press the eyeballs. Press gently, curving the fingers to the shape of the eyeballs and touching the outer corners of the eyes with the second phalanges of the middle and the index fingers. Do not press the cornea.
5. Place the ends of the ring fingers at the root of the nose, near the nasal passages. Allow the breath to move slowly, by controlling the fingers on the nasal passages.
6. Rest the little fingers just above the upper lip and under the nostrils and let them feel the regulated and rhythmic flow of breath.
7. Pressure on the eyes as well as on the nasal passages must be equal on both sides (Figure 211).
8. Observe the following points:
   (a) As the eyeballs are closed and pressed, draw the sight inwards;
   (b) relax the skin of the body, though the trunk is erect;
   (c) relax the brain.

9. Listen to the humming sound in the ears. Your mind will be at peace due to this inner sound and inner vision.
10. Stay in this position as long as possible, then remove the fingers gently from the eyes, but keep the eyes closed. Loosen the thumbs in the earholes so that external sounds do not hit the eardrums immediately. Lower the hands and rest the back of the palms on the knees.
11. Experience the light and the darkness which take place in front of the closed eyes, the colourful patterns and the humming sound in the ears. Stay for a minute or two. When everything is peaceful and normal, open the eyes gently without disturbing the calmness of the brain. If the sight is blurred due to pressure on the eyes, close the eyes again. Do not be alarmed. This happens when the pressure on the eyeballs is too hard; therefore, next time do not press so much.
12. Keep the eyes open and still, look straight ahead. Do not move the pupils of the eyes. Release the legs from *Padmāsana* and stretch them gently.
13. If you are tired or weak, practise *Ṣaṇmukhī Mudrā* in *Śavāsana*. If you cannot do *Padmāsana* (Figure 52) sit in any posture and do *Ṣaṇmukhī Mudrā*.

Effects: The sense organs are drawn inwards and are thus controlled. Breathing is rhythmic; this calms the mind and one experiences Joy.

Ṣaṇmukhī Mudrā calms the brain and the nervous system and is excellent for removing irritation, tension, loss of temper, dizziness, burning in the eyes, blurred vision and brain fatigue due to intellectual work.

91. *ŚAVĀSANA*

In this āsana one lies motionless like a corpse, with the mind calm and still. This conscious relaxation of the body and the mind removes all tensions and invigorates both. The process is like re-charging the battery of a car.

Although this āsana appears simple, it is most difficult to master.

The body and the mind are interdependent and interconnected. They are inseparable in the art of introspection. *Śavāsana* is a link connecting the body and the mind; it connects āsana and prāṇāyāma and leads one to the spiritual path.

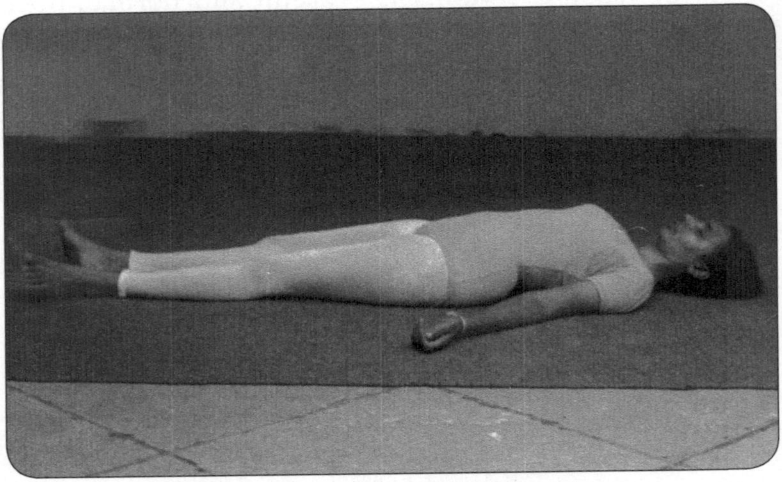

Fig. 212: *Savāsana* (Final Stage)

Technique

Adjustment of the body.

1. Spread a blanket on the floor and sit in *Daṇḍāsana* (Figure 23). Broaden and flatten the buttocks so that the flesh in this area does not become tight, especially in the small of the back.

2. Lean the trunk backwards and start lowering it by placing the elbows and the forearms on the blanket.
3. While lowering the spine to the floor make it convex so that the vertebrae come closer towards the floor one after another. During this movement do not move the buttocks or the legs. Both the sides of the trunk should be spreading outwards, from the centre of the spine towards the sides of the body. Now the body will be lying flat on the blanket, from heels to head. The flesh of the buttocks should not move towards the sacrum.
4. Keep the chest relaxed but do not cave it in.
5. Now, relax the legs and drop the feet sideways to the ground, without disturbing the position of the legs.

Head

6. Move the hands towards the head to adjust it and place the back of the head centrally on the floor. Do not let the back of the ears move towards the neck. Keep the pebble-like projection at the base of the back of the skull down. Observe the following points:
   (a) do not tense the neck and the throat;
   (b) do not press the chin against the throat.

Eyes and Ears

7. Close the eyes. Bring the upper eyelids downwards without disturbing the pupils.
8. Keep the ears and the eardrums relaxed. This can be adjusted by relaxing the lower jaw.

Arms

9. Broaden the shoulder-blades sideways but keep the shoulders away from the neck so that the shoulders remain flat on the floor.

10. Bend the elbows and bring the palms towards the chest.
11. Extend the upper arms from their sockets outwards and place them on the floor without disturbing the position of the elbows. Extend the forearms up to the wrists and place them on the floor so that the arms are at an angle of 15° to 20° from the sides of the trunk. Observe the following points:
    - (a) if the angle between the sides of the body and the arms is more than this, the shoulders come off the floor and are contracted; this contraction also causes constriction of the neck;
    - (b) if the arms are too close to the sides of the trunk, the armpits of the chest remain in contact with the inner upper arm; this hinders the broadening of the chest and disturbs relaxation.
12. Keep the fingers relaxed and the skin of the palms passive.

Nose

13. Keep the nose in a straight line, without tilting it to the side. Keep the tip of the nose facing the middle of the chest.
14. The movement of breathing should not disturb the trunk, the limbs and the brain.
15. Remain in this final position of *Śavāsana* for at least 10 to 15 minutes. Observe the following points:
    - (a) relax the skin of the forehead, the cheeks, the lips, the hands, the sides of the trunk, the buttocks and the thighs;
    - (b) keep the skin soft everywhere;
    - (c) relax all muscles;

(d) drop the sides of the sacrum towards the floor to relax the buttocks;

(e) do not lift the lumbar vertebrae too much away from the floor;

(f) both the sides of the trunk near the spinal column should rest evenly on the floor;

(g) one half of the body tends to tilt to one side; see that this does not happen and that both the sides are evenly placed;

(h) rest the scapulae on the blanket but do not press them down, as pressure creates tension in the brain;

(i) see that the palms are thin and soft;

(j) relax the fingers;

(k) relax the skin of the facial muscles which in turn relaxes the organs of the perception;

(l) any disturbance in the sense organs is immediately reflected in the face and spreads throughout the body via the nerves, tensing the entire system; the source of such a disturbance should be located and relaxed;

(m) if the brain is not at rest but is engaged in thinking, the front of the head moves up from the chin as if the head and the trunk are separate; in *Śavāsana* one has to train oneself not to allow the thought process to arise;

(n) if the brain is active, the eyeballs become hard and disturb the focal point of the eyes;

(o) direct the brain and the eyes towards the heart centre;

(p) the interrelation of the eyes, the mind, and the brain is very important; if the mind wanders, the brain moves upward and the eyes too become unsteady; therefore, it is important to keep the eyes still;

(q) draw in the eyes and ears, draw them inwards and fuse them at a point inside the centre of the chest where external sounds cease to disturb;

(r) surrender yourself, your body and mind to Mother Earth so that you are calm and passive. This is total relaxation.

Respiration

16. Do not do deep breathing. Breathing in *Śavāsana* should be as subtle, smooth, and quiet as the quiet flow of water in a river so that the mind remains undisturbed.

Observe the following points in inhalation (puraka):

(a) do not jerk the head;
(b) do not tighten the throat;
(c) do not jerk the diaphragm;
(d) do not disturb the muscles at the back of the trunk;
(e) do not cave in the sternum or the chest;
(f) do not inflate the abdomen; and
(g) do not tense the palms while inhaling.

Observe the following points in exhalation (rechaka):

(a) relax the brain during exhalation;
(b) do not allow the air to touch the walls of the throat, causing irritation;
(c) do not suddenly release the diaphragm;
(d) keep the mind passive, let it watch the flow of exhalation and regulate its flow;
(e) correct exhalation results in a feeling of quiet surrender of the mind and the body to Mother Earth, bringing a feeling of peace and oneness within oneself.

17. In perfect relaxation, the mind remains unperturbed and an inward flow of energy is experienced. A new state of consciousness, with no movement and so no waste of energy, arises. There is a feeling as if the body has been elongated by several inches. This is freedom of the mind and freedom of the body.
18. Remain in this state of total relaxation as long as you can. From this state of silence come back gradually to the active state. Do not disturb the silence of the mind nor jolt the body suddenly and break its silence.
19. Gradually bring your intellect, mind, and sense organs which have been submerged in a quiet, blissful state, to come in contact with the world around you.
20. Open the eyelids but do not move the pupils of the eyes up or down. Look passively and continue experiencing the serene state while establishing contact with the external world.
21. Now turn to the right side, and slowly get up.

Note: It may take some time for the mind to become steady and the body to become silent. By regular practice you learn to release tensions to experience the blissful state. In the beginning one may fall asleep when silence is experienced, but later one will learn to be silent without falling asleep.

In the beginning you may find it hard to adjust everything consciously, but gradually it becomes easy to observe and to adjust everything simultaneously so that the mind and the body rest quicker.

Later, as one masters this āsana one experiences the non-existing state of the body, the mind, the intellect, and the ego, and the Self is realised. The external world is there, but in this state it seems non-existent.

SPECIAL INSTRUCTIONS

1. If suffering from cold, cough, or asthma, place a pillow or a folded blanket about 3 to 4 inches thick on which the head and the back of the trunk can rest; in this way the chest is raised and the diaphragm remains a little lower than the chest, facilitating easy breathing (Figure 200).
2. If it is difficult to relax the eyes in the beginning, wrap a soft black bandage or cloth around the head, covering the eyes, the ears, and the back of the head. The cloth should be folded fourfold, lengthwise.

Effects:

uttānam śavavadbhūmau śayanam tacchavāsanam
śavāsanam śrāntiharam cittaviśrāntikārakam

H.P. I, 32

[To lie flat on the ground like a corpse is *Śavāsana*; it is the remover of fatigue and gives peace of mind.]

In *Śavāsana* all parts of the body, skin, muscles and nerves are relaxed. Energy which flows outward from the body is deflected to flow inwards. It thus becomes harnessed instead of dissipated.

Śavāsana is like an experience of death in a living state. For a brief period the body, the mind and the speech are still. The āsana is also called *Mṛtāsana*, because one experiences the gross and subtle body as a corpse. Unlike in the dead body, however, the soul exists—it exists in a pure state.

Śavāsana is invigorating and refreshing. It helps the body and the mind to recuperate after long and serious illnesses. Asthmatic patients and those suffering from other respiratory diseases, heart trouble, nervous tension, and insomnia derive tremendous benefits from it as it soothes the nerves and calms the mind. Practice of *Śavāsana* brings a sound and refreshing sleep devoid of dreams. It is not simply lying flat on the back. It is a state of meditation.

Śavāsana is control over the inner world and surrender to the Supreme Being.

CHAPTER XIV

Hints and Suggestions for the Practice of Prāṇāyāma

The Beginning

1. *athāsane dṛḍhe yogī vaśī hitamitāśtanaḥ*
   gurūpadiṣṭamārgeṇa prāṇāyāman samabhyaset

   H.P. II, 1

   [The Yogi, having perfected himself in the āsanas should practise prāṇāyāma according to the instructions of a Guru, with his senses under control and observing throughout a nutritious and moderate diet.]

   Some simple variations of prāṇāyāma are described in this book, with elaborate hints and techniques. Study these carefully before commencing practice, to avoid injury.

2. *yathā simho gajo vyāghro bhavedvaśyah śanaiḥ śanaiḥ*
   tathaiva sevito vāvuranyathā hanti sādhakam

   H.P. II, 15

   [As the lion, the elephant, and the tiger are tamed gradually, so also breath has to be tamed, otherwise it can be harmful to the sādhaka.]

   Practise prāṇāyāma systematically and regularly. Carefully note the subtleties described below in your practice.

3. First a beginner should master the āsanas and gain control over the body. Four to six months' practice of āsanas is essential before starting prāṇāyāma. Those sādhakas who are slow to grasp the technique of the āsanas may take a little longer.

Personal Hygiene

4. Prāṇāyāma should be practised after the morning chores of cleaning the teeth, washing and answering the calls of nature are completed.
5. Those who are constipated may without any fear practise *Ujjāyī Prāṇāyāma I*, *Viloma Prāṇāyāma* and *Sūrya Bhedana Prāṇāyāma*, but not *Kumbhaka*. This will not upset their health.
6. If a bowel movement is felt during prāṇāyāma practice, complete the cycle, answer the call of nature, then continue prāṇāyāma practice. On no account should the bowel movement be suppressed.

Food

7. Prāṇāyāma is best practised on an empty stomach. If this is not possible, a cup of tea, coffee, or milk may be taken before the practice.
8. Meals may be taken one hour after practising prāṇāyāma. Not less than four hours should elapse after a full meal before starting prāṇāyāma practice.

Time

9. The best time to practise is morning before sunrise, or evening after sunset. If this is unsuitable one may practise after doing the āsanas, or whenever convenient.
10. (a) If prāṇāyāma is practised first, allow a minimum of half an hour to pass before practising the āsanas.
    (b) If āsanas are practised first, allow an interval of a minimum of 15 minutes and then do prāṇāyāma. In this case, however, the duration of prāṇāyāma may be shorter than when it is practised first.
    (c) If you are exhausted after practising the āsanas, only do *Ujjāyī Prāṇāyāma I*. When exhausted, do not force the lungs to do prāṇāyāma.
    (d) Prāṇāyāma should preferably be performed at a chosen time each day. This will give the maximum benefit to the practitioner.

Place

11. The place should be airy, clean, free of insects and the ground should be level.

Āsana

12. Prāṇāyāma should be practised while sitting on the floor with a blanket or a deer-skin spread on it, according to Yoga texts.
13. Any of the three āsanas, *Siddhāsana* (Figure 48), *Vīrāsana* (Figures 49, 50), or *Padmāsana* (Figure 52) may be chosen for sitting.
14. Choose any of the above postures which give you physical steadiness and mental tranquility. The āsana should be physically firm and mentally soothing, in accordance with the sūtra "*Sthirasukhamāsanam*" a steady, calming posture is necessary for prāṇāyāma.
15. However, *Padmāsana* (Figure 52) is the best because the legs are crossed to give the body firmness and stability. In *Padmāsana* it is easy to keep the spine erect and the mind alert. The base of the spine and the perineum remain off the ground giving a feeling of weightlessness in the body and a steady, thoughtful state of the mind. The base of the trunk becomes light giving freedom to the thoracic region to expand in prāṇāyāma. The body remains compact, self-contained and undistracted by the external world and leads us inward in prāṇāyāma and dhyāna. The posture should not disturb the prāṇāyāma processes. If this occurs, sit in an easier posture until *Padmāsana* is perfected.
16. While practising prāṇāyāma, the facial muscles, ears, eyes, neck, shoulders, arms and thighs get tight or strained. It is essential to keep these parts completely relaxed.

17. Whatever the posture you choose for prāṇāyāma, see that the spine is well stretched and concave and that the body is kept erect.
18. The legs should stay immovable like the root so that the trunk above remains firm and strong. Stretch the thigh muscles in the direction of the spine, to assist the body to maintain an erect position. See that the weight of the body does not fall on the thighs.
19. Balance the coccyx and the cervical vertebrae on each other and maintain them at right angles to the ground so that the trunk does not lean forward or backward.
20. Rest the seat, balancing the trunk in between the anus and the perineum.
21. Stretch the spine vertebra by vertebra and extend it upwards, in the direction of the head. The extension from the base to the top has to be felt as though one is climbing a ladder step by step. First correct the position of the spine and then adjust the other portions of the body.
22. Normally the sacrum sags and sticks out, which affects the flow of energy at the base. So the sādhaka has to take it in, to lift it up, thus reversing the process of sagging energy. The lumbar spine caves in, resulting in convex dorsal and collapsed chest; it must be reeducated by observation and by creating space between the waist and the chest to enable the torso to extend vertically up. The dorsal spine is usually convex, keeping the lungs dropping within the thoracic cavity. It must be made concave so that the inner organs function well. The cervical region must be taken slightly back and then extended up for proper alignment of the body and integration of the mind. Otherwise dullness sets in. The spine, with all its natural curvatures, has to remain erect without undue concavities or convexities so that energy and life force may flow freely throughout the body.

Shoulders

23. The lower portion of the scapulae (shoulder-blades) should be pushed into the chest and away from the spine. This will broaden the thoracic cavity.
24. The shoulders should be extended sideways away from the neck and should not be tensed up nor pulled towards the ears.

Chest

25. Tuck in and roll up the back ribs so that the frontal ribs lift and broaden, creating space for the intercostal muscles to extend and expand the chest.
26. The sternum should be lifted up from its lower extremity.
27. The floating ribs should expand towards the sides so that the diaphragm can move with ease.
28. One has to learn to extend the intercostal muscles upwards and to expand them sideways during inhalation and to relax them towards the centre in exhalation. These movements are to be performed without any jerk or aggressiveness and without sudden shrinking or contraction.

Jālandhara Bandha

29. While practising prāṇāyāma in a sitting posture *Jālandhara Bandha* is essential. Jāla means net and bandha means bondage or binding. This bandha regulates the flow of blood and prāṇa to the heart as well as to the glands in the neck and the brain.
30. In *Jālandhara Bandha* the neck and the throat are contracted and the chin rests in the notch between the collarbones and at the top of the breast bone (Figure 213). When mastery is gained in *Sālamba Sarvāṅgāsana* (Figure 85) this bandha becomes easy to practise. Till then one should not force the neck muscles to rest the

chin between the collar bones, but the neck should be lowered as far as it can reach comfortably.

From the physical point of view, *Jālandhara Bandha* prevents strain on the heart in the practice of prāṇāyāma. From the psychological point of view, *Jālandhara Bandha* has a deeper significance. The brain is considered to be the seat of the ego. In *Jālandhara Bandha* the brain is lowered, thereby reducing its dominance over the practitioner during prāṇāyāma. The brain is made to bow down in salutation to one's own Soul, which is part of the Universal Soul. The breath becomes quiet and subtle and one experiences a state of impersonality.

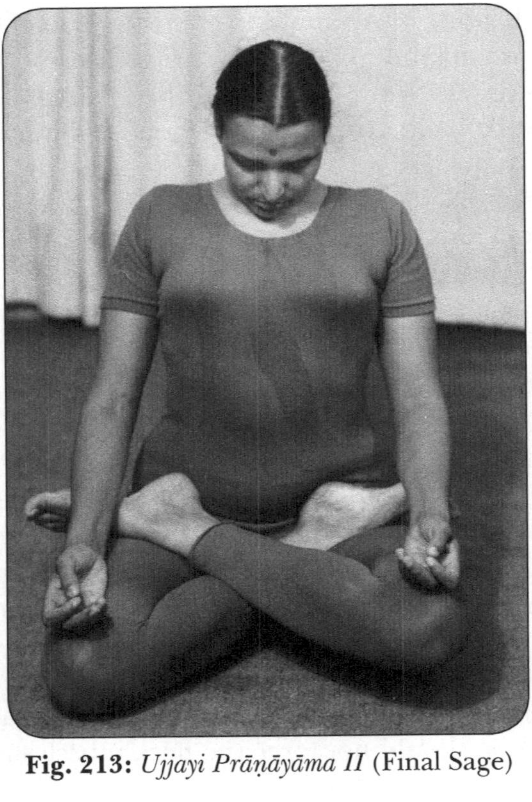

Fig. 213: *Ujjayi Prāṇāyāma II* (Final Sage)

During inhalation the head has a tendency to lift up. Care must be taken with every inhalation in prāṇāyāma that it does not lift up.

31. The head should be lowered from the nape of the neck and at the same time the sternum should be lifted. Do not cave in the chest when lowering the head.

Eyes

32. The eyes should be kept completely closed, but not shut tight. The eye-lids should be lightly closed and the pressure of the lids on the eyeballs should be very light. Keeping the eyes open in prāṇāyāma is disturbance in one's practice and causes burning sensation in the eyes.
33. The eyes should look inwards and watch the subtle movements. If the pupils turn upwards towards the forehead, the thought process begins. Hence the pupils should be focused on the seat of the Self.
34. To keep the eyes steady and not tensed, one has to master *Ṣaṇmukhī Mudrā* (Figure 211).

Ears

35. Keep the ear-drums relaxed. If they contract or are subjected to tension, the lower jaw will also contract and the temples will be tensed. Prāṇāyāma performed in this state causes headache and heaviness in the head.
36. During prāṇāyāma listen to the sound of inhalation and exhalation. The sound should be smooth, clear, steady and long. The inhalation and the exhalation should have equal tempo and rhythm. The sound should be pleasant to hear. The ears should remain alert throughout practice so that the moment the sound becomes ruffled or harsh it can be immediately

corrected. Sometimes jerky and forceful inhalation causes irritation and bleeding. Watch and rectify this.

Nose

37. Prāṇāyāma has to be practised through the nose alone. There are some variations where the mouth is used. But they have not been described in this book as they are not as effective for the average sādhaka as those given here.
38. The septum (made of bone and cartilage) which divides the nose should always be kept straight. It should not be tilted to the right or to the left with the fingers during practice.
39. The mucous membrane should be soft and not tensed to enable the sensations of inhalation and exhalation to be registered. If the membrane is tough and hard, sufficient air does not pass through. This reflects on the lungs making them inactive.
40. During inhalation and exhalation the membrane is adjusted against the current of air-flow. During inhalation the membrane is massaged downwards and in exhalation it is massaged upwards. This has to be learned by adjusting the fingers correctly and skillfully on the nose as well as by keeping the membranes soft and sensitive.

Tongue

41. The tongue should be relaxed and rested on the lower jaw. It tends to touch the upper jaw, but this habit has to be broken. If the tongue is not relaxed, saliva accumulates in the mouth and this hinders the flow of breath.
42. Saliva does ooze out in the beginning. It should be swallowed only after exhalation and not during the process of breathing, nor after inhalation.

Mouth

43. Do not press the teeth tight. Loosen the lower jaw from the upper jaw. Keep the lips relaxed.
44. Relax the throat.

Arms

45. Relax the arms in the sockets so that they remain loose.

Jñāna Mudrā

46. Rest the back of the wrists on the knees. Join the tips of the thumb and the index finger, forming them into a circle. Loosen the other three fingers. (Normally when *Jñāna Mudrā* is shown these three fingers are extended; in prāṇāyāma, however, they should be kept loose.) *Jñāna Mudrā* is indicative of knowledge; it symbolises the union of the Individual Soul (represented by the index finger) with the Supreme Being (represented by the thumb). The Mudrā indicates the experience of Supreme Knowledge (Figure 214).
47. The hand on the knee should be in *Jñāna Mudrā*, with the fingers loose. The palm should remain soft and the back of the wrist should rest on the thigh.

Fingers

48. Adjustment of the fingers on the nostrils in prāṇāyāma:

    It is necessary to have the nails cut for prāṇāyāma. In *Sūrya Bhedana Prāṇāyāma* and *Nāḍī Śodhana Prāṇāyāma* the inflow of breath is controlled by the fingers of the right hand by carefully manipulating the nostrils.

    Bend the index and the middle fingers inwards towards the palm and keep them passive. Form a circle by joining the tip of the thumb with the tips of the little fingers and the ring finger. Bend the right arm at the elbow, raise the hand and bring the fingers towards the nose.

While holding the nose with the fingers, curve the right wrist outwards so that its weight is not felt on the nose. Do not curve it inwards.

Control the right nostril with a gentle pressure by the tip of the thumb and the left nostril by the ring finger and the little finger. Place the tips of the fingers on the soft cartilage of the nose, a little below the nasal bone (Figure 214). Both the tips should be at the same level.

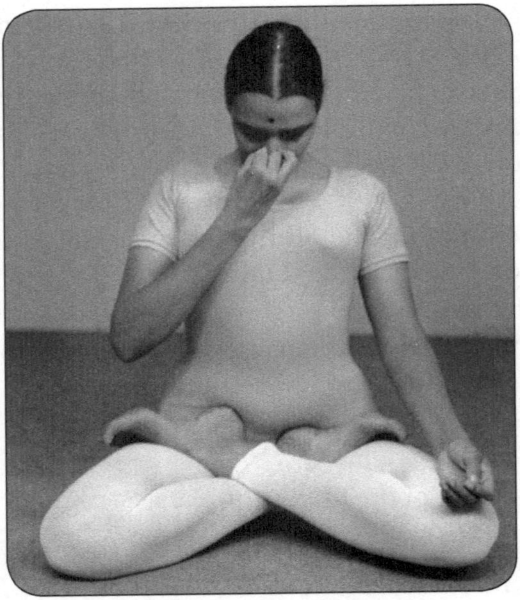

Fig. 214: *Nāḍī Śodhana Prāṇāyāma, Sūrya Bhedana Prāṇāyāma* (Final Sage)

Brain

49. Keep the brain calm and passive, at the same time alert, throughout the practice of prāṇāyāma. Do not tighten the skin covering the skull, nor the brain. Let the brain be the controller and the receiver of signals.

50. The function of the brain is to watch closely the subtle movements of breath, adjustments, and actions of the body; to send messages to those parts of the body where adjustments are needed (here it is acting as the controller); and to get those adjustments done by the various parts (here it is acting as the receiver).

51. Now the question arises as to how to keep the brain passive as well as alert to perform certain actions, for surely these two qualities are mutually contradictory. However, during prāṇāyāma, by regular persistent effort it is possible to adjust and perform these apparently contradictory actions with ease.

    Once learned, no extra energy is essential to achieve these actions as they become automatic and the brain, the trunk, the chest, and the mind all function spontaneously.

Regulation of Breath

52. *yuktam yuktam tyajedvāyum yuktam yuktam ca pūrayet*
    yuktam yuktam ca badhnīyādevam siddhimavāpnuyāt

    H.P. II, 18

    [One should learn to inhale, exhale and retain the breath slowly by regulating it. Thus one attains success.]

    The breath should not be fast and forceful.

53. In the beginning stage of prāṇāyāma one should not be too strict with the duration or the retention of breath by keeping a watch on time. For many months or even years, one has to train the body to be perfectly balanced and steady as described above and one has to train the flow of breath to be soft, smooth, and quiet. This means that one has to improve the quality of breath. This in turn leads to the extension of the breath without exertion and thus one achieves quantity

in its length. It is more important and beneficial to do a few cycles correctly than to be strict with duration.

54. The breath should be steady, long, and resonant and it should have a rhythm. If the rhythm or the sound changes, it is an indication that one's capacity is over. Then prāṇāyāma should be discontinued for that day as otherwise it is harmful. If you exert beyond your capacity, the brain cells will be taut and tension is created throughout the body. If the volume of sound is increased, the brain gets irritated. These are the indications of overexertion in prāṇāyāma. Thus, one has to learn to balance both quality and quantity in prāṇāyāma.
55. The sādhakā should first understand her limits for prāṇāyāma by the following method: Suppose a cycle of breath consists of inhalation lasting 10 seconds and exhalation lasting 10 seconds, one may continue with this cycle for, say, 5 minutes. Later, when one finds that the breath is shorter than 10 seconds and that the sound of inhalation and exhalation has also changed, it means that one has to stop prāṇāyāma for that day. It is a warning signal. Exertion in prāṇāyāma is harmful to the lungs and the heart. One should not be out of breath after prāṇāyāma practices.
56. The minimum number of cycles to be practised has been mentioned in the various prāṇāyāma given in Chapter XV. Though this may differ slightly according to individual capacity, some people can easily do more cycles than others without exerting, while others may find even the given minimum too much—one should know that capacity can only be increased by training the lungs through practice. Therefore, first of all one should attain steadiness in the minimum number of cycles, paying attention to maintaining their quality and quantity.

57. The duration of inhalation and exhalation should be equal. In the beginning, however, it may vary and this variation has to be gradually corrected. Suppose you inhale for 10 seconds and exhale for 8 seconds, then you have to adjust the inhalation to 9 seconds and the exhalation also to 9 seconds, with practice. Some people have a longer inhalation and some exhalation. One has to shorten whichever is the longer to bring the other process to the same duration. After the two have become equal, increase the duration of inhalation and exhalation, adding even time for both. See that there is no tension in the forehead, the neck, the throat and the chest.
58. When coming to the end of prāṇāyāma, in the sitting posture, the right hand which is used for regulating the breath should be brought down from the nostrils after the completion of the last cycle and should be placed on the knee in *Jñāna Mudrā*. The head, which is bent down in *Jālandhara Bandha*, should not be lifted up immediately with a jerk and the eyes also should not be opened suddenly.

    After completion of prāṇāyāma, do *Śavāsana* for at least five minutes. The poise and quietness gained during prāṇāyāma is thus retained.
59. ***Menstruation***
    (a) If one is tired during the menstrual period, *Ujjāyī Prāṇāyāma I* and *Viloma Prāṇāyāma I* and *II* are beneficial as they remove fatigue. They also check the menstrual overflow.
    (b) Young girls should practise *Ujjāyī Prāṇāyāma I* and *II* and *Viloma Prāṇāyāma I* and *II* in adolescence, as these promote physical strength, emotional stability and mental peace.
    (c) The other varieties of prāṇāyāma may be practised according to the time at one's disposal. It is

advisable to practise *Sūrya Bhedana Prāṇāyāma* and *Nāḍī Śodhana Prāṇāyāma* after the age of 20 but not before, as this would make a young person look prematurely old.

Pregnancy

(d) During pregnancy all the various types of prāṇāyāma may be practised. *Ujjāyī Prāṇāyāma I* and *Viloma Prāṇāyāma I* and *II* are particularly helpful for relaxation, removing tension and for making delivery easy.

(e) For further details refer to Chapter X and to Chapter XII, Section IX.

After Delivery

(f) After delivery one should start with the practice of *Ujjāyī Prāṇāyāma I* and *Viloma Prāṇāyāma I* and *II*.

(g) Three months after delivery one may practise all the types of prāṇāyāma described in this course.

Menopause

(h) At this time, the practice of *Ujjāyī Prāṇāyāma I* and *II*, *Viloma Prāṇāyāma I* and *II*, and *Sūrya Bhedana Prāṇāyāma* is soothing to the nerves and calms the mind.

(i) Avoid *Ujjāyī Prāṇāyāma II* and *Nāḍī Śodhana Prāṇāyāma* if you are subject to hot flushes.

(j) When one becomes strong and healthy, gradually all the different types of prāṇāyāma which have been described in this book may be practised.

General

(k) For those suffering from coronary conditions do only *Ujjāyī Prāṇāyāma I*.

(l) In case of high blood pressure, avoid *Ujjāyī Prāṇāyāma II*.

(m) For those with low blood pressure, all types of prāṇāyāma mentioned here are of great help.

Harmful Effects due to Faulty Practice

60. If the lungs and the diaphragm are made to work beyond their normal capacity, the respiratory system is liable to be injured.

prāṇāyamena yuktena sarvarogakśayo bhavet
ayuktābhyāsayogena sarvarogasamudbhavah
hikkā śvāsaśca kāsaśca śiraḥkarṇākśivedanāḥ
bhavanti vividhā rogāḥ pavanasya prakopataḥ

H.P. II, 16, 17

[If prāṇāyāma is done correctly, all diseases are eradicated. Faulty practice can invite all diseases. Faulty practice of prāṇāyāma will result in hiccups, asthma, cough, pain in the eye, the ears and the head.]

The effects of prāṇāyāma are observed not only on the gross body but also on the subtle plane.

Benefits of Correct Practice

61. The brain experiences a coolness after prāṇāyāma. The mind becomes calm and exhilarated. The body feels light, the nerves are calm and without tremors. The chest feels strong. An energetic feeling in the body and a freshness in the mind are the immediate results of correct prāṇāyāma.

62. *yadā tu nāḍīsuddhiḥ syāttathā cihnāni bāhyataḥ*
kāyasya kṛśatā kāntistadā jāyeta niścitam
yatheṣṭam dhāraṇam vāyoranalasya pradīpanam
nādābhivyaktirārogyam jāyate nāḍīśodhanāt.

H.P. II, 19, 20

[When the nerves are purified by prāṇāyāma the following effects are observed: The body becomes slender and lustrous, gastric fire increases; Inner sound is heard: excellent health is attained.]

63. After regular and long practice of prāṇāyāma the sādhaka scores a victory over the mind, the emotions, and the senses. Being stable-minded, she does not move from her determination. Concentration of the mind improves and she becomes a Sthita Prajña—one who is not swayed by conflicting emotions and thoughts.

64. Practice of prāṇāyāma leads to discrimination and attainment of knowledge. Thoughts and actions become clear and pure. Like the āsana, prāṇāyāma too becomes a stepping-stone to meditation.

Chapter XV

Prāṇāyāma— Techniques and Effects

Section-XII

After mastering Section XI the practice of prāṇāyāma may be commenced, following the hints given in Chapter XIV.

Before going into the right method in the art of deep inhalation and deep exhalation, given below are two stages which are preparatory to deep breathing. It is advisable to start with these two stages before proceeding further.

Although breathing is a natural process for all, astonishingly enough, many people have faulty inhalation and exhalation. Therefore the basis of prāṇāyāma, which is correct inhalation and exhalation, should first be mastered. Variations of prāṇāyāma can then be learned later with ease.

1. Normal Inhalation

In normal breathing the middle ribs expand more than the top and bottom ribs; the chest extends and expands as fully and naturally as possible without tension or pressure on the brain, nor on the intercostal muscles, or the diaphragm; the sternum is held up.

2. Normal Exhalation

The diaphragm is kept soft so that it does not condition the outflow of breath by volitioning the lungs and the muscles of the chest.

3. Normal Retention

The gap between inhalation and exhalation and between exhalation and inhalation is retention. It is such a natural process that it takes place unconsciously.

4. Deep Inhalation (Pūraka)

Deep inhalation is a conscious effort to breathe in fully by expanding the chest deliberately and gradually from bottom to top and outwards like a fountain spreading up and sideways.

While taking a deep breath do not inflate the abdominal area but keep it in contact with the spine.

In deep inhalation the chest moves up like a hill and the abdomen remains like a valley.

5. Deep Exhalation (Recaka)

In deep exhalation the breath is allowed to go out slowly, steadily, and deeply to synchronise with the gradual release of the chest.

In order to breathe out deeply the top ribs and the diaphragm are gripped and made to release rhythmically.

However the sternum is not allowed to cave in during exhalation.

I. PREPARATION FOR DEEP BREATHING

Stage I: Here the emphasis is laid on the art of deep exhalation.

Technique

1. Lie on a blanket in *Śavāsana* (Figure 212).
2. Exhale whatever breath is in the lungs.
3. Take a normal inhalation, observing the following points:
   (a) do not inhale with an effort;
   (b) see that the position of the head is not disturbed while inhaling.

4. Grip the diaphragm and exhale slowly, rhythmically, quietly, and deeply, observing the following points:
   (a) do not exhale suddenly or force the breath to come out;
   (b) exhale till the lungs feel empty and the abdominal organs are relaxed;
   (c) see that the duration of the outgoing breath is two to three times longer than that of the incoming breath;
   (d) at the end of exhalation a small pause is indicating the completion of experienced, exhalation.
5. This is one cycle. Repeat 15 to 20 cycles at a stretch and then relax in *Śavāsana*.

Stage II: Here the emphasis is on deep inhalation.

Technique

1. Lie on a blanket as in *Śavāsana* (Figure 212).
2. Exhale completely whatever breath is in the lungs.
3. Now, inhale slowly, steadily, and deeply, observing the following points:
   (a) gradually broaden the chest from the floating ribs to the top ribs, with the incoming breath;
   (b) do not tighten the throat nor make a rough sound in the throat;
   (c) keep the sternum up;
   (d) do not inflate the abdominal organs;
   (e) fill the lungs from bottom to top and see that the incoming breath is two to three times longer than the outgoing breath;
   (f) at the end of inhalation a small pause is experienced, indicating the completion of inhalation.
4. Exhale normally, without effort. Though the exhalation is normal, it effortlessly becomes slightly deeper than

normal in Yoga practice. Observe the following points:
   (a) do not exhale with undue haste;
   (b) do not cave in the chest.
5. This completes one cycle. Repeat 15 to 20 cycles at a stretch and then relax in *Śavāsana*.

Effects: These two types of breathing prepare the lungs for the advanced practice of prāṇāyāma.

Stage I is very soothing and helpful for those who suffer from high blood pressure, coronary disorders, nervous tension, headache, migraine and hot flushes during menopause.

Stage II is a boon for those who suffer from low blood pressure, depression, inferiority complex, fear complex, low vitality and general weakness.

II. *UJJĀYĪ PRĀṆĀYĀMA I* (*Figure 212*)

Uḍ means upwards or superior in rank. It also means expanding or blowing, indicating a sense of power. Jaya means victory or conquest, in other words restraint. In *Ujjāyī Prāṇāyāma* the chest and the lungs are fully expanded like those of a hero or a conqueror.

Technique

1. Lie on a blanket in *Śavāsana* (Figure 212).
2. Exhale completely whatever breath is in the lungs.
3. Relax the diaphragm so that it is soft. Deflate the abdominal organs and keep them in contact with the spine. Exert no pressure on the chest. The thoracic cavity will thus be separated from the abdominal cavity. The abdominal organs must not be forcibly pressed in.
4. Inhale slowly, quietly, deeply and steadily.

5. Fill the lungs with air completely, from the floating ribs to the top brim of the chest. This is called pūraka. Observe the following points:
   (a) keep all other parts of the body relaxed;
   (b) let the abdomen remain like a valley; the chest is filled with air and expanded;
   (c) when the lungs are full and no more breath can be taken in, a natural pause will be experienced for a second or two;
   (d) do not allow the ribs to collapse and do not let loose the grip on the diaphragm suddenly;
   (e) keep the chest as though tucked up without tightening the throat.
6. Exhale slowly, quietly, steadily and rhythmically. If the exhalation is sudden there will be tremors of the body.
7. Exhale quietly but fully, till the lungs are empty. This is called recaka.
8. This completes one cycle.
9. In the beginning start with 8 to 10 cycles and gradually increase the number of cycles to 15 or 20.
10. After completing the last cycle, lie in *Śavāsana* with normal breathing.

Respiration in *Ujjāyī Prāṇāyāma I*

Pūraka (Inhalation)

(a) Breathe through the nose. Feel the touch of the breath on the upper palate. If it is soothing the sound is like the syllable 'sssa'. If it is irritating to the throat, it causes coughing and also does not allow the lungs to fill properly;

(b) while inhaling, fill the lower part of the lungs first, then the middle, and lastly the upper part. Do not puff the muscles of the chest. Intake of breath and opening of the chest should synchronise;

(c) expand and extend the intercostal muscles from the sternum to the sides of the trunk as well as upwards, from the floating ribs to the top of the chest simultaneously so that the chest is broadened circumferentially;

(d) raise the back ribs slightly towards the front ribs;

(e) open the chest from the centre outwards gently as if it were a flower opening, the pressure of incoming air being the centrifugal force;

(f) inhalation, extension and expansion of the chest should be simultaneous;

(g) after inhalation the head and the chin tend to lift up; see that this does not happen.

(h) During inhalation make sure that the ribs below the top of the breasts are lifted and expanded. Generally, the intercostal muscles between these ribs do not open efficiently due to the heaviness of the breasts.

Recaka (Exhalation)

(a) Keep the brain, the throat and the sense organs relaxed before exhaling. The expelled air will make a sound 'Huuum' at the base of the throat.

(b) Do not drop the intercostal muscles and the sternum suddenly. Exhale gently through the nose without straining the throat. In the beginning of exhalation the top ribs remain firm. Relaxation of the top intercostal muscles takes place only after one reaches the middle of exhalation.

(c) Inhalation causes a certain amount of tension on the diaphragm. Stretch it sideways to remove the tension and to make it soft; tension on the diaphragm strains the heart.

(d) During exhalation do not collapse the chest suddenly. The abdominal organs should be maintained parallel to the spine.

(e) While exhaling, the sides of the trunk should not be pressed. The chest should deflate slowly and gradually, from the sides to the centre with centripetal force, like a lotus closing its petals after sunset;

(f) Do not allow the chest to contract inwards during exhalation;

(g) Both pūraka and recaka should be done consciously with alertness.

Note: Those who are flabby or have weak ribs should place a folded blanket 3 to 4 inches thick under the shoulder-blades before doing *Śavāsana*, The blanket should extend from the lumbar vertebrae to the top of the dorsal so that the chest is lifted up and the abdominal organs remain at a lower level. The head has to be raised a little higher than the chest by placing a blanket below the back of the head. This will facilitate the free functioning of the diaphragm, without creating tension in the head. This method is useful for those whose intercostal muscles near the breastbone do not lift or stretch. For beginners also, who are unable to expand the chest, this method is ideal (Figure 200).

Effects: This is the basis of prāṇāyāma, beneficial to all, as it aerates the lungs and tones the nervous system. Among the āsanas, *Sālamba Śīrṣāsana* and *Sālamba Sarvāṅgāsana* are the ideal ones. Likewise, *Ujjāyī Prāṇāyāma* is ideal among the different types of prāṇāyāma. It should always be practised, even if other variations cannot be practised for the lack of time.

It soothes the nervous system, the wandering mind becomes steady and exhaustion, burning in the chest, insufficient breathing, blockage in respiration, shortness of breath are all cured by its practice. It generates vital energy.

III. *VILOMA PRĀṆĀYĀMA*

'Vi' denotes negation, 'loma' means hair. Viloma means against the hair, or against the natural order of things.

Viloma Prāṇāyāma (Figure 212) has two variations. The first variation is done with interrupted inhalation—this is Stage I; the second variation is done with interrupted exhalation—Stage II.

Stage I

Technique

1. Lie down in *Śavāsana* (Figure 212). This should be done correctly, as described in the technique for *Śavāsana*.
2. Exhale, empty the lungs.
3. Inhale through both the nostrils, feeling the touch of air on the outer membranes. Follow all the instructions given for *Ujjāyī Prāṇāyāma I* under Pūraka, but remember that here inhalation is with interruptions.
4. Inhale for two seconds, hold the breath for two seconds; again inhale for two seconds, hold the breath for two seconds, and continue with this process until the lungs are full.
5. After the last inhalation, retain the breath for 3 to 5 seconds.
6. Exhale slowly and deeply, without a halt, until the lungs are emptied, following the instructions given in *Ujjāyī Prāṇāyāma I*.
7. This completes one cycle. In the beginning practise 6 to 8 cycles. Gradually the number of cycles can be increased to 15 or 20.
8. The complete cycle of *Viloma Prāṇāyāma*, Stage I, is thus as follows: (a) Inhalation-Retention; Inhalation Retention; Inhalation-Retention; Inhalation-Retention (the last retention is a little longer than the previous ones); (b) complete exhalation without a break.

9. After the first two seconds of inhalation the chest expands and extends. The diaphragm remains firm. During retention one should not release the chest, the diaphragm, or the sternum, and this holds good for each inhalation. Retention should not cause any pressure or tension in the brain. The abdomen should not be puffed in retention.
10. This prāṇāyāma can also be done in sitting posture—in *Siddhāsana* (Figure 48), *Vīrāsana* (Figure 49), or *Padmāsana* (Figure 52). However, one should first master it in *Śavāsana*.
11. In the sitting postures keep the spine erect. Lower the head and do *Jālandhara Bandha* (Chapter XIV). Follow the same techniques as above.
12. Usually an average woman can do 4 to 5 retentions. Later, when the inhalation time increases, the retention time also increases. However, all the interrupted inhalations and retentions should be of even duration. Do not make one longer and the other shorter.
13. In the beginning one finds it difficult to do retention with each cycle. Therefore, do one cycle of *Viloma Prāṇāyāma* and one cycle of *Ujjāyī Prāṇāyāma I* (deep breathing), that is to say, the cycles of *Viloma Prāṇāyāma* and *Ujjāyī Prāṇāyāma I* should be performed alternately. The number of cycles of each should be equal. Later, one has to do all the cycles of *Viloma Prāṇāyāma* at a stretch.

Stage II

Technique

1. After completing Stage I allow one or two minutes to pass while breathing normally.
2. Exhale, empty the lungs.

3. Inhale slowly, steadily, deeply and rhythmically. After complete inhalation pause for a while, observing the following points:
   (a) do not raise the head up;
   (b) keep the sternum up;
   (c) keep the diaphragm firm so that you do not exhale suddenly.
4. Exhale for two seconds, pause for two seconds; again exhale for two seconds, pause for two seconds; continue in this manner until the lungs are completely emptied.
5. After the last exhalation retain the breath for 2 to 3 seconds. This completes one cycle.
6. In the beginning practise 6 to 8 cycles. Gradually increase to 15 or 20.
7. The complete cycle of *Viloma Prāṇāyāma*, Stage II, is thus as follows: (a) Complete inhalation; (b) Exhalation-Retention; Exhalation-Retention; Exhalation-Retention; Exhalation-Retention, and so on.
8. In each retention there is firmness in the chest, but it does not expand or constrict. After complete exhalation relax the head, the chest and the diaphragm, before starting the inhalation.

Special Instructions

1. Stage II can also be done in a sitting position, as mentioned in Stage 1, but only after it has been mastered in *Śavāsana*,
2. In sitting postures *Jālandhara Bandha* must be performed, otherwise there is a strain on the heart. Follow the same techniques as above.
3. The number of pauses in inhalation (Stage I) and exhalation (Stage II) should be equal. The interrupted exhalations and retentions in Stage II should be evenly divided as far as duration is concerned.

4. Here also, if it is difficult to perform the several cycles of *Viloma Prāṇāyāma* Stage II at one stretch, the cycles of Stage II and *Ujjāyī Prāṇāyāma I* can be performed alternately. The same number of each should be performed. Later, all the cycles of Stage II have to be done at a stretch.

Effects: Stage I of *Viloma Prāṇāyāma* is effective in low blood pressure, but both can be practised as they do not harm. If the mind has not attained poise in deep breathing, these two variations will achieve it.

Viloma Prāṇāyāma cures shallow breath, asthma, tuberculosis and diabetes.

The effects on the mind are particularly discernible and this prāṇāyāma is ideal for women who have moods and are disturbed.

IV. *UJJĀYĪ PRĀṆĀYĀMA II*

Ujjāyī Prāṇāyāma II (Figure 213) is similar to I, but here it is done in a sitting position and with Kumbhaka (Retention).

Technique

1. Sit in *Siddhāsana*, *Vīrāsana,* or *Padmāsana* (Figures 48, 50, 52).
2. Keep the spine erect, raise the sternum, lower the head, and perform *Jālandhara Bandha* (Chapter XIV).
3. Place the back of the wrists on the knees and the palms in *Jñāna Mudrā* (Figure 214). Keep the fingers loose (Chapter XIV, Nos. 46 and 47).
4. Close the eyes and draw them inwards (Figure 213).
5. Exhale slowly and completely.
6. Take a slow, deep and steady inhalation through the nose. The touch of the incoming air is felt on the roof of the upper palate and makes a sound 'sssssa'. Keep the tongue loose, resting on the lower palate.

7. Fill the lungs fully with an inward breath, extending and expanding the chest as explained at the beginning of this chapter.
8. Hold the breath for 3 to 5 seconds, observing the following points:
   (a) keep the abdominal organs pulled in towards the spine and the spine extended upwards;
   (b) do not tense the brain, the eyes, and the temples;
   (c) the diaphragm should be firm.
9. Release the pressure on the abdominal organs. Exhale slowly, deeply, and completely, observing the following points:
   (a) do not release the tension on the intercostal muscles, the sternum and the diaphragm suddenly;
   (b) after one or two seconds of exhalation only, gradually release them, otherwise the heart and the lungs get injured.
10. Before inhaling again, wait for a second (normal retention). This completes one cycle.
11. The complete cycle of *Ujjāyī Prāṇāyāma II* is thus as follows:
    (a) Pūraka (inhalation)—full and complete.
    (b) Kumbhaka (retention)—3 to 5 seconds.
    (c) Recaka (exhalation)—full and complete.
    (d) Kumbhaka (normal retention)—1 second.
12. Inhale again, as described above and practise a few cycles for 5 to 10 minutes. The retention period should be increased from 3 to 10 seconds.
13. After completing the last cycle, breathe normally and remain still in this position for some time. Then slowly raise the head, open the eyes quietly and lie down in *Śavāsana*.

Special Instructions

1. If it is difficult to perform Kumbhaka with every cycle, perform the cycles of *Ujjāyī II* and *Ujjāyī I* alternately, with an equal number of cycles of each. When this has been mastered, perform all the cycles of *Ujjāyī II* at a stretch.
2. If you do not recover by the method explained in the Special Instructions (1), then perform cycles of normal inhalation and normal exhalation as explained in the beginning of this chapter, until you recover and feel fresh to do the cycle of *Ujjāyī II*.

Effects: *Ujjāyī Prāṇāyāma II* removes phlegm, improves the appetite, cures dropsy, builds endurance and soothes the nervous system. It gives courage by removing fear complexes.

V. *SŪRYA BHEDANA PRĀṆĀYĀMA*

Sūrya denotes the Sun. Bhedana is derived from the root 'bhid' meaning to pierce or pass through. The nerve on the right side of the nose is called *Pingalā Nāḍī* or *Sūrya Nāḍī*. The one on the left is known as *Iḍā Nāḍī* or *Candra Nāḍī*.

In *Sūrya Bhedana Prāṇāyāma* (Figure 214), one inhales through the right nostril and exhales through the left nostril.

Technique

1. Sit in *Siddhāsana*, *Vīrāsana*, or *Padmāsana* (Figure 48, 50, 52).
2. Extend the spine from the coccyx to the cervical region upwards and keep the trunk lifted up.
3. Lower the head from the nape of the neck and perform *Jālandhara Bandha* (Chapter XIV, Nos. 29 to 31).
4. Close the eyes and draw them inwards.

5. Place the back of the left wrist on the left knee and keep the palm in *Jñāna Mudrā*. Keep the fingers loose (Figure 214).
6. Bend the right arm at the elbow, adjust the fingers on the nostrils as explained in Chapter XIV, No. 48.
7. Press the right nostril gently with the tip of the thumb so that the passage remains half-open. Do not remove the thumb from the nose. Close the left nostril with the ring and the little fingers so that the air may not move in it. Inhale slowly and fill the lungs to the brim.
8. After complete inhalation, close the right nostril with a gentle pressure from the tip of the thumb. Now both nostrils are blocked. Wait for one second.
9. Now, partially release the pressure of the fingers on the left nostril and exhale through the left nostril. The exhalation should be slow, steady and complete.
10. This is one cycle. Complete minimum 3 cycles in the beginning. Later do 8 to 10 such cycles, gradually increasing the number as experience is gained.
11. The complete cycle of *Sūrya Bhedana Prāṇāyāma* is thus as follows:
    (a) Inhalation through the right nostril;
    (b) Small pause to adjust the fingers on the nose—1 second;
    (c) Exhalation through the left nostril.
12. After completion of the last cycle, lower the right arm and place the hand in *Jñāna Mudrā* on the right knee. Stay for a while, experiencing the peace and quietness that has come from this practice. Then gently raise the head, open the eyes and lie down in *Śavāsana*.

13. The following points have to be observed while practising this prāṇāyāma:
    (a) When the fingers are on the nose, the septum should not be tilted to the side with the pressure of the fingers. When the right nostril is closed the septum should not be tilted to the left, and when the left nostril is closed it should not go to the right;
    (b) do not take the thumb or the fingers off the nostril which is half-open;
    (c) the pressure of the tips of the fingers and the thumb on the nose should be manipulated in such a way that a narrow passage is formed for the incoming or the outgoing air to pass through slowly and steadily—however, it should be neither too narrow nor too wide. In the beginning adjust the passage for the breath to move easily. As practice progresses make it narrower;
    (d) while paying attention to one nostril the other nostril should not be let loose; thus, while inhaling with the right nostril the left should not be let loose, otherwise air will pass in and vice versa.

Special Instructions

1. If the right nostril is blocked due to cold or for other reasons, inhale through the left nostril and exhale through the right one. This is known as *Candra Bhedana Prāṇāyāma*. It can be done on alternate days.
2. If you have migraine or heaviness on one side of the head, exhale through the same side nostril and do all inhalations through the other nostril.

Effects: As the nostrils are controlled by the fingers, the air goes in more slowly and steadily. Consequently the lungs are filled more fully than in *Ujjāyī Prāṇāyāma*.

This *prāṇāyāma* increases digestive power, calms the brain and increases vitality. It is good for those who suffer from tremors, burning eyes, fears, restlessness, profuse discharge and leucorrhoea.

VI. *NĀḌĪ ŚODHANA PRĀṆĀYĀMA*

Nāḍī denotes a tubular organ which carries prāña or energy through our body. Śodhana means purifying. Nāḍī Śodhana is purifying the blood vessels and nerves so that they function effectively.

Nāḍī Śodhana Prāṇāyāma should be practised after gaining some mastery over *Sūrya Bhedana Prāṇāyāma* and *Ujjāyī Prāṇāyāma II*. *Nāḍī Śodhana Prāṇāyāma* is a difficult variation of prāṇāyāma. In the initial stages perspiration, slight increase in body temperature, and tremors may be experienced. When control is gained, the above sensations do not occur.

Technique

1. Sit in *Siddhāsana*, *Vīrāsana*, or *Padmāsana* (Figures 48, 50, 52).
2. Lower the head from the nape of the neck and perform *Jālandhara Bandha* (Chapter XIV, Nos. 29 to 31; Figure 214).
3. Place the left palm on the left knee in *Jñāna Mudrā* (Chapter XIV, No. 47).
4. Raise the right hand and adjust the fingers on the nostrils as explained in Chapter XIV, No. 48 (Figure 214).
5. Loosen the tip of the thumb slightly, but do not remove it from the right nostril. Exhale fully through the half open right nostril and begin the cycle of *Nāḍī Śodhana*.
6. Now, inhale slowly, steadily and rhythmically through the right nostril, keeping the left nostril blocked.
7. Fill the lungs to the brim.

8. After full inhalation, close the right nostril with the pressure of the tip of the thumb. Release the pressure of the other two fingers and slightly open the left nostril; exhale slowly, steadily and rhythmically through the left half-open nostril. Empty the lungs but do not allow the trunk to sag.
9. Pause for a moment then inhale slowly through the same nostril, keeping the right nostril closed.
10. After full inhalation, close the left nostril open the right nostril partially by lessening the pressure of the tip of the thumb and exhale.
11. This completes one cycle. Then again inhale through the right nostril and continue with the next cycle. Complete minimum 3 cycles in the beginning. Later do 8 to 10 cycles in this manner, increasing the number gradually.
12. The complete cycle of *Nāḍī Śodhana Prāṇāyāma* is thus as follows:
    (a) inhalation through the right nostril;
    (b) exhalation through the left nostril;
    (c) inhalation through the left nostril;
    (d) exhalation through the right nostril.
13. After completing the last cycle, inhale fully through the right nostril, remove the fingers from the nose, and place the palm on the right knee. Stay quietly for a while, then slowly and carefully raise the head up, open the eyes, and lie down in *Śavāsana*.

Special Instructions

1. All the instructions given in Technique No. 13 of *Sūrya Bhedana Prāṇāyāma* are applicable in the case of *Nāḍī Śodhana Prāṇāyāma* also.
2. Avoid jerking the neck or opening the eyes suddenly. The nerves which have become quiet through the practice of prāṇāyāma should not be jolted. Experience

the peace and quietness within as described in *Ṣaṇmukhī Mudrā* (Figure 211). Then slowly open the eyes.

3. The inhalation and exhalation should not be done with force, nor with roughness or harshness of sound.

Note:

(a) The sound of inhalation should be rhythmic and smooth. If it is irregular, the brain is disturbed. The sound must therefore be controlled by the fingers.

(b) If one is thirsty and drinks water slowly and gradually, the coolness is felt deep inside. Inhalation should bring a similar sensation—the touch of air should be felt in the lungs.

(c) In deep breathing, inhalation and exhalation make the sounds 'sssssa' and 'huuuum' respectively, but in the nasal prāṇāyāma the sound, though not pronounced, is subtle and is experienced by membranes of the nostrils.

(d) In nasal Prāṇāyāma, the arrangement and the dexterous manipulation of the fingers on the nostrils and the response of the nostrils play an important part. Every movement has to be cautiously and minutely examined to see that the pressure of the fingers, the sound of the air, the expansion of the lungs are correct.

(e) The variations of Kumbhaka (retention), Āntara Kumbhaka (inhalation retention), and Bāhya Kumbhaka (exhalation retention) have not been described as the techniques given here are sufficient for the average practitioner. Students who are keen to study further may refer to the *Light on Yoga* and *Light on Prāṇ āyāma*.

Effects: The effect of *Nāḍī Śodhana Prāṇāyāma* on the body and the mind is more intense than in *Sūrya Bhedana*. It develops the strength of will-power, determination and stability. Further, it helps control the senses and leads towards self-knowledge.

CHAPTER XVI

Dhyāna (Meditation)

THE NATURE OF MEDITATION

In Chapter III an account of what meditation is has been given; hence repetition is not necessary. The experience is beyond description, it has to be personally experienced. Sugar has to be tasted to understand its sweetness, and its sweetness cannot be explained in words. Here an attempt shall be made to help the sādhaka taste the sweetness of meditation, or experience that which cannot be described in words.

The body is often considered to be an insignificant factor in the practice of meditation. This is an erroneous view. Our body is our vāhana—our vehicle. Without this vehicle we cannot experience anything. It is the body that carries us to our destruction or to Self-realisation. A vehicle that does not function well cannot take its owner anywhere. So also we are sometimes at the crossroads in our journey when our vehicle, the body, does not work properly. When the body is weak, shaky, or in pain, meditation is impossible and we have first to put it right by the practice of āsana and prāṇāyāma before proceeding further in the path of Yoga.

A sound and healthy body is thus the very first stage in meditation. It is the beginning of the journey. The end of the journey is realisation of the Supreme. In between are stopping-places—mental development, intellectual growth, self-knowledge. Each stage has to be perfected before the final goal is reached. Just as, during a journey, we see various scenes which are stored in memory and new experiences await in the future, likewise the journey for Self-realisation comprises a constant search—from bodily perfection to the Ultimate Goal. During the course of the journey all minute details have to be observed with an introspective eye.

The first four of the eight limbs of Yoga—yama, niyama, āsana and prāṇāyāma—are conducive to and inseparable from the art of meditation. They are preparatory stages. The next two limbs—pratyāhāra and dhāraṇā—are directly and intimately connected with meditation, leading onwards to Samādhi. Yet this stage, meditation, defies description. It is a philosophy beyond words which has to be experienced personally. Meditation is not bound by place and time—it can be experienced any time, anywhere. The scope of its preparation is as the horizon.

The preparation for a literary pursuit, too, has its beginning with the alphabet. Meditation also must have its humble beginning which finally leads to supreme joy.

The first four limbs of Yoga develop such qualities as health, cleanliness, moral discipline, stability, courage, mental peace and concentration. The inner and outer cleanliness leads the sādhaka towards a spiritual quest. The ground is prepared for dhāraṇā, dhyāna and samādhi.

A safe technique for meditation is given below. It should be practised every day for 5 to 10 minutes with a peaceful frame of mind. Later, the duration should be increased. The time for meditation should be the same every day. Early morning is the best. Meditation should be practised before prāṇāyāma. This is because at the time of starting the mind is fresh and free from wants and anxieties. If prāṇāyāma is done first, by then the āsana may irk the muscles and the nerves and disturb a serene state. When prāṇāyāma is done after meditation, attention is focused on the flow and the rhythm of breath and so one forgets the body pain. prāṇāyāma should follow immediately after meditation.

Technique

Āsana

1. Sit still in *Siddhāsana, Vīrāsana,* or *Padmāsana*. *Padmāsana* is preferable (Figure 52).

2. Sitting still in any position for meditation does not mean that the position should be lifeless and limp. It should be perfectly tuned for meditation. Even a slight headache makes us uneasy. Such impediments are not conducive to good meditation. A collapsed and loose body is an indication of inertia of the body and the mind. It leads to lassitude and indolence of the intellect. Meditation in such a state leads into darkness. An erect and alert body is indicative of a pure illuminating intellect. Hence keep the body erect and alert during meditation. Meditation in a pure state will be productive of inner Light.

Spine

3. An erect and alert spine results in an alert position. A straight, strong spine is conducive to concentration—the mind desists improper thoughts.
4. A correct spine position is essential. Follow the instructions given in Chapter XIV, Nos. 17 to 21. The spinal column controls the body.

Head and Brain

5. The next important factor is the head and its position. The trunk should not feel the weight of the head, nor should its weight be felt on the spine. The feeling should be as though the head is a weightless mass floating above the spine. The head should be straight, still and motionless. One should feel as if a thread is tied from the ceiling to the centre of the crown of the head. The position of the brain should be likewise. According to Yoga, the brain is divided into two main portions—the frontal brain and the back brain. The front brain always thinks of the external world and thought processes begin there. We shall call this portion the active or the creative brain. When the ego and the intellect are withdrawn from outside stimulus and become

introverted, existence is felt in the back portion of the brain. We shall call this portion the meditative brain. Both these, the front and the hindbrain, have to be balanced evenly for dhyāna.

Throat

6. When the mind runs after external influences, this reflects on the throat which tends to harden. When the throat is loose and free from contraction, the brain is bound to be calm and peaceful. Therefore, the throat is considered to be the seat of the Purifying Wheel (Viśuddhi Cakra).

Ātmāñjali

7. Now, when the entire body from the anus (Mūladhāra Cakra) to the top of the skull (Brahmaraṅdhra) is made weightless and free of tensions by extension and inner expansion, fold the hands in namaskāra (salutation). Broaden the shoulders sideways so that the sternum does not sink in, before folding the palms. Let the upper arms be free and tensionless, right from the shoulder-blades. See that the side ribs do not collapse and that the sternum is erect. Bring the palms to the centre of the chest with the thumbs pointing towards the middle of the chest and the other fingers touching each other (Figure 215). Though the physical heart is on the left, the spiritual heart is in the centre, behind the base of the sternum. Here, the wheel or the Cakra of the Heart controls the intelligence of the active mind.

   This sacred symbol of the folded hands is called Ātmāñjali, saluting or paying respect to the Inner Self. By tradition it is considered that namaskāra is the highest tribute one can pay to the Soul.

   Any deviation of the folded palms from the centre of the chest will lead to absence of alert watchfulness. A

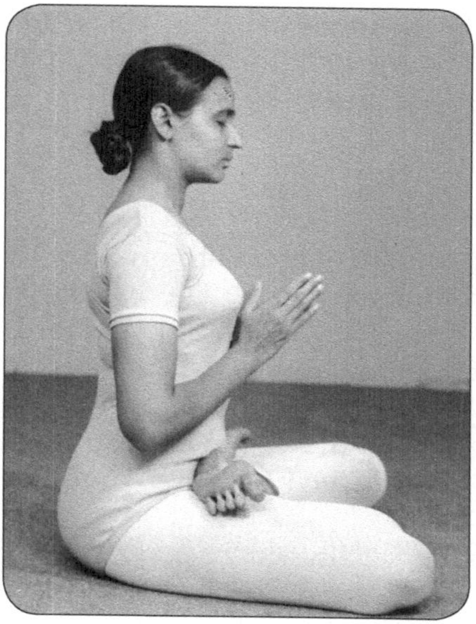

Fig. 215: *Dhyāna* (Meditation)

stable brain and stable mind go together. Both the palms are subject to the magnetic influences of the body. Any variation in the pressures of the palms is an indication that intellectual alertness is disturbed. Similarly, energy which flows on both the sides of the body is gauged by the hands. Any variation is registered by the palms, which in turn act on the mind and the intellect.

Poise

8. The poise that has to be attained is described in the Gita thus:

samam kāyaśirōgrīivam dhārayannacaḷam sthirah

B.G. VI, 13

[Hold the body, the head and the neck erect and still, with eyes steady and remain motionless within.] (Figure 215)

9. Now we shall examine the sense-organs:
   Tongue: Rest the tongue on the lower palate.
   Skin: Keep the skin all over the body free from tautness and tension.

Eyes, Ears and Nose

10. These organs are of great importance. The eyes should be kept completely closed. There is always a temptation to keep them half-closed, and it should be avoided. Gently drop the upper lids of the eyes and look inwards. Keep the ears and the eardrums receptive and the apertures of the ears parallel to each other. Look inwards towards the heart. Here one experiences:

    samprekṣya nāsikāgraṁ svaṁ diśaścānavalokayan
    B.G. VI, 13

    [Look fixedly at the tip of the nose, without looking around, with eyes closed.]

    This makes one look at the seat of the heart.

    One experiences pratyāhāra and dhāraṇā (withdrawal of the senses and concentration). The emotional centre and the intellectual centre should be brought together as one single thread of intelligence. When both these are united one experiences a cool, peaceful and quiet state within.

11. Respiration becomes slow and subtle, as the diaphragm remains light. Its stimulus is not felt by the navel, the heart and the head. The gentle act of inhalation and exhalation keeps the nerves quiet.
12. This is the stage when the presence of the gross body is not felt; one experiences a quiet flow of peace towards the seat of the Soul near the cakra of the heart. This state of mind is not an emptiness, but a fullness. It is both alert and inert.

However, to achieve this state, complete control is essential and the following self-examination has to take place:

Self-examination

1. If the spine is not firm and erect, the intellect collapses, leading to a dull and tāmasic state. From the Yogic point of view this is unethical practice and it must be corrected. Therefore, keep your spine firm, alert and erect.
2. If a thought process starts, this disturbs the flow of peace from the brain to the heart, and the eyes and the ears are in turn disturbed and forced towards the external world. The chain of reaction is thus as follows: disturbed thought-disturbed mind disturbed eyes and ears-renewed contact with the external forces of the outer world-disturbed meditation.
3. If the sense organs are disturbed, the direction of the flow changes and they run towards the external world; the spine loses its firmness, the brain its concentration; the existence shifts from the meditative brain to the active one and the chain of thoughts begins. Tremors of the body and disturbed respiration set in. The stillness and firmness felt at the heart, the emotional centre, is lost. Therefore, one must constantly watch and be on guard and be wakeful to see that the sense organs are kept under control.
4. Find out whether the control of senses is leading to peace dominated by tamas (darkness) or peace dominated by sattva (purity). Peace dominated by tamas will lead to sensuality; only peace in a sāttvic state will lead towards spirituality.
5. See whether the organs of sense are drawn inwards or whether they are merely passive because the body is free from tension.
6. See whether the thought process has begun and the mind has started wandering; whether the sense organs,

the mind, and the intellect are introspective or running towards the outer world. Find out and experience the pure and serene peace.

7. Check at frequent intervals whether the position of the folded hands at the centre of the chest, near the heart, has shifted. If the hands are out of alignment, then the alignment of the mind and the intellect with the Soul is also disturbed.

When the mind is still and stable, respiration is still and calm and the body becomes stable and quiet along with the emotions. The mind is the controller and the king of the senses, prāṇa is the king of the mind, and rhythm is the king of prāṇa. This rhythm is the sound (nāda) of inner peace.

That is the supreme stage in which one gets the answer to the question raised by Arjuna to Lord Kṛṣna in the Bhagvad Gīta:

sthita prajñasya ka bhāṣā
samādhisthasya keśava
sthitadhīḥ kiṁ prabhāṣeta
kimāsīta vrajeta kiṁ

B.G. II, 54

[What is the mark of one who is stable of mind, who is merged in Supreme Consciousness, Oh Lord? How does the stable-minded speak, sit and walk?]

When the senses are disciplined, the mind becomes stable. Such a mind becomes free from anger, passion, infatuation, and fear. It remains unperturbed in the state of sorrows as well as of pleasures and makes one free from confusion, delusion, undeterminate reason and egoism. The tranquility of mind fixes the discriminating intellect firmly in the Supreme and remains constantly awake in that state and attains the Brahmic state.

Om Śāntiḥ, Śāntiḥ, Śāntiḥ

Index

A

Abhyāsa 13
Ādhibhautika 42
Ādhidaivika 42
Adho Mukha Śvānāsana 85, 88, 91, 93, 98, 99, 103, 115, 120, 121, 125, 151, 153, 301
Ādhyātmika 42
Advanced Course 113, 120
Āgama 12
Aham 30
Ahaṃkāra 63, 76
Ahiṃsā 21
Ajapahamsa Vidyā 31
Amṛtanādopaniṣad 16
Amenorrhoea 54, 92
Ānandamaya 45
  Kośa 81
Annamaya 45
  Kośa 81
Antaraṅga Sādhanā 17, 18, 34
Antarātma Sādhanā 17, 19, 34
Anumāna 12
Aparigraha 23
Ardha,
  Baddha Padma Paścimottānāsana 93, 99, 103, 111, 115–118, 122, 159
  Candrāsana 103, 107, 112, 138, 339, 342, 364
  Halāsana 89
  Matsyendrāsana 88, 106, 112, 113, 116–120, 285, 290, 295
Ārjava 24
Āsanas,
  Abdominal and Lumbar 105, 262
  Advanced 102, 366
  Backbends 106, 297
  Forward Bends 103, 154
  Inverted 104, 208
  Pregnancy 107
  Sitting and Supine 104, 187
  Standing 103, 125
  Twists 106, 283
  Yoga, Kuruṇṭa 106, 315
Art of Yoga 35
Assimilation 41, 70
Aṣṭāṅga Yoga 16
  Eight Branches of Yoga 14
Asteya 22
Āstikya 26
Aśvatara Nāgarāja 36
Atrisamhitā 8
Austerity 24, 25
Avyakta 63
Āyāma 29
Āyurveda 7, 40–42, 45, 63, 64, 84

B

Baddha Koṇāsana 58, 84, 90–95, 104, 105, 108, 111, 112, 116, 118, 119, 121, 122, 173, 176, 219, 227, 344, 364, 365
  in Śīrṣāsana 91, 94, 105, 112, 118, 219, 227
Bahiraṅga Sādhanā 17, 18, 34
Bāhya Kumbhaka 30
Bhagavad Gītā 7, 38
Bhakti, Mārga 81
  Sādhanā 30, 31
Bhāradvājāsana 92, 96, 106, 108, 112, 115–120, 283, 286, 360, 364
Bhedana Prāṇāyāma 88, 92–95, 98, 109, 113, 118, 120–122, 363, 365, 388, 395, 396, 400, 415–418, 419
  Candra Bhedana Prāṇāyāma 417
  Sūrya Bhedana Prāṇāyāma 88, 92–95, 98, 109, 113, 118, 120–122, 363, 365, 388, 395, 396, 400, 415, 416, 418, 419

Bhujaṅgāsana 106, 107, 317, 320, 324
Blood, circulation 45, 47, 57, 69, 141, 168, 207, 219, 261
Pressure 88
Supply 141, 218, 231
Vessels 41, 70, 83, 191, 418
Brahmacaryāsana 165
Brahmānanda 28
Brahmaraṅdhra 424
Brain 47, 51, 65, 68, 72, 77, 125, 127, 391, 392, 396–398, 401, 403, 408, 411, 414, 418, 423–425, 427
Breath control 18, 25, 29, 30, 187, 188, 194
Buddhi 63, 76

C

Caesarean 97
Caraka Samhitā 39
Circulatory System 45, 66, 70
Citta 11, 31, 33, 40
Cleanliness 21, 24, 40, 422
Climacteric 60
Clothing 85
Compassion 21, 23, 26
Concentration 10, 32, 188
Constipation 58, 83, 238, 334
Contentment 10, 24
Cosmic Energy 31

D

Daṇḍāsana 86, 92–94, 98, 103, 106, 111, 112, 114–116, 118, 119, 154, 156, 157, 159, 160–166, 169–173, 178–180, 183, 184, 188, 192, 193, 197, 202, 207, 267, 268, 283, 285–287, 289, 290, 292–295, 309, 343–345, 349, 374, 375, 380
Dānam 26
Darśanopaniṣad 21
Deep Breathing 93, 108, 109, 112, 116, 117, 362, 365, 404
Exhalation 403, 404
Inhalation 404
Dhṛti 23
Dhanurāsana 106, 114, 302
Ūrdhva 92, 106, 113, 118, 119, 304
Ūrdhva Hasta 107, 324
Dhāraṇā 15, 32, 187, 422, 426
Dhātu 41, 64
Dhyāna 15, 19, 30, 32, 33, 100, 102, 109, 123, 187, 361, 363–365, 373, 389, 421, 422, 424, 425
Diet and cleanliness 21
Digestive System 45–47, 66, 70, 153, 165, 205, 418
Discipline,
of the senses 15, 18, 80, 188
of Yoga 8, 76
Doṣa 41, 64
Dvi Pāda Viparīta Daṇḍāsana 86, 92–94, 98, 106, 112, 114, 116, 118, 309
Dysmenorrhoea 54, 92

E

Ear Fungus 89
Ego 11, 19, 32, 40, 76, 385, 392, 423
Eka Pāda Rājakapotāsana 109, 369
Elementary Course 111, 113, 115, 123
Endocrine System 45, 47, 52, 55, 72, 98, 261, 296, 369
Excretory 45, 66, 71, 186, 221
Exhalation 29–31, 88, 144, 375, 384, 391, 393, 394, 398, 399, 403–405, 407–410, 412, 414–416, 419, 420, 426

F

Five-Faceted Mind 12

G

Glandular 45, 66, 95
Goddess Pārvatī 35
Guṇas 41, 42, 63, 218

H

Haṭhayoga Pradīpikā 19, 21, 25, 27, 28, 290
Halāsana 47, 58, 82, 83, 85, 87–89, 91, 93, 95–98, 105, 107, 108, 111, 112, 115–122, 125, 154, 208, 235, 238, 239, 241–249, 253, 272, 315, 327, 328, 330, 356, 364, 365
Heart Disease 89
Hrī 26
Human body 7, 64
Hygienic Habits 83
Hypomenorrhoea 55, 92
Hysteria 47

I

Iṣṭa Devatā 32
Illumination 41
Individual discipline 14
Inhalation 29–31, 88, 129, 375, 384, 391, 393, 394, 398, 399, 403–405, 407, 408, 410–416, 419, 420, 426
Insomnia 60, 238, 261, 386
Intellectual Faith 26
Intelligence 37, 40, 46, 75, 76, 79, 80, 110, 125, 182, 424, 426
Intensive Course 123
Intermediate Course 112, 118
Introductory Course 115
Īśopaniṣaḍ 6
Īśvarapraṇidhāna 25

J

Jñāna,
  Mudrā 395, 399, 413, 416, 418
  Yoga 34
Jñāneśvar 77
Jaṭhara Parivartanāsana 105, 113, 118, 121, 269
Jālandhara Bandha 236, 375, 376, 391, 392, 399, 411–413, 415, 418
Jānu Śīrṣāsana 56, 85, 89, 93, 96–99, 103, 108, 111, 112, 115–119, 121, 122, 156, 169, 343, 364, 365, 374
Japa Sādhanā 26, 30, 81
Jathara Parivartanāsana 94
Jīvātmā 63
Jnāna Mārga in Sādhanā 81
Jnānendriya 63

K

Kaṭhopaniṣaḍ 8, 20
Kālidāsa 22, 37, 132
Kṣama 23
Kāma 22
Kapotāsana 109, 369
Karṇapīḍāsana 105, 107, 111, 116–118, 243–245, 330
Karma Mārga 81
Karmendriya 63
Kidneys 71
Kumbhaka 30, 388, 413–415, 420
Kūrmāsana 90, 91, 104, 112, 113, 118, 120, 121, 180, 182
Kuruṇṭa 102, 106, 112–114, 116–119, 120, 121, 232, 235, 297, 301, 315, 333

L

Lactation 59
Lepana 41
Leucorrhoea 55, 91
Light on,
  Prāṇāyāma 420
  Yoga 277, 287, 290, 366, 420

M

Madālasā 36
Mṛtāsana 386

Mahābhārata 21, 35
Mahābhūta 63, 64
Mahā Mudrā 92, 93, 95–97, 109, 112, 116, 117, 119, 373, 374, 376
Mahat 63
Mala 64
Mālāsana 90, 92, 104, 111, 112, 116, 118, 121, 184, 332
Manana 80, 81
Manas 63, 77
Manomaya 45
Manusmṛti 36
Marīcyāsana 93, 99, 103, 106, 111, 113, 116–120, 122, 163, 287
Mati 26
Matsyāsana 84, 89–91, 93, 98, 104, 111, 116, 117, 119–122, 187, 206
Menopause 50, 60, 98, 400
Menorrhagia 54, 92
Menstrual Disorder 53, 55
Menstruation 50, 51, 53, 54, 56, 60, 90, 91–93, 207, 399
Mental Attitude 55, 74
Metrorrhagia 54
Mitahāra 24
Moderation in Diet 24
Modern medical science 48
Modesty 24
Mudrā and Śavāsana 97, 109, 373
Mūla Bandha 376
Mūladhāra Cakra 424
Muscular system 68, 186, 231

N

Nāḍī Śodhana Prāṇāyāma 109, 114, 121, 122, 363, 365, 395, 396, 400, 418–420
Naṭarājāsana 109, 370
Nature of Health 39
Nāvāsana 111
Nervous system 5, 29, 43, 45, 54, 55, 60, 66, 71, 79, 86, 96, 97, 153, 238, 261, 314, 334, 373, 379, 386, 406, 409, 415
Neurasthenia 47
Nididhyāsana 80, 81
Nidrā 12
Niyama 14, 16, 18, 24, 27, 74, 422
Non, Acquisitiveness 20
  Covetousness 20, 21
  Violence 20, 21

O

Oligomenorrhoea 55, 92

P

Pacana 41
Padmāsana 84, 104, 105, 108, 111–113, 116, 120, 122, 123, 159, 187, 192–194, 201–207, 219, 229–231, 256–258, 260, 286, 359, 364, 368, 378, 379, 389, 411, 413, 415, 418, 422
Pañca Tanmātra 32
Paripūrṇa Nāvāsana 94, 96, 105, 111, 116–118, 121, 267
Parivṛttaikapāda Śīrṣāsana 83, 104, 108, 112, 118, 219, 221, 228, 353, 364
Parivṛtta,
  Jānu Śīrṣāsana 103, 112, 118, 121, 169
  Paścimottānāsana 103, 113, 121, 171
  Trikoṇāsana 103, 111, 115, 140
Pārśva,
  Halāsana 83, 105, 107, 112, 118, 245, 249, 330
  Kukkuṭāsana 109, 368
  Piṇḍāsana 83, 105, 113, 259, 260
    in Sarvāṅgāsana 105, 113, 259
  Śīrṣāsana 83, 104, 108, 112, 118–221, 228, 352, 363, 364
Pārśvaika Pāda,
  Sarvāṅgāsana 105, 107, 111, 116–118, 249, 330

Śīrṣāsana 104, 112, 118, 219, 224, 228
Pārśvottānāsana 99, 103, 107, 111, 115, 125, 142, 150, 153, 340, 342, 364
Parvatāsana 57, 96, 97, 104, 108, 111, 116, 120, 122, 187, 197, 201, 349, 364
Pāśāsana 106, 114, 285, 294, 295
Paścimottānāsana 82, 85, 87, 88, 91, 93, 96, 98, 99, 103, 106, 107, 111, 113–122, 159, 165, 168, 171, 272, 320, 322, 332
  Ūrdhva Mukha 106, 107, 114, 120, 121, 272, 320, 322, 332
Patañjali 11, 13–17, 20, 21, 23, 24, 27–29, 32, 43, 75, 80, 124
  Yoga Sutras 27, 28
Path of,
  Action 6, 34
  Devotion 6, 34
  Knowledge 6
  Yoga 6–9, 22, 27, 37, 187, 421
Pīñcha Mayūrāsana 109, 368
Piṇḍāsana 83, 105, 113, 219, 230, 259, 260
  in Sarvāṅgāsana 105, 113, 257, 259
  Śīrṣāsana 105, 113, 230
Pitta 41
Polymenorrhoea 55, 92
Prajnā 76
Prakṛti 6, 37, 63
Pramāṇa 12
Prāṇamaya 45
Prāṇavaha 41
Prāṇa-vāyu 30
Prāṇāyāma 15, 18, 29, 30, 35, 37, 38, 40, 44–47, 50, 51, 55, 57–59, 74, 76, 80, 88–90, 92–95, 97–102, 107–110, 112–114, 116–123, 125, 187, 334, 335, 361–365, 373, 376, 380, 387–403, 406, 407, 409–422
Prāṇāyāma and Dhyāna 109, 363
Prasārita Pādottānāsana 91, 98, 99, 103, 108, 111, 115, 125, 145, 150, 341, 342, 364, 365
  Ūrdhva Prasārita Pādāsana 91, 94, 105, 111, 113, 116–118, 121, 235, 262
Pratyāhāra 15, 18, 31, 32, 182, 422, 426
Pratyakṣa 12
Pregnancy 50, 56, 94, 107, 334, 363, 400
  and Delivery 50
Premenstrual Tension 55, 93
Preparation for Deep Breathing 108, 109, 112, 116, 117
Prerequisites 16, 74, 217
Psychoneurosis 47
Psychophysiological 46
Puberty 51, 54, 56
Purāṇas is Āstikya 26
Pūraka 30, 404, 407, 409, 410, 414
Pursuit of,
  External Purity 17, 18
  Inner Purity 18, 19
  the Soul 19
Puruṣa 6, 63
Puruṣārthas 22
Pūrvottānāsana 107, 323

Q

Queen Mother of Belgium 53

R

Raghuvamśa 22
Rajoguṇa 28
Recaka 30, 384, 404, 408, 414
Recitation of Mantras 26
Religious Observances 26
Reproductive Systems 45, 72
Respiratory System 45, 47, 66, 69, 386, 401
Retention 30, 31, 375, 397, 404, 410–413, 414, 420

Retina 89
Rope Arrangement 315
Running Ear 89

S

Sādhaka 25, 29–33, 74–77, 80, 81, 100, 110, 114, 122–124, 334, 370, 376, 390, 394, 402, 421, 422
Sādhanā 17–19, 27, 30, 31, 34, 42, 74, 78–81, 100–102, 124, 217
Saguṇa and Nirguṇa 33
Saint Baḥinābai 37
Sāṃkhya Yoga 37, 63, 64
Sālamba
 Sarvāṅgāsana 82, 83, 85, 88, 89, 91, 93–98, 105, 107, 108, 111, 115–122, 125, 154, 208, 209, 232, 235, 239, 327, 333, 354, 364, 365, 391, 409
 Śīrṣāsana 82, 83, 85, 86, 88, 91, 93–96, 98, 104, 108, 111, 115–122, 208, 312, 350, 363–365, 409
Samādhi 15, 16, 19, 27, 28, 33, 187, 422
Śankarāchārya 77
Ṣaṇmukhī Mudrā 93, 109, 113, 118, 373, 377, 379, 393, 420
Santoṣa 25
Śāṅḍilyopaniṣaḍ 32, 33
Śarīra 78
Sarvāṅgāsana 47, 56, 57, 82, 83, 85, 87–89, 91, 93–98, 105, 107, 108, 111, 113, 115–122, 125, 154, 208, 209, 232, 235–239, 242, 243, 246–252, 254–257, 259, 260, 261, 315, 327, 328, 330, 333, 354, 358, 359, 364, 365, 391, 409
 Setu Bandha 47, 56, 82, 87– 89, 91, 93, 94, 96–98, 105, 111, 117, 118, 122, 125, 251, 252, 254, 255
 Ūrdhva Padmāsana 105, 108, 113, 256, 359, 364
Sati 36
Sauca 24
Śavāsana 59, 84, 86, 88–90, 92, 93, 95, 97, 100, 102, 108, 109, 112, 115–123, 125, 187, 361, 362, 364, 365, 373, 379, 380, 382–384, 386, 399, 404–407, 409–412, 414, 416, 419
 Ūrdhva Mukha 106, 112, 116, 300
Self,
 confidence 255, 261, 313
 control 19, 182
 realisation 6, 11, 14, 15, 17–19, 25, 29, 40, 43, 81, 100, 187, 188, 421
Siddhānta Vākya Śravaṇam 26
Siddhāsana 84, 104, 111, 116, 123, 187, 188, 193, 194, 389, 411, 413, 415, 418, 422
Śīrṣāsana 47, 53, 56, 57, 82, 83, 85, 86, 88, 89, 91, 93–96, 98, 99, 103–105, 108, 111–113, 115–122, 153, 156, 169, 208, 209, 212, 213, 215, 217–231, 237, 309, 312, 343, 350–353, 355, 363–365, 374, 409
 Eka Pāda 105, 107, 108, 111, 116–118, 330, 358, 364
 Ūrdhva Pādāsana 105, 113, 219, 229
Skeletal system 66
Sleṣma 41
Śloka 28
Smṛti 12, 37
Social discipline 14
Spiritual knowledge 6
 sādhanā 27, 124
Standing āsanas 52, 135, 335
Steady intellect 21, 23
Sthira 27
Sthirasukhamāsanam 389

Sthiratā 28
Straightforwardness 24
Sukhatā 27, 28
Sunshine 85
Supta,
Baddha Koṇāsana 84, 90–95, 104, 112, 118, 119, 121, 122, 176, 345, 364
Koṇāsana 91, 105, 107, 111, 116–118, 244–246, 330
Kūrmāsana 104, 113, 121, 182
Pādāṅguṣṭāsana 94, 106, 113, 114, 119, 121, 273
Vīrāsana 57, 84, 89–93, 98, 104, 108, 111, 116, 117, 119, 121, 122, 177, 187, 198, 200, 207, 348, 364
Suśruta Saṃhitās 45
Svādhyāya 25
Śvānāsana 85, 88, 91, 93, 98, 99, 103, 106, 111, 112, 115, 116, 120, 121, 125, 151, 153, 300, 301

T

Tanmātra 63
Tāḍāsana 103, 111, 115, 126–142, 144–152, 154, 317, 319, 320, 322–325
Tapas 25
Triang Mukhaikapāda Paścimottānāsana 93, 99, 103, 111, 116, 117, 119, 161
Truthfulness 20, 21

U

Ujjāyī Prāṇāyāma 58, 59, 89, 94, 97, 98, 108, 109, 112, 113, 116–122, 362, 363, 365, 388, 399–401, 406, 407, 409–411, 413–415, 417, 418
Universal Spirit 7
Uḍḍīyāna Bandha 376
Upaniṣad 16, 40
Upaviṣṭha Koṇāsana 57, 58, 90–92, 94, 95, 104, 108, 111, 112, 116, 118, 120, 121, 178, 219, 226, 345, 364, 365
in Śīrṣāsana 91, 94, 104, 112, 118, 226
Ūrdhva Kukkutāsana 109, 367
Uṣṭrāsana 106, 107, 113, 118, 119, 298, 326
Uttānāsana 85, 87, 88, 91, 93, 96, 98, 99, 103, 111, 115, 125, 149–152, 317, 319, 320
Utthita Hasta Pādāṅguṣṭāsana 106, 111, 114, 116, 119, 121, 277
Utthita Pārśvakoṇāsana 90, 96, 103, 107, 111, 115, 125, 130, 337, 363, 364
Utthita Trikoṇāsana 90, 96, 103, 107, 111, 115, 125, 128, 336, 363, 364

V

Vāgbhata 5
Vairāgya 14
Vāta 41
Vedas in the Gurukula 36
Vijñānamaya 45
Vikalpa 12
Viloma Prāṇāyāma 58, 88–90, 92–95, 97, 98, 109, 112, 118–120, 362, 365, 388, 399, 400, 410–413
Viparyaya 12
Vīrabhadrāsana 96, 103, 107, 111, 112, 115, 132, 134, 136–339, 364
Vīrāsana 57, 84, 89–93, 98, 104, 108, 111, 115–123, 177, 187, 190, 194–198, 200, 207, 209, 286, 290, 347–349, 364, 365, 389, 411, 413, 415, 418, 422
Cycle 91, 92, 104, 108, 111, 115, 116, 118–122, 195, 347
Viśuddhi Cakra 424

Vrata 26
Vṛkṣāsana 96, 103, 111, 115, 127, 149, 197, 324
Vṛścikāsana 109, 370
Vṛttis 12, 13
Vyāsa 13

W

Weekly schedule 115
Womanhood 50–52, 60
Women, Eligible for Yoga 35
  Yoginis 36

Y

Yājñavalkya 35
Yama 8, 14, 20, 27, 74
Yoga,
  an Art 10
  a Philosophy 11
  Āsanas 3
  As naturopathic process of treatment 48
  a Science 10
  Definition 9
  Ideal for Women 44, 76
  Importance 8
  in Yogabīja 8
  Kuruṇṭa Variation 112–114, 117
  Mudrāsana 104, 112, 118, 120–122, 187, 205
  Philosophy 27, 63
  Sādhanā 74, 81
  Six-Sided Yoga 16
  Sūtra of Patañjali 16
Yogaḥcittavṛtti nirodhaḥ 11
Yogacūḍāmaṇi 16
Yogāngāṇuṣṭhāna 34
Yoganidrāsana 109, 366
Yogāsanas and Prāṇāyāma 44–46, 51, 55–58, 60, 115, 315
Yogayāgñavalkya 35
Yogopaniṣaḍs 21